NEONATAL JAUNDICE
New Trends in Phototherapy

NEONATAL JAUNDICE
New Trends in Phototherapy

Edited by

Firmino F. Rubaltelli
Department of Pediatrics
University of Padua
Padua, Italy

and

Giulio Jori
Department of Biology
University of Padua
Padua, Italy

Plenum Press • New York and London

Library of Congress Cataloging in Publication Data

Meeting on New Trends in Phototherapy (1983: Padua, Italy)
   Neonatal jaundice.

   "Proceedings of a meeting on New Trends in Phototherapy, held June 9–11, 1983,
in Padua, Italy."—T.p. verso.
   Includes bibliographical references and index.
   1. Jaundice, Neonatal—Treatment—Congresses. 2. Phototherapy—Congresses. I.
Rubaltelli, Firmino F. II. Jori, Giulio. III. Title. [DNLM: 1. Jaundice, Neonatal—
Therapy—Congresses. 2. Phototherapy—In infancy and childhood—Congresses.
WH 425 M495n 1983]
RJ276.M43   1983   618.92′01   84-3365
ISBN 0-306-41669-7

Proceedings of a meeting on New Trends in Phototherapy, held
June 9–11, 1983, in Padua, Italy

©1984 Plenum Press, New York
A Division of Plenum Publishing Corporation
233 Spring Street, New York, N.Y. 10013

Printed in the United States of America

PREFACE

Hyperbilirubinemia of the neonate and the related risk of brain damage with consequent important alterations in motor development, particularly in sick preterm babies, remains a major problem in nurseries throughout the world.

Since its introduction in the 1950's phototherapy has been used for reducing serum bilirubin concentrations in the newborn with hyperbilirubinemia; however, only recently the photoprocesses invoked by light on various substrates including bilirubin have been clarified in sufficient detail. Light treatment actually exemplifies the intimate relationship between the clinical and basic sciences: the better understanding of the mechanism of phototherapy as a result of investigations initiated in the laboratory has been extended to the bedside as new types of lamps or new schedules of treatment. As a consequence, phototherapy of hyperbilirubinemia has emerged as a well-established branch of photomedicine, based on molecular photobiology, scientific method, and creative use of physics and sophisticated electrooptical capabilities. The collaboration and exchange of information between workers in different basic and clinical disciplines is likely to stimulate a further optimization of phototherapy.

The purpose of this monograph is to discuss some of the new aspects of bilirubin metabolism and phototherapeutic treatment. Bilirubin conjugation in the fetal and early neonatal life, the mechanism of bilirubin entry into the brain, the measurements of bilirubin concentration in the skin and serum bilirubin binding capacity are discussed by a number of prominent neonatologists. The chemistry and photochemistry of bilirubin, as well as novel developments in the phototherapy of neonatal jaundice are presented by distinguished scientists from the clinical and basic sciences.

We hope that the present monograph will contribute to a more precise understanding of the possible risk of bilirubin encephalopathy, especially in preterm newborn infants, and the appropriate treatment.

Firmino F. **Rubaltelli**, M. D.
Giulio **Jori**, Ph. D.

ACKNOWLEDGEMENTS

This symposium was sponsored by the National Research Council (CNR), the University of Padova, the Province Administration of Padova, and the Regional Government of Veneto. The organization of the symposium was made possible by the financial support obtained from Nestle-Guigoz, Monico Farmaceutici, Olympic Medical Corporation, Cassa di Risparmio di Padova and Banca Popolare di Padova.

CONTENTS

CONTENTS

BILIRUBIN METABOLISM IN THE NEWBORN:

ITS MECHANISMS AND RELATIONSHIP TO KERNICTERUS

Leo Stern

Professor and Chairman of Pediatrics
Brown University
Providence, R.I., U.S.A.

INTRODUCTION

Although jaundice as a sign of disease was known to both Galen and Hippocrates, the earliest record of its mention in relationship to the newborn is in Bartholomeus Metlinger's[1] book Ein Regiment der Jungen Kinder, published in 1473. In 1708 Michael Ettmuller[2], in his treatise De Infantum Morbis, mentioned jaundice which appeared shortly after birth. He recommended feeding the affected infant saffron with breast milk several times daily. In 1751 John Burton's[3] An Essay Towards a Complete New System of Midwifry, Theoretical and Practical contained the following description and therapeutic annotation:

"The want of Respiration to squeeze forward the Bile, and the Resistance made to its Entry into the Guts of Foetuses by the tough Slime which lines the Intestinal tube make the Effusion of their Bile very slow, and therefore their Gallbladder is generally full of green Bile. Hence at birth or soon after, Children are often observed to have the Jaundice, the thick Slime produces the same Effect in them, as if Stones or the Gravel obstructed the Neck of the Gallbladder. The Jaundice generally yields to any gentle Purgative, and very often is carried away by any Medicine that increases the Contraction of the Gut, which is no more than might be expected from understanding the cause of the disease."

Ylppo[4] in 1913 first introduced the concept of neonatal icterus as a manifestation of hepatic immaturity when he wrote that "...the liver at birth is functionally incomplete and with the physiologic increase of the bile towards the end of the fetal

period and after birth bile flows into the general circulation."
In the same year, Hirsch[5], in his study of 180 newborns, established
a relationship between the level of bilirubin in cord serum and
subsequent jaundice in the infant. Goldbloom and Gottlieb[6], who
found an increased level of bilirubin in the cord sera of infants,
proposed that this was hemolytic, that it occurred in all newborns,
but that jaundice was visible only if the serum bilirubin exceeded
4 van den Bergh units of bilirubin (2 mg/100 ml). Davidson and
colleagues[7] suggested that icterus neonatorum was related to
hemolysis of excessive red blood cells at birth and to immaturity
of liver function, and that the degree of hyperbilirubinemia determined the severity and duration of the visible jaundice. In his
Bela Schick Lecture of 1946, Weech[8] elegantly presented this view of
physiologic icterus in the newborn--a description which remains a
classic to this day.

Although the liver had been implicated as the focal point of
the problem, our understanding of the mechanisms involved in this
"immaturity" is only relatively recent. Most of the early theories
regarding bilirubin transport in plasma and the splitting off of the
"bilirubin-globin" complex by the liver are now known to be incorrect. Modern concepts of the hepatic handling of bilirubin stem
from the work of Schmid who demonstrated that bilirubin is excreted
in its conjugated form as a glucuronide[9,10]. This observation led
to the concept that the hepatic cell transfers the free, fat-
soluble, unconjugated bilirubin from plasma to the liver, conjugates
it there into a water-soluble diglucuronide, and subsequently
excretes it as such into the biliary tract.

MEASUREMENT OF BILIRUBIN

In 1916, Van den Bergh and Muller[11] observed that serum from
patients with hemolytic jaundice did not react promptly with
diazotized sulfanilic acid except in the presence of alcohol,
whereas serum from patients with obstructive jaundice reacted
immediately in aqueous solution, thus establishing the concept of
"direct" and "indirect" reacting bilirubin. Current methods which
record these two fractions are basically modifications of the method
of Malloy and Evelyn[12], which determines "direct" acting and "total"
bilirubin, with the subtraction product serving as the "indirect"
acting fraction. The "indirect" acting fraction represents unconjugated bilirubin, while the "direct" acting fraction is conjugated
bilirubin diglucuronide.

The differences in toxicity of the two fractions with respect
to the brain, (i.e., kernicterus) appear to be a function of their
different physical properties. Bilirubin itself (indirect acting,
unconjugated) is insoluble in water but soluble in lipids, which

accounts for its entry into the lipid-rich central nervous system.
In contrast, glucuronidated bilirubin (direct acting, conjugated) is
soluble in aqueous solution and insoluble in lipids. Thus the elevation of the indirect fraction represents a distinct hazard for
kernicterus while even extreme elevations of the direct acting frac-
do not. In addition, direct acting (conjugated) bilirubin may be
found in urine in the presence of an elevated serum bilirubin level,
whereas indirect (unconjugated) bilirubin will not appear even in
the face of extreme serum elevations (cf. acholuric jaundice).

BINDING OF BILIRUBIN TO ALBUMIN

Unconjugated bilirubin is bound to albumin in plasma. The
resulting complex is non-diffusible, and the binding to albumin
thus plays a vital role both in transporting the bilirubin to the
liver and in preventing the egress of bilirubin from serum into
tissues. The amount of "free" and "bound" bilirubin at any given
time is thus a function of the quantity of albumin in the circulation, as well as the capacity of the albumin to bind any bilirubin
present.

The binding process is pH dependent, and the complex tends to
dissociate with acidosis. Moreover, the presence of one or more
anions, which may compete with bilirubin for common binding sites
on the albumin molecule, may give rise to large amounts of "free",
unconjugated, bilirubin despite the presence of sufficient albumin
to bind all the bilirubin in the system. Thus, by displacing
bilirubin from its binding site, these anions will promote the
development of kernicterus at relatively low levels of serum
bilirubin.

Since Silverman et al.[13] reported that the administration of
sulfisoxazole to premature infants provoked the development of
kernicterus at low levels of serum bilirubin, other workers have
identified a number of endogenous and exogenous substances that
compete with bilirubin for one or more albumin-binding sites.
Hematin, which is present in increased amounts in hemolytic conditions, explains the higher risk of kernicterus in hemolytic as
compared to non-hemolytic hyperbilirubinemias. The non-esterified
fatty acids are elevated in plasma under conditions of both hypothermia and hypoglycemia. In addition to sulfisoxazole, salicylates,
and caffeine sodium benzoate will displace bilirubin from its
albumin-binding sites, and other drugs, singly or in combination,
may also share this capacity[14]. Not only should these agents be
avoided in the newborn who is jaundiced, but they should also be
withheld from a nursing mother who can transmit them to the newborn
in her milk.

ENZYME INDUCTION

Drugs, steroids, thyroxin and bilirubin are metabolized to glucuronides by UDPGA dependent glucuronyl transferases in hepatic microsomes. Inscoe and Axelrod were the first to demonstrate enhancement of hepatic glucuronyl transferase by administration of a foreign chemical[15]. They showed that treatment of newborn rats with 3,4, benzpyrene stimulated o-aminophenol-glucuronyl transferase activity in hepatic microsomes, but no such stimulation was observed when the mothers were treated with this agent during pregnancy. However, treatment of pregnant rats with chloroquine or chlorcyclizine did stimulate hepatic glucuronide formation in the newborn[16]. Subsequently it was shown that administration of barbiturates to animals enhanced enzymatic glucuronidation of bilirubin by hepatic microsomes, stimulated bile flow, and accelerated the metabolism of bilirubin in vivo[17,18]. Other studies revealed that barbiturates and other microsomal enzyme inducers increased the concentration in hepatic cytoplasm of a bilirubin binding protein (ligandin) important for the uptake of bilirubin by the hepatic cell[19].

Phenobarbital has been shown to effectively lower serum bilirubin in newborn infants when administered either to the infants themselves[20,21] or to their mothers in the latter weeks of gestation[22]. Agents other than phenobarbital appear to be capable of a similar effect. Sereni et al. have obtained a bilirubin reduction in newborns using diethylnicotinamide (coramine)[23]. Both ethanol[24] and dicophane (DDT)[25] appear to lower serum bilirubin effectively and show similar enhancement of microsomal activity, an effect shared by several other insecticides and herbicides.

BREAST MILK JAUNDICE AND OTHER HEPATIC INHIBITORS OF
BILIRUBIN METABOLISM

Clinically, breast-fed infants tend to have higher bilirubin levels than do bottle-fed infants. This difference persists even if one corrects for any increase in hematocrit in the breast-fed infant who may have a lower fluid intake. Experimentally some breast milks markedly inhibit an in vitro conjugating system, suggesting that they contain a factor which can depress glucuronyl transferase activity. Arias and his colleagues[26] have suggested that the factor responsible is pregnane-3α,20β-diol; others doubt that this particular steroid plays any role[27,28]. However, there is general agreement that breast milk contains such a factor and that it is probably a steroid derivative. Clinically, this factor expresses itself as hyperbilirubinemia only in the presence of the inhibitor and an inadequate conjugating system. Because the conjugating capacity of normal infants varies up to 6-fold, breast milk containing a specific concentration of inhibiting substance

may not produce hyperbilirubinemia, depending upon the conjugating
capacity of the infant's liver. Similarly, cessation of breast
feeding may produce a fall in serum bilirubin, which does not
become elevated again when breast feeding is resumed. Since the
liver matures progressively in the immediate neonatal period, time
alone will permit the enzyme system to cope with a partial inhibitor,
which a day or two earlier might have provoked a rise in bilirubin.
Despite this adaptation, a few infants will show recurrent elevation
of bilirubin with breast-milk feeding for several months, suggesting
that the milk they are consuming contains a more powerful type or a
greater amount of inhibiting substance.

OTHER INHIBITING SUBSTANCES

    Arias and his colleagues [29] have described a familial transient
neonatal hyperbilirubinemia associated with an inhibiting factor
present in the plasma. In addition, it has been demonstrated that
a number of other endogenous and exogenous substances can suppress
glucuronyl transferase activity in vitro and in vivo, namely, one
or more of the steroids of the estrogen progesterone groups[30,31].
Experimental evidence exists to support the ability of novobiocin
to reduce enzyme activity[32]. Other agents suspected of having this
effect include the phenothiazines and their derivatives and the
ester proprionate preparation of erythromycin. It has also been
suggested that pitocin and its analogues used in the induction of
labor may have a similar effect thereby accounting for a higher
incidence of jaundice in newborns born to induced as opposed to
non-induced parturient women. Recently inhibition of other enzymes
in the haem-bilirubin conversion chain has been demonstrated with
potentially beneficial effects. Thus the experimental administration of tin protoporphyrin IX has been shown to lower bilirubin
levels in newborn rats by virtue of its inhibitory effect on the
haem oxygenase system and subsequent slowing of the rate of haem
to bilirubin conversion[33].

REABSORPTION OF BILIRUBIN FROM THE GUT
(ENTEROHEPATIC CIRCULATION)

    Bilirubin sequestered in meconium in the gut of the newborn
makes a contribution to the total bilirubin pool. The concentration of bilirubin in meconium is approximately 1 mg/g. The
average neonatal gastrointestinal tract contains 200 g of meconium
and thus can contribute 200 mg of bilirubin to the enterohepatic
circulation, contrasted with an endogenous bilirubin production of
10 to 20 mg/kg/day. Meconium differs from adult feces (which contains very little, if any, bilirubin) because the newborn gut contains no intestinal bacteria to reduce bilirubin to urobilinogen.
The fetal and neonatal intestine also contains β-glucuronidase,

which hydrolyzes bilirubin diglucuronide excreted into the gut to bilirubin, thereby making possible its reabsorption into the blood stream via the enterohepatic circulation.

More than a century ago, Condie[34] commented that jaundice in the newborn was related to "want of a free evacuation of the meconium." In 1937, Ross and his colleagues[35] demonstrated that anicteric infants excreted more bilirubin in their stools during the first few days of life than icteric ones. This finding has been confirmed clinically. Unconjugated hyperbilirubinemia has been noted in newborns with high intestinal obstruction and those with delayed passage of meconium[36,37].

INTESTINAL BINDING AND EXCRETION OF BILIRUBIN

Attempts to block the re-entry of bilirubin from the intestinal tract by absorbing bilirubin in the gut on medicinal charcoal or cholestyramine have met with only minimal success[38,39]. More recently, Poland and Odell[40] employed orally administered agar for this purpose. Their results show a reduction in serum bilirubin levels and an enhancement of bilirubin excretion in the meconium of agar-fed versus control infants. Agar stabilizes bilirubin in aqueous solution and prevents its bacterial conversion; it also possesses the properties of a colloid laxative. This work suggests a further method of reducing serum bilirubin level by "immobilizing" and removing bilirubin from the gut, thus preventing its re-entry into the enterohepatic circulation. In this connection it appears reasonable to assume that the reported beneficial effects of early versus delayed feeding in lowering serum bilirubin in the newborn reflect an increase in bacterial flora as well as earlier expulsion of meconium in the infants fed earlier. Both result in a reduction of the available intestinal content of reabsorbable bilirubin.

PHOTOTHERAPY

The North American Indians were apparently aware of the beneficial effects of the sun in reducing the yellow color of a baby exposed to its light. A sample of serum left in the light will show a fall in measurable serum bilirubin levels compared to one stored in a dark cupboard. Biochemically, this change reflects a partial breakdown of bilirubin with a shift in the absorption spectrum of the serum[41].

Phototherapy for neonatal hyperbilirubinemia, first proposed by Cremer and his colleagues[42] in England, has been used extensively in South America[43] and subsequently on this continent[44], both for the reduction of elevated serum bilirubin levels and for the "prophylactic" prevention of hyperbilirubinemia in prematures.

Theoretically, the photodecomposition of bilirubin is most effective in blue light whose peak emission at 480 nm is close to the absorption maximum of bilirubin in serum (460 to 465 nm). In vitro, the by-products of photodecomposition comprise biliverdin, with an absorption maximum at 650 nm (resulting from the loss of two hydrogen atoms from bilirubin--photo-oxidation) and at least two dipyrroles, with absorption maxima at 380 and 280 nm. The latter are water soluble and would, therefore, not diffuse readily into the central nervous system and also be easily excreted into both bile and urine. In vivo, however, photodecomposition yields only small amounts of the dipyrroles and little or no biliverdin. The by-products of in vitro photodecomposition show no neurotoxicity in brain-tissue culture media or in vivo in animal experiments. Moreover, their absorption maxima are well below those of bilirubin, making it exceedingly unlikely that they would displace bilirubin from its albumin-binding sites.

As a clinical observation, Giunta and Rath[45] reported that serum bilirubin levels in infants kept in a brighter nursery were lower than those kept in a darker one in the same hospital. Studies of the natural variations in environmental lighting, depending on the amount of sunlight, time of day, and location of the infants within the nursery, reveal a wide range of variability in illumination intensity for all three of these parameters[46]. These variations suggest an environmental explanation for the seasonal variations in bilirubin levels within any given geographic area, and for the lower incidence of hyperbilirubinemia reported in areas with more sun. Moreover, in any nursery, the position of the baby in relation to the sources of external light may play a major role in determining the amount of illumination received.

Although photo-oxidation of bilirubin is clearly apparent in in vitro studies of bilirubin solutions, the consistent failure to demonstrate any significant amounts of either biliverdin or dipyrroles in photo-irradiated infants has led to an alternative more-acceptable explanation of the bilirubin light effect as resulting from an internal isomerization and rotation of the bilirubin molecule which permits its conversion at an unconjugated stage to a water soluble form; thereby allowing for its detoxification and for the appearance of unconjugated bilirubin in the bile[47,48].

KERNICTERUS

Although the toxicity of bilirubin to the central nervous system was originally described by Schmorl in 1903[49], the term kernicterus refers to the pathological finding of yellow staining of the nuclei of the brain. The term bilirubin encephalopathy was first proposed by Zetterstrom and Ernstner as being more appropriately reflective of a gradual and progressive degree of impairment, a feature which might explain the incidence of high-tone deafness in premature infants as a reflection of the earliest site of bilirubin deposition as being the auditory nucleus of the eighth cranial nerve. They attempted to explain the mechanism of CNS toxicity by virtue of the uncoupling of oxidative phosphorylation of brain mitochondria[50], a finding which was refuted a decade later by Diamond and Schmid[51]. The factors that promote the occurrence of central nervous system toxicity at lower levels of bilirubin are clinically associated with acidosis, hypothermia, hypoxia, and hypercapnea[52], but the precise mechanisms by which the injurious effect occurs is still a subject of both study and speculation. In addition to its dissociation effects on bilirubin albumin binding[53], acidosis also results in an increased affinity for bilirubin on the part of brain mitochondria[54]. As to what the bilirubin does when it arrives at the CNS cell, recent studies using an isolated fat cell preparation have suggested that the water insolubility rather than lipid solubility of unconjugated bilirubin is involved in the mechanism of cell toxicity with an aggregation of bilirubin at the margins of the cell and a subsequent inhibition of adenylate cyclase in the cell membrane as a reflection of the compromise of cellular integrity[55]. In this regard we can formulate the questions to be posed for future examination as relating to a better understanding of the CNS toxicity of bilirubin and the mechanisms by which it occurs. We have historically been exposed to the view that there is a blood brain barrier other than that governed by the differing solubilities of the conjugated vs. unconjugated bilirubin molecule. Is this in fact the case, and if so, what precisely does the barrier consist of? Clearly the original supposition that the barrier somehow "matured" in the first week of life is incorrect. It represents an inversion of the fact that as hepatic conjugating capacity improves, the serum bilirubin levels tend to fall, but the risk for bilirubin CNS injury given the appropriate conditions and levels of bilirubin and albumin is not altered. We need to know more about the factors governing the increased risk of hemolytic vs. non-hemolytic causes of hyperbilirubinemia, i.e., are there factors other than the enhanced displacement of bilirubin from albumin by haem involved; perhaps the anemia and the presence of antibodies do play a role after all? We need also to abandon the term "physiologic jaundice". There is nothing physiologic about it, and a commonly occurring event is not less dangerous because it is not rare.

In the final analysis the brain and bilirubin need to be looked at as the answer to an overall encompassing question--"How does the bilirubin get into the brain, and what does it do once it gets there?" In the answers to this problem lie the directions of future studies in a search for specific and clinically relevant solutions.

REFERENCES

1. B. Metlinger, Ein Regiment der Jungen Kinder, G. Zainer, Augsberg, (1473).

2. M. Ettmuller, De Infant Morbis, Frankfurt, (1708).

3. J. Burton, An Essay Towards a Complete New System of Midwifry, Theoretical and Practical, J. Hodges, London, (1751).

4. A. Ylppo, Icterus neonatorum (incl. I.n. gravis) und gallenfarbstoffsekretion bein foetus und neugeboren, Z. Kinderheilkd, 9:208, (1913).

5. A. Hirsch, Die physiologische icterusbereitschaft des neugeborenen, Z. Kinderheilkd., 9:196, (1913).

6. A. Goldbloom and R. Gottlieb, Icterus neonatorum, Am J. Dis. Child., 38:57, (1929).

7. L. T. Davidson, K. K. Merritt, A. A. Weech, Hyperbilirubinemia in the newborn, Am. J. Dis. Child., 61:958, (1941).

8. A. A. Weech, The genesis of physiologic hyperbilirubinemia, Adv. Pediatr., 2:346, (1947).

9. R. Schmid, Direct-reacting bilirubin, bilirubin glucuronide, in serum, bile, and urine, Science, 124:76, (1956).

10. R. Schmid, L. Hammaker, and J. Axelrod, The enzymatic formation of bilirubin glucuronide, Arch. Biochem. Biophys., 70:285, (1957).

11. A. A. H. Van Den Bergh and P. Muller, Uber eine direkte und eine indirekte diazoreaktionen auf bilirubin, Biochem. Z., 77:90, (1916).

12. H. T. Malloy and K. A. Evelyn, Determination of bilirubin with the photoelectric colorimeter, J. Biol. Chem., 119:481, (1937).

13. W. A. Silverman, D. H. Anderson, W. A. Blanc, and D. N. Crozier, A difference in mortality rate and incidence of kernicterus in premature infants allotted to two prophylactic bacterial regimens, Pediatrics, 18:614, (1956).

14. D. Schiff, G. Chan, and L. Stern, Fixed drug combinations and the displacement of bilirubin from albumin, Pediatrics, 48:139, (1971).

15. J. K. Inscoe and J. Axelrod, Some factors affecting glucuronide formation in vitro, J. Pharmacol. Exptl. Ther., 129: 128-131, (1960).

16. I. M. Arias, L. Gartner, M. Furman, and S. Wolfson, Effect of several drugs and chemicals on hepatic glucuronide formation in newborn rats, Proc. Soc. Exp. Biol., 112:1037-1040, (1963).

17. C. Catz and S.J. Yaffe, Barbiturate enhancement of bilirubin conjugation and excretion in young and adult animals, Pediat. Res., 2:361-370,(1968).

18. R. J. Roberts and G. L. Plaa, Effect of phenobarbital on the excretion of an exogenous bilirubin load, Biochem. Pharmacol., 16:827-835, (1967)

19. H. Reyes, A. J. Levi, R. Levine, Et Al., Bilirubin, a model
    for studies of drug metabolism in man, Ann. N.Y. Acad.
    Sciences, 179:520-528, (1971).

20. D. Trolle, Decrease of total serum bilirubin concentration in
    newborn infants after phenobarbital treatment, Lancet,
    2:705, (1968).

21. L. Stern, N. Khanna, G. Levy, and S. J. Yaffe, Effect of
    phenobarbital on hyperbilirubinemia and glucuronide
    formation in newborns, Amer. J. Dis. Child., 120:26, (1970).

22. C. Ramboer, R. P. H. Thompson, and R. Williams, Controlled
    trial of phenobarbitone therapy in neonatal jaundice,
    Lancet, 1:966, (1969).

23. F. Sereni, L. Perletti, and A. Marini, Influence of diethyl-
    nicotinamide on the concentration of serum bilirubin in
    newborn infants, Pediatrics, 40:466, (1967).

24. R. Waltman, F. Bonura, G. Nigrin, and C. Pipat, Ethanol in the
    prevention of hyperbilirubinemia in the newborn, Lancet,
    2:1265, (1969).

25. R. P. H. Thompson, C. W. T. Pilcher, J. Robinson, G. M.
    Stathers, A. E. M. McLean, and R. Williams, Treatment of
    unconjugated jaundice with dicophane, Lancet, 2:4, (1969).

26. I. M. Arias, L. M. Gartner, S. Seifter, and M. Furman,
    Prolonged neonatal unconjugated hyperbilirubinemia associated
    with breast feeding and a steroid, pregnane-3α,20β-diol, in
    maternal milk that inhibits glucuronide formation in vitro,
    J. Clin. Invest., 43:2037, (1964).

27. A. Ramos, M. Silverberg, and L. Stern, Pregnanediols and
    neonatal hyperbilirubinemia, Am. J. Dis. Child., 111:353,
    (1966).

28. B. P. F. Adlard and G. H. Lathe, Breast milk jaundice: Effect
    of 3α,20β-pregnanediol on bilirubin conjugation by human
    liver, Arch. Dis. Child., 45:186, (1970).

29. I. M. Arias, S. Wolfson, J. F. Lucey, and R. J. McKay, Jr.,
    Transient familial neonatal hyperbilirubinemia, J. Clin.
    Invest., 44:1442, (1965).

30. D. Y. Y. Hsia, R. M. Dowben, R. Shaw, and A. Grossman,
    Inhibition of glucuronosyl transferase by progestational
    agents from serum of pregnant women, Nature, 187:693, (1960).

31. M. Z. Sas and J. Herczeg, Serum bilirubin level and steroid
    excretion following progesterone loads in newborn infants,
    Acta Paediatr. Acad. Sci. Hung., 11:35, (1970).

32. H. Lokietz, R. M. Dowben, and D. Y. Y. Hsia, Studies on the
    effect of novobiocin on glucuronyl transferase, Pediatrics,
    32:47, (1963).

33. G. S. Drummond and A. Kappas, Prevention of neonatal hyper-
    bilirubinemia by tin protoporphyrin IX, a potent competitive
    inhibitor of haem oxidation, Proc. Nat. Acad. Sciences,
    78:6466-6470, (1981).

34. D. F. Condie, A Practical Treatise on the Diseases of Children, Ed. 4, Blanchard & Lea, Philadelphia, 698, (1854).

35. S. G. Ross, T. R. Waugh, and H. T. Malloy, The metabolism and excretion of bile pigment in icterus neonatorum, J. Pediatr., 11:397, (1937).

36. T. R. Boggs, Jr. and H. Bishop, Neonatal hyperbilirubinemia associated with high obstruction of the small bowel, J. Pediatr., 66:349, (1965)

37. J. Rosta, Z. Makoi, and A. Kertesz, Delayed meconium passage and hyperbilirubinaemia, Lancet, 2:1138, (1968).

38. R. A. Ulstrom and E. Eisenklam, The enterohepatic shunting of bilirubin in the newborn infant, J. Pediatr., 65:27, (1964).

39. R. Lester, L. Hammaker, and R. Schmid, A new therapeutic approach to unconjugated hyperbilirubinaemia, Lancet, 2: 1257, (1962).

40. R. L. Poland and G. B. Odell, Physiologic jaundice: the enterohepatic circulation of bilirubin, N. Engl. J. Med., 284:1, (1971).

41. S. H. Blondheim, D. Lathrup, and J. Zabriskie, The effect of light on the absorption spectrum of jaundiced serum, J. Lab. Clin. Med., 60:31, (1962).

42. R. J. Cremer, P. W. Perryman, and D. H. Richards, Influence of light on hyperbilirubinaemia of infants, Lancet, 1:1094, (1958).

43. J. Obes-Polleri, La fototerapia en las hiperbilirubinemiae neonatales, Arch. Pediatr., Uruguay, 38:77, (1967).

44. J. F. Lucey, M. Ferreiro, and J. Hewitt, Prevention of hyper-bilirubinemia of prematurity by phototherapy, Pediatrics, 41:1047, (1968).

45. F. Giunta and J. Rath, Effect of environmental illumination in prevention of hyperbilirubinemia of prematurity, Pediatrics, 44:162, (1969).

46. L. Stern, N. R. Khanna, and P. MacLeod, Nouvelles methodes de traitement de l'hyperbilirubinemie du nouveau-ne, Union Med. Can., 100:506, (1971).

47. J. D. Ostrow, Photocatabolism of labelled bilirubin in the congenitally jaundiced (Gunn) rat, J. Clin. Invest., 50: 707, (1971).

48. R. Brodersen, Free bilirubin in blood plasma of the newborn: effect of albumin, fatty acids, pH, displacing drugs, and phototherapy; in Intensive Care of the Newborn, Volume II, Stern, L., Oh, W., and Friis-Hansen, B., (eds.), Masson USA, New York, 331-347, (1978).

49. G. Schmorl, Zur kentus des icterus neonatorum, Verh. Deutch Ges. Path., 6:109, (1903).

50. R. Zetterstrom and L. Ernstner, Bilirubin, an uncoupler of oxidative phosphorylation in isolated mitochondria, Nature, 178:1335, (1956).

51. I. Diamond and R. Schmid, Oxidative phosphorylation in experi-
     mental bilirubin encephalopathy, Science, 155:1288, (1967).
52. L. Stern and B. Doray, Hypothermia, acidosis, and kernicterus
     in small premature infants, Proc. 12th Int. Cong. of Ped.,
     Mexico City, p. 512, (1968).
53. G. B. Odell, The dissociation of bilirubin from albumin and
     its clinical significance, J. Ped., 5:268, (1959).
54. G. B. Odell, The distribution of bilirubin between albumin
     and mitochondria, J. Ped., 68:164, (1966).
55. R. E. Shepherd, F. J. Moreno, W. J. Cashore, and J. N. Fain,
     Effects of bilirubin on fat cell metabolism and lypolysis,
     Am. J. Physiol., 237:E-504-508, (1979).

SERUM BILIRUBIN MONO- AND DICONJUGATES

IN HUMAN NEWBORNS

Maurizio Muraca, Norbert Blanckaert and Johan
Fevery
Laboratory of Hepatology, Catholic University
of Leuven, Belgium

Firmino F. Rubaltelli, Virgilio Carnielli and
Gianna Pettenà
Neonatal Intensive-Care Unit, University of Pa-
dova, Italy

INTRODUCTION

Several alterations of bilirubin metabolism are present during the neonatal period, all essentially leading
to an increased load of unconjugated bilirubin and a decreased hepatic handling of the pigment. The resulting
neonatal jaundice is a classical example of unconjugated
hyperbilirubinemia(1). The presence of conjugated bilirubin in neonatal plasma has often been investigated, and
considered as an index of function of hepatic conjugation
or secretion(2-5). Unfortunately, several methodological
problems are met when trying to measure serum conjugated
bilirubin in the presence of high concentrations of the
unconjugated pigment. Most procedures for measurement of
bilirubins in biological samples rely on diazo-cleavage,
resulting in splitting of the tetrapyrrole moiety and producing dipyrrolic red azoderivatives. After the discovery
that bilirubin in bile reacts rapidly, without requiring
the presence of an "accelerator", the distinction between
direct-reacting and total bilirubin was introduced. However, "direct-reacting" bilirubin is just operationally
defined, and it is therefore dependent on reaction conditions and sample composition, while it does not accurately reflect conjugated bilirubin(6). The ethyl-anthrani-
late method is more specific, and allows to separate and
identify the dipyrrole azoderivatives(6). However, it is
impossible to relate the sugar-conjugated azodipyrroles

13

to the parent rubins. A similar problem is present with
the isotope-dilution method(2). Direct analysis of the
tetrapyrroles has been tried by various solvent-partition
and chromatographic procedures, but none of these methods
proved to be truly specific and accurate(6).

The Alkaline-Methanolysis procedure constitutes a
significant improvement for direct tetrapyrrole analysis
(7). Bilirubin mono- and disugar conjugates are converted
to the corresponding mono- and dimethyl esters, which are
then extracted into an organic solvent together with the
unconjugated bilirubin. The pigments can then be separated by High Performance Liquid Chromatography (HPLC) and
individually quantified, using an internal standard(8).
This normal-phase liquid chromatographic procedure, however, was not sensitive enough to measure the concentration of bilirubin conjugates in normal human serum and in
serum of patients with unconjugated hyperbilirubinemia.
Such a limitation was recently eliminated by the development of a new reverse-phase HPLC procedure(9). Some preliminary investigations, performed by this method on serum of healthy adults and of patients with unconjugated
hyperbilirubinemia, support the concept that conjugated
bilirubin present in serum is in equilibrium with the
amount of conjugates formed in the liver, and is therefore dependent on bilirubin production rate(10). The absolute concentration of conjugated bilirubin was found to
be about 0.3 μmol/L in serum of normal adults, which corresponds to about 4% of total serum bilirubin in these
subjects(9). The concentration of conjugates was increased
in patients with hemolytic disease, but the conjugated
fraction relative to total bilirubin was comparable to
normal adults(10). These findings suggest that, when a
higher load of bilirubin reaches the liver, more conjugates will be formed and more will exchange with plasma;
the fractional exchange of this pigment between liver and
plasma should however be constant, provided bile secretion is not affected. The absolute concentration of conjugates was normal in patients with Gilbert's syndrome, who
exhibit decreased hepatic UDP-glucuronyltransferase acti-
vity(10). Since unconjugated bilirubin concentration was
high in these sera, the conjugated fraction was lower than
in normal adults. The finding that, in conditions associated with decreased hepatic conjugation, the concentration
of conjugated bilirubin in plasma is normal, suggests that
also in these situations a normal amount of conjugates is
formed in the liver, which equals bilirubin production.
Such an equilibrium is however reached at higher concentrations of the substrate unconjugated bilirubin.

From these preliminary results, we conclude that the absolute concentration of conjugated bilirubin in plasma, in the presence of a normal secretory function, is dependent on bilirubin production rate, while a low conjugated fraction relative to total bilirubin seems to be an index of decreased hepatic UDP-glucuronyltransferase activity. On the basis of these results, we decided to investigate the more complex situation in the newborn.

PATIENTS AND METHODS

The pattern of serum bilirubins was evaluated by Alkaline Methanolysis and reverse phase HPLC(9) in 9 full-term healthy newborns and in 3 newborns affected by erythroblastosis fetalis, two full-term and one pre-term (32 weeks of gestational age).

RESULTS AND DISCUSSION

In the full-term healthy newborns, the concentration of unconjugated bilirubin in serum ranged between 19 and 115 μmol/L on the first day of life (fig.1).

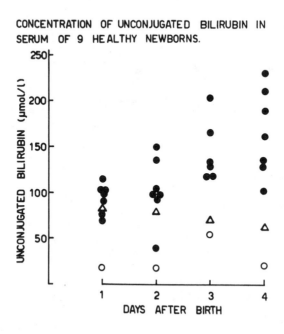

Fig. 1.

This concentration increased during the next three days
in all the children except in two (identified by open symbols in the figure), who exhibited rather constant and relatively low values during the period of observation.

Conjugated bilirubin was present in all the serum
samples tested (fig.2). Its concentration was very variable on the first day of life, while it was more uniform
on the second day, ranging from 0.5 to 1 µmol/L, with the
exception of one child. During the next two days, the concentration increased in all the children,with the exception
of the two children in wich also unconjugated bilirubin was
relatively constant (open symbols in the figure).

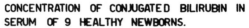

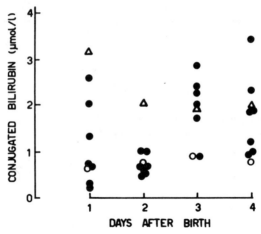

Fig. 2

The serum fraction of conjugated bilirubin (expressed as percent of total bilirubin in fig. 3) was also very variable on the first day of life, while it was rather
constant during the following days, with a mean value
around 1% of total bilirubin. The two children with low
unconjugated bilirubin behaved again differently, their
conjugated fraction being relatively high, and comparable
to the values found in serum of healthy adults. These findings suggest that the increased serum concentration of
conjugated bilirubin during the first days of life is not
the result of deficient biliary excretion, since the con-

jugated pigment fraction remains low. The increased bilirubin load present in the neonate could be responsible
for the parallel rise of both the unconjugated and conjugated pigment in serum.

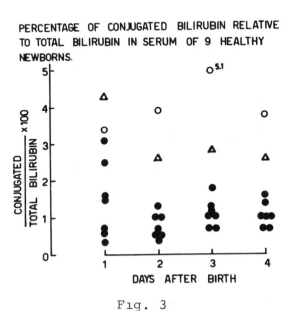

Fig. 3

As mentioned previously, we were able to identify
both bilirubin mono- and diconjugates in serum. In adult
serum, about 60% of the esterified pigment was found as
diconjugate(9). This fraction was decreased to 20% in the
newborn, and it did not change significantly during the
first days of life (fig.4).

The concentration of bile acids is increased in newborn serum, when compared to adult serum(11,12). This phenomenon is considered as an index of "physiologic cholestasis". Also in the children of the present series, serum
bile acids concentration usually exceeded 5 μmol/L, considered as the upper limit of normal range in adults with
the enzymatic-fluorimetric method used for the assay (fig.
5). No correlation could be demonstrated between the concentration of total bile acids and of conjugated bilirubin
in these sera, suggesting that the increased concentration
of these two organic anions originate from different mechanisms.

PERCENTAGE OF BILIRUBIN DICONJUGATES RELATIVE
TO TOTAL CONJUGATES IN SERUM OF 9 HEALTHY
NEWBORNS.

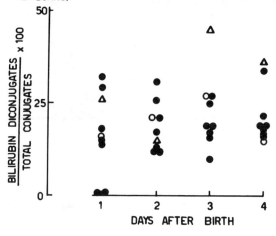

Fig. 4

CONCENTRATION OF TOTAL BILE ACIDS (ENZYMATIC-
FLUORIMETRIC DETERMINATION) IN SERUM OF 9
HEALTHY NEWBORNS.

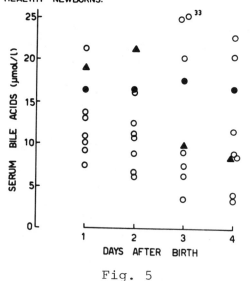

Fig. 5

In two full-term babies affected by erythroblastosis
fetalis, the absolute concentration of conjugated bilirubin was respectively around 1 and 3 µmol/L during the first
days of life, and therefore in the range of values found
in healthy newborns (fig.6). These concentrations corres-
ponded respectively to about 1 and 2% of total bilirubin,
again in the range of values found in normal babies.

SERUM CONCENTRATIONS OF CONJUGATED BILIRUBIN IN 2
BABIES AFFECTED BY ERITHROBLASTOSIS FOETALIS.

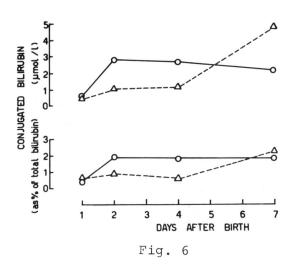

Fig. 6

The pre-term baby affected by erythroblastosis fetalis included in our study developped cholestasis. The serum concentrations of conjugated bilirubin and of total
bile acids during the first week of life of this child
are shown in fig. 7. Numbers in parenthesis refer to the
percent of conjugated bilirubin relative to total bilirubin. On the second day of life, the unconjugated fraction
was 6.4%, the highest of our series, while the serum bile
acids were still in the range of values found in normal
babies. Both the concentration of conjugated bilirubin
and of bile acids became clearly pathological during the
following days.

From these preliminary results, we conclude that conjugated bilirubin is normally present in neonatal serum.
Its average concentration in the present series of healthy children was between 1 and 2 µmol/L, or about 1.3-1.5%

of total bilirubin. About 80% of the esterified pigment
is monoconjugated.

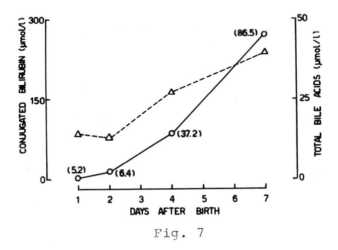

CONCENTRATIONS OF CONJUGATED BILIRUBIN (o—o) AND OF TOTAL
BILE ACIDS (Δ—Δ) IN SERUM OF A BABY AFFECTED BY SEVERE
ERYTHROBLASTOSIS FOETALIS.

Fig. 7

The concentration of conjugated bilirubin is higher
in newborn than in adult serum. Our data do not provide
any clear evidence for the presence of a relative secretory deficit of conjugated bilirubin in the healthy newborn. We suggest that the high concentration of this pigment in serum during the first days of life might be the
result of the high bilirubin load presented to the neonatal liver, leading to the formation of high amounts of
conjugates which equilibrate between liver and plasma.
Since the plasma conjugated fraction remains low, the bile
secretory system of the neonatal liver seems to be able
to transport into bile a load of pigment which is at least
twice as high as in healthy adults.

In two babies affected by erythroblastosis fetalis,
the serum pattern of conjugated bilirubin did not differ
from the one found in healthy newborns. Therefore, exposure to high loads of bilirubin already in utero did not
alter the composition of bilirubins in serum at birth.
The finding of a high fraction of conjugated bilirubin
in an erythroblastic child could be an early sign of cholestasis.

This work was supported by the Grant n° CT82.00187.04 from the Consiglio Nazionale delle Ricerche, Rome, Italy.

REFERENCES

1. G. B. Odell, Neonatal Jaundice, in: "Progress in liver disease", H. Popper and F. Schaffner eds, Grune and Stratton, New York (1976).
2. J. Jacobsen, R. Brodersen and D. Trolle, Patterns of bilirubin conjugation in the newborn, Scand. J. clin. Lab. Invest., 20:249(1967).
3. A. Bakken, Bilirubin excretion in newborn human infants. I. Unconjugated bilirubin as a possible trigger for bilirubin conjugation, Acta Paediat. Scand., 59:148 (1970).
4. A. Bakken, Bilirubin excretion in newborn human infants. II. Conjugated bilirubin as a possible trigger for bilirubin excretion, Acta Paediat. Scand., 59:153 (1970).
5. A. Winsnes and D. Bratlid, Unconjugated and conjugated bilirubin in plasma from patients with erythroblastosis and neonatal hyperbilirubinaemia, Acta Paediat. Scand., 61:405(1972).
6. K. P. M. Heirwegh and N. Blanckaert, Analytical chemistry of rubins, in: "Bilirubin", volume I, K. P. M. Heirwegh and S. B. Brown eds, CRC Press, Boca Raton (1982)
7. N. Blanckaert, Analysis of bilirubin and bilirubin mono- and di-conjugates. Determination of their relative amounts in biological samples, Biochem. J., 185:115 (1980).
8. N. Blanckaert, P. M. Kabra, F. A. Farina, B. E. Stafford, L. J. Marton and R. Schmid, Measurement of bilirubin and its monoconjugates and diconjugates in human serum by alkaline methanolysis and high performance liquid chromatography, J. Lab. Clin. Med., 96:198(1980).
9. M. Muraca and N. Blanckaert, Identification and measurement by high-performance liquid chromatography of mono- and diester conjugates of bilirubin in human serum of healthy adults, Clin. Chem., in the press.
10. M. Muraca and N. Blanckaert, unpublished observations.
11. L. Barbara, R. Lazzari, A. Roda, R. Aldini, D. Festi, C. Sama, A. Moselli, A. Collina, F. Bazzoli, G. Mazzella and E. Roda, Serum bile acids in newborns and children, Pediat. Res., 14:1222(1980).
12. F. J. Suchy, W. F. Balistrieri, J. E. Searcy and R. S. Levin, Physiologic cholestasis: elevation of the primary serum bile acids concentration in normal infants, Gastroenterology, 80:1037(1981).

MECHANISM OF BILIRUBIN ENTRY INTO THE BRAIN IN AN ANIMAL MODEL

Dag Bratlid

Department of Pediatrics
Rikshospitalet
Oslo, Norway

INTRODUCTION

Hyperbilirubinemia is still one of the most common problems in the newborn, particularly in the premature infant. Kernicterus may occur when unconjugated bilirubin enters the brain and produces toxic effects on the nerve celes(1). Although the mechanism is not fully understood, it has been assumed that the toxicity is caused by the entry of the non-albumin bound fraction of the unconjugated bilirubin into the brain. As long as the molar concentration of serum bilirubin is less than that of serum albumin, the bilirubin molecule is usually firmly bound to the albumin molecule, and only insignificant levels of free or unbound bilirubin can be detected (2, 3). Several studies have, however, shown that multiple factors can affect the binding of bilirubin to albumin and thus increase the serum level of free bilirubin in the newborn and thereby probably also the risk for bilirubin toxicity (3, 4). A large number of tests have therefore been developed to measure the free bilirubin concentration in the blood of the newborn (5) as a way of assessing the potential risk of kernicterus.

One of the risk factors thought to increase the possibility of bilirubin toxicity in the newborn is acidosis (5). However, in vivo experimental results to date do not conclusively characterize the role of acidosis on bilirubin entry into the brain. When measured by Sephadex technique (6) or fluorescent dye method (7), a low pH produces a decrease in albumin binding capacity for bilirubin. However, similar studies using the fluores-

cense-quenching method (8) or the peroxidase technique (9)
have not demonstrated any change in bilirubin-albumin
binding with changes in pH. This "free bilirubin theory"
has provided a basis for understanding the risk factors
in neonatal hyperbilirubinemia and for several years has
been used as the basis and rationale for the treatment
of neonatal jaundice. A number of studies, however, failed
led to show any significant correlation between the ac-
nowledged risk factors and the occurrence of kernicterus
in the newborn infants (10-12). In addition, the "free
bilirubin theory" as the sole explanation of kernicterus
in low birth weight infants has also been challenged (13).

More recently, Levine and coworkers (14) presented
evidence that reversible opening of the blood-brain
barrier in rats could cause yellow staining of the brain
when it was perfused with albumin bound bilirubin. The
present study was designed to further assess the role of
the blood-brain barrier in the mechanism of bilirubin
penetration into the brain.

MATERIALS AND METHODS

Male Sprague Dawley rats (150-250 g) were used for
the study. Two to 6 days before the experiments the external jugular vein was catherized under intraperitoneal
ketamine anesthesia by a slight modification of the method
described by Davis and Campbell (15). On the day of the
experiment the rats were placed in a harness but were
allowed to move freely around in their cage with access
to food and water. At the beginning of the experiment
10-20 μCi of ^{125}I bovine albumin (New England Nuclear)
was infused into the jugular vein. Following this infusion,
a buffered bilirubin solution at a concentration to
deliver 30 mg/kg/hour was infused at a rate of 0.028ml/min
for 180 minutes. This buffered bilirubin solution was
constituted by mixing 5 ml of unconjugated bilirubin
(Sigma Chemical Corporation) dissolved in 0.1 N NaOH
with 10 ml solution of bovine albumin (Cohn fraction V)
in a phosphate buffer. The final pH of the infusate was
adjusted to 8.0.

At 120 minutes following the start of the bilirubin
infusion, urea (Fisher Scientific Corporation) was infused
ed in 3 different groups of rats at a dose of 50 (n=6),
75 (n=6) and 100 mmoles/kg (n=9), respectively, as a bolus
over a two minute period. A fourth group of control rats
(n=11) was infused with a similar volume of isotonic
saline at the same rate.

In a second series of experiments the effects of acidosis and hypercarbia were studied. All groups of rats

received the same bilirubin infusion throughout the period of 180 minutes, but at 120 minutes of the study period, two different manipulations were done to induce acidosis: One group (n=8) was made metabolically acidotic by infusion of 0.5 N HCl at a rate of 0.02 ml/g/hour for the last 60 minutes of the study period. A second group (n=8) was made respiratory acidotic by exposing the rats to 20% CO_2 in 21% O_2 and balanced nitrogen. This was achieved by placing the rats in a restrainer inside a closed plexiglass container with a volume of 2.3 liters and delivering the gas mixture into the container at a flow rate of 5 L/min. To allow for blood sampling, the tail of the rat was kept outside the container through a hole which also allowed for gas flow out of the container. A third group (n=8) served as a control and were given only 0.02 ml/g/hour of saline in addition to the bilirubin infusion.

Finally, a third series of experiments were performed where the animals were given a bolus injection of sulfisoxazole 50 mg/kg at 120 minutes of the study period.

Blood samples were obtained at baseline, 60, 120, 135 and 180 minutes of the study period. Serum bilirubin was measured by Martinek's modification of the method of Malloy and Evelyn (16), free bilirubin by peroxidase method (17), osmolality by vapor pressure (18) and albumin by the bromcresol green method (19). Blood gas analysis and pH determinations were done on a Corning 168 blood gas analyzer. Colorimetric determinations were done on a Gilford spectrophotometer 240 with an automatic recorder 6051.

At the end of the infusion period the rats were euthanized by a rapid injection of a saturated solution of potasium chloride. The chest was immediately opened, a catheter placed in the ascending aorta and the brain perfused in situ with 20 ml of cold saline at a rate of 6.1 ml/min. The rats were then decapitated and the brain was removed. The brain was then divided into equal parts by a sagittal section. One half of the brain was used for counting of $_I$125 albumin content. The albumin concentration in the brain was then calculated from the specific activity of the serum albumin. The other half of the brain was used for determination of bilirubin concentration by chloroform extraction after homogenization.

In a fourth series of experiments regional distribution of bilirubin in the brain was studied in piglets. The piglets 1-2 days old were made hyperbilirubinemic by bilirubin infusion of 12 mg/kg as a bolus and maintenance infusion of 10 mg/kg for 3 hours. Hypercarbia was induced at 120 minutes by letting the piglets breathe 15% CO_2 in a closed cardboard box. After 180 minutes of the study period the piglets were killed by injection of sodium thiamylal, the brain flushed by carotic perfus-

ion, and bilirubin concentrations were measured in the
brainstem, midbrain, cerebellum, thalamus and cerebrum by
chloroform extraction as in the rats.
     Statistical evaluation of the results was done by
unpaired t-test. A p-level of less than 0.05 was chosen
as the limit of significance.

RESULTS

     Hyperosmolality. The serum bilirubin levels at steady
state varied between 149 and 187 /uM/L in most of the
groups studied. No difference was found in unbound bilirubin, albumin, blood-gases or pH. The serum osmolality
levels remained stable throughout the study period in the
control group. In the groups given urea, the serum osmo-
lality was raised from $293\overset{+}{-}4$ mOsm/L (mean$\overset{+}{-}$S.E.M.) in the
control group to $345\overset{+}{-}1$, $383\overset{+}{-}5$ and $400\overset{+}{-}4$ mOsm/L in the
rats who were given 50, 75 and 100 mmoles/kg of urea
respectively. The elevated osmolality levels decreased
only slightly for the rest of the study period.
     As shown in Figure 1, significant increases in bili-
rubin concentrations were found in the brains of the rats

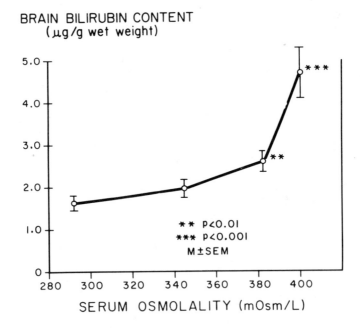

Fig. 1. Brain bilirubin in hyperosmolar rats

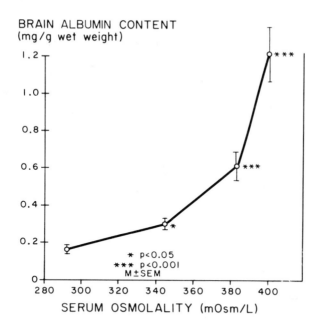

Fig. 2. Brain albumin in hyperosmolar rats

in the hyperosmolar groups. The group with the highest
serum osmolality of 400 mOsm/L thus showed a more than
threefold increase in brain bilirubin concentration compared to the control group. Most of the animals in this
group had brains that were clearly yellow stained.
　　A significant finding in the present study is also
the demonstration that leakage of albumin into the brain
is related to the degree of hyperosmolality. As shown in
Figure 2, the albumin leakage was moderate with an increase in serum osmolality from 293 mOsm/L to 345 mOsm/L,
but then increased rapidly. The group with a serum osmolality of 400 mOsm/L thus had an albumin leakage about
6 times higher than the control group.
　　Acidosis. The results are shown in Table 1. The
serum bilirubin levels were as in the hyperosmolar study.
No differences were found in in ubound bilirubin, serum
albumin or osmolality . All three groups had normal and
comparable pH, pCO_2 and Base Excess levels at 120 minutes. The control group showed normal values at 180 minutes of the study period. The group given an infusion
of hydrochloric acid showed a significant and steady
decrease in pH (data not shown) and reached a level of
7.03 ± 0.01 at 180 minutes, with a pCO_2 level of 38.6 ± 1.6
mmHg and a Base Excess of -20.3 ± 1.9 meq/L. The animals
breathing the high CO_2 gas mixture showed a more rapid

Table 1. Total and unbound serum bilirubin , pH, Base
Excess, pCO_2, brain bilirubin and brain albumin in rats
made acidotic (see text). Values given are mean$\pm$s.e.m.

STUDY GROUPS

	Control	Metabolic acidosis	Respiratory acidosis
Serum bilirubin 180' /uM/L	149$\pm$16	150$\pm$18	179$\pm$14
Unbound bilirubin 180' nM/L	12.0$\pm$1.7	13.0$\pm$2.6	13.5$\pm$1.7
Blood pH 180'	7.40$\pm$0.01	7.03$\pm$o.01*	7.04$\pm$0.01*
Blood Base Excess 180' meq/L	1.3$\pm$0.7	-20.3$\pm$1.9*	-8.0$\pm$0.9*
Blood pCO_2 180' mmHg	40.6$\pm$1.6	38.6$\pm$1.6	100.4$\pm$2.3*
Brain bilirubin /ug/g wet weight	1.25$\pm$0.12	1.39$\pm$0.14	3.01$\pm$0.36*
Brain albumin /ug/g wet weight	114$\pm$21	123$\pm$20	216$\pm$20*

*p less than 0.05

decrease in pH (data not shown) but had values at 180
minutes very comparable to the other group with a pH of
7.04$\pm$0.01, pCO_2 of 100.4$\pm$2.3 mmHg, and a Base Excess of
-8.0$\pm$0.9 meq/L. The brain bilirubin and albumin content
in the metabolic acidotic group were similar to the
control group. In the respiratory acidotic group,
however. a significant increase in both brain bilirubin
and brain albumin was found, with more than double the
levels found in the control animals.

Sulfisoxazole. Results from preliminary experiments
are shown in Figure 3. Infusion of sulfisoxazole 50mg/kg
as a bolus caused a significant increase in brain bilirubin concentration without any increase in the brain
albumin concentration. A significant increase in the
concentration of unbound bilirubin was found in the
animals given sulfisoxazole (data not shown).

Regional distribution of bilirubin. Figure 4. shows
preliminary results from studies in the piglet. In
control animals (given only the bilirubin infusion) the
brainstem, midbrain and cerebellum contained more bilirubin than thalamus and cerebrum. In the animals made
hypercarbic (pCO_2 about 70 mmHg) a significant increase
in bilirubin concentration was found in the brainstem,
midbrain, cerebellum and thalamus, while the concentration in the cerebrum only increased slightly.

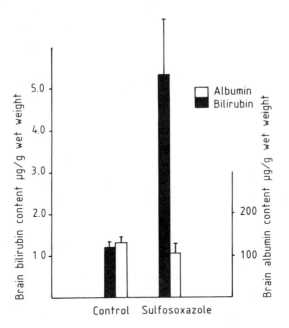

Fig. 3. Brain bilirubin and brain albumin in control and sulfisoxazole treated rats.

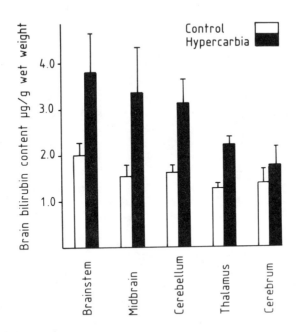

Fig. 4. Regional distribution of bilirubin in brain of control and hypercarbic newborn piglets.

DISCUSSION

The present investigation confirms the recently published study by Levine and coworkers (14) that serum
hyperosmolality can cause leakage of albumin into the
brain and thereby give a yellow staining of the brain if
hyperbilirubinemia is present simultaneously. Furthermore,
data on the rate of bilirubin entry into the brain at
different degrees of hyperosmolality has been provided.

Although the magnitude of bilirubin increase in the
brain was not entirely proportional to that of albumin,
this does not invalidate the conclusion that bilirubin is
able to enter the brain in the form of albumin bound
bilirubin. The brain is known to contain a very active
bilirubin oxidase (21) which could possibly cause some
bilirubin destruction during the study period. In addition,
if separation of the bilirubin-albumin complex would occur
after entering the brain, the bilirubin molecule of lower
molecular weight could diffuse out of the brain to the
cerebrospinal fluid, leaving the albumin molecule behind.
Both these factors could account for a lower bilirubin
concentration in the brain at the time of the assay than
would have been expected.

In the present study neither acidosis nor hypercarbia
altered the level of apparent unbound or "free" bilirubin
in the serum. These results are contrary to the general
belief that acidosis may reduce the bilirubin binding
capacity of albumin and predispose the newborn to kernicterus (22). The present results indicate that the danger
of acidosis and hypercarbia in the hyperbilirubinemic
infant is not caused by reduced albumin binding or increased cellyular binding of unbound bilirubin, but by increased entry of albumin bound bilirubin into the brain because
of opening of the blood-brain barrier by hypercarbia.
Acidosis alone did not seem to have any effect on brain
bilirubin. This is in agreement with other studies not
involving bilirubin showing that severe hypercarbia
damages the blood-brain barrier (23).

On the other hand, the results in the sulfisoxazole
group confirm the view that bilirubin might also get
access to the brain by displacement from the albumin
molecule. Since no increase in brain albumin was found
in this group, the sulfonamides does not seem to influence upon the blood-brain barrier, as has been
suggested (14).

As presented in Figure 4, great differences exist
in bilirubin concentrations within different regions of
the brain, both in control animals and during hypercarbia-
At least in the hypercarbic animals the regions with the
highest bilirubin concentrations correspond to the reg-

ions with the highest blood flow (24). this might indicate that the cerebral blood flow or bilirubin delivery
to the brain also might play a role in determining the
amount of bilirubin that might gain access to the brain.

The results of the present study may finally be
summarized as illustrated in Figure 5. Bilirubin may
enter the brain under at least three different conditions.
Under normal low-grade hyperbilirubinemia, most of the
bilirubin is strongly bound to serum albumin, and this
bilirubin-albumin complex is normally excluded from the
brain by the blood-brain barrier. However, some unbound
bilirubin also exists, and this small fraction can pene-
trate into the brain, as in all the control animals in
the present study, who had significant bilirubin levels
in their brains. Under normal conditions this low bilirubin level in the brain is probably not toxic. However,
one might speculate how much bilirubin can gain access
to the brain if the hyperbilirubinemia is of long duration.

In some clinical situations high levels of unbound
bilirubin can be found in the blood, as indicated in the
middle part of the figure. This is possible with markedly elevated bilirubin concentrations exceeding the binding capacity of the albumin molecule, or by displacement of bilirubin from the albumin binding site by a displacing agent, as in the present study. Under such circumstances high levels of unbound bilirubin are deposited

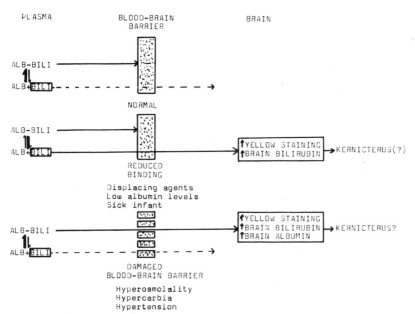

Figure 5.   Mechanisms of bilirubin entry into the brain.

in the brain. This is probably the mechanism by which the classical kernicterus as seen for instance in Rh-disease develops.

Finally, bilirubin might also gain access to the brain as the bilirubin-albumin complex, as indicated in the lower part of the figure. This is possible when breakdown of the blood-brain barrier occurs, as for instance in hyperosmolality or hypercarbia. It is not, however, obvious that demonstration of entry of unconjugated albumin bound bilirubin into the brain due to blood-brain barrier breakdown necessarily equates to kernicterus as seen in the newborn infant. It is possible that when breakdown of the blood-brain barrier occurs, the yellow staining of the brain is a secondary phenomenon without any clinical or pathological significance. On the other hand, demonstration of bilirubin entry into the brain at relatively low serum bilirubin concentrations because of breakdown of the blood-brain barrier, might explain some of the cases of unexpected kernicterus in the small premature infants with low serum bilirubin concentrations.

REFERENCES

1. W. B. Karp, Biochemical alterations in neonatal hyper-bilirubinemia and bilirubin encephalopathy: A review, Pediatrics, 64:361, (1979).
2. J. Jacobsen, Binding of bilirubin to human serum albumin - determination of the dissociation constants, FEBS lett., 5:112, (1969).
3. R. Wennberg, M. Lau, and L. F. Rasmussen, Clinical significance of unbound bilirubin, Pediatr. Res., 10:434, (1977).
4. W. J. Cashore, A. Horwich, E. P. Karotkin, and W. Oh, Influence of gestational age and clinical status on bilirubin binding capacity in newborn infants, Am. J. Dis. Child., 131:898, (1977).
5. K-S. Lee and L. M. Gartner, Bilirubin binding by plasma proteins. A critical evaluation of methods and clinical implications, Rev. Perinat. Med., 2:319, (1979).
6. F. Chunga and R. Lardinois, Separation by gel filtration and microdetermination of unbound bilirubin, I. In vitro albumin and acidosis effects on albumin bilirubin binding, Acta Pediatr. Scand., 60:27, (1971).
7. K-S. Lee, L. M. Gartner, and I. Zarafu, Fluorescent dye method for the determination of the bilirubin binding capacity of serum albumin, J. Pediatr., 86:280, (1975).

8. R. L. Levine, Fluorescence-quenching studies of the
    binding of bilirubin to albumin, Clin. Chem.,
    23:2292, (1972).
9. J. Jacobsen and R. Brodersen, The effect of pH on
    albumin-bilirubin affinity, Birth Defects Original
    Articles Series, 12:175, (1976).
10. S. B. Turkel, M. E. Guttenberg, D. R. Moynes, and J.
    E. Hodgman, Lack of identifiable risk factors for
    kernicterus, Pediatrics, 66:502, (1980).
11. M. H. Kim, J. J. Yoon, J. Sher, and A. K. Brown, Lack
    of predictive indices in kernicterus. A comparison
    of clinical and pathological factors in infants
    with or without kernicterus, Pediatrics, 66:852,
    (1980).
12. D. A. Ritter, J. D. Kenny, H. J. Norton, and A. J.
    Rudolph, A prospective study of free bilirubin and
    other risk factors in the development of kern-
    icterus in premature infants, Pediatrics, 69:260,
    (1982).
13. R. L. Levine, Bilirubin. Worked out years ago?,
    Pediatrics, 64:380, (1979).
14. R. L. Levine, W. R. Fredericks, and S. I. Rapoport,
    Entry of bilirubin into the brain due to opening
    of the blood-brain barrier, Pediatrics, 69:225,
    (1982).
15. J. D. Davis and C. S. Campbell, in:"Physiological
    Techniques in Behavioral Research," D. Sing and D.
    P. Avery, eds., Brooks/Cole Publishing Company,
    Monterey, (1975).
16. R. G. Martinek, Improved micromethod for determination
    of serum bilirubin, Clin. Chim. Acta. 13:161, (1966).
17. J. Jacobsen and R. P. Wennberg, Determination of
    unbound bilirubin in serum of newborns, Clin. Chem.
    20:783, (1974).
18. D. Bratlid, W. J. Cashore, and W. Oh, Effect of serum
    hyperosmolality on opening of blood-brain barrier
    for bilirubin in rat brain, Pediatrics, 71:909,
    (1983).
19. B. T. Doumas, W. A. Watson, and H. G. Biggs, Albumin
    standards and the measurement of serum albumin
    with bromcresol green, Clin. Chim. Acta, 31:87,
    (1971).
20. D. Bratlid and A. Winsnes, Determination of conjugated
    and unconjugated bilirubin by methods based on
    direct spectrophotometry and chloroform extraction.
    A reappraisal. Scand. J. Clin. Lab. Invest. 28:41,
    (1971).
21. R. Brodersen and P. Bartels, Enzymatic oxidation of
    bilirubin, European J. Biochem. 10:468, (1969).
22. J. Maisels, Neonatal jaundice, in: "Neonatology,

    Pathophysiology and management of the newborn,"
    G. B. Avery, ed., J. B. Lippincott Company,
    Philadelphia, (1981).
23. B. Johansson and B. Nilsson, The pathophysiology of
    blood-brain barrier dysfunction induced by severe
    hypercarbia and by electric brain activity, Acta
    Neuropath. 38:153, (1977).
24. N. B. Hansen, A-M. Brubakk, D. Bratlid, W. Oh, and B.
    Stonestreet, Brain blood flow response to CO_2 in
    newborn piglets, Pediatr. Res. 17:316A, (1983).

THE IMPORTANCE OF SERUM BINDING AND THE BLOOD BRAIN BARRIER IN

THE DEVELOPMENT OF ACUTE BILIRUBIN NEUROTOXICITY

Richard P. Wennberg, A. J. Hance and Jorgen Jacobsen

University of California, Davis, School of Medicine
Davis, CA, 95616

Several recent studies have created considerable confusion about the cause and prevention of kernicterus.[1,2,3] In 1982, Levine et al[1] demonstrated in rats that "kernicterus" could be produced by osmotic opening of the blood brain barrier. Using a technique described by Rapoport et al,[4] a hypertonic solution of arabinose was infused into one carotid artery, producing a temporary osmotically induced disruption of the blood brain barrier in the ipsilateral hemisphere. Subsequent intravenous infusion of bilirubin resulted in yellow staining of the affected region. Levine proposed that movement of albumin bound bilirubin across a disrupted barrier was the principal cause of kernicterus, and presented this as "an alternative hypothesis" to the "free bilirubin theory." However, he provided no evidence that the yellow staining produced brain damage, either by histological examination or behavioral consequences. These observations, together with other studies which failed to confirm any predictive indices for kernicterus in premature infants,[2,3] prompted Lucey[5] to editorialize that current concepts of the pathogenesis of kernicterus should be abandoned in search for a "more attractive hypothesis."

The present study was undertaken to establish, at least in principle, the relative contributions of free bilirubin and blood brain barrier permeability to the pathogenesis of bilirubin toxicity and staining. We used a rat model similar to that of Levine et al, but, in addition, implanted electrodes to monitor cortical electrical activity as a sign of bilirubin toxicity. The level of free bilirubin was varied by infusing some rats with human serum albumin (HSA) before administering arabinose and bilirubin. HSA binds bilirubin more tightly than does rat albumin. Our results indicate that disruption of the barrier potentiates acute neuro-

35

toxicity as measured by changes in the electroencephalogram, but
only if the free bilirubin reaches a critical level.

MATERIALS AND METHODS

Young male Wistar rats, 300-350 gm, were anesthetized with
pentobarbital sodium (50 mg/kg ip). The calvarium was exposed and
cleaned of periosteum and 3/16 inch stainless steel electrodes were
placed through burr holes drilled anteriorally and posteriorally
3-4 mm on each side of the midline. A similar ground electrode was
placed overlying the frontal sinus. Bipolar anterior to posterior
recordings were made from the right and left pairs of cortical
electrodes on a Grass Model 7D Polygraph. Temperature was monitored
by rectal thermometer. A femoral artery catheter was placed for
blood sampling and blood pressure monitoring, and a femoral vein
catheter was placed for infusion of bilirubin, albumin, and drugs.
A tracheostomy was performed to insure a patent airway, and a PE10
catheter was placed in the right external carotid artery with the
tip lying near the branch of the internal carotid artery for
infusion of a hyperosmolar arabinose solution.

Ten minutes prior to arabinose infusion the animal was given
1.5 gm/kg human serum albumin (25% HSA, Cutter Laboratories) or an
equivalent volume of saline intravenously. A solution of arabinose,

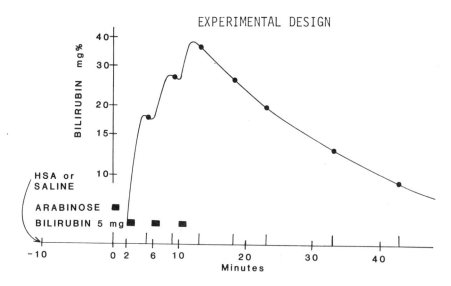

Figure 1 Schematic of the experimental protocol demonstrating a
typical serum bilirubin response in a control rat.

approximately 1.6 molal, was infused at a rate of 1.0 to 5.0 ml/min for 30 to 40 seconds or until changes in the EEG appeared over the ipsilateral hemisphere. Two minutes later, 5 mg bilirubin dissolved in one ml of 0.1 N NaOH in saline, pH 9-10, was infused intravenously over a 60 second period (figure 1). The bilirubin infusion was repeated at 4 minute intervals until the rat either received a total dose of 15 mg (45 mg/kg) or developed a change in the EEG. Blood samples were obtained for bilirubin determinations (direct spectroscopy) two minutes after each infusion and 5, 10, 20 and 30 minutes thereafter. Arterial blood pH and apparent unbound bilirubin concentration (peroxidase method[6]) were determined within two minutes of an EEG change. The rats were sacrificed following the 30 minute blood sample, and the brain was immediately removed, examined for external staining and fixed in 10% formalin for future histological examination. Preliminary studies indicated good agreement between superficial and deep staining, so only atypically stained brains were cut fresh.

RESULTS

In total, 57 rats were studied. A transient decrease in amplitude in the ipsilateral EEG and occasionally contralateral EEG developed during the arabinose infusion if successful opening of the barrier occurred. A typical response can be seen in figure 2 (A-C). In such cases subsequent infusion of bilirubin usually resulted in staining of the ipsilateral hemisphere, particularly the base of the temporal lobes, olfactory bulb and mammillary bodies. Some animals developed bilateral EEG changes in response to bilirubin even though arabinose infusion did not affect the EEG. These animals usually had generalized staining involving both hemispheres and cerebellum without evidence of lateralization. Three control rats who did not receive arabinose, as well as most rats who demonstrated no change in EEG following arabinose, failed to develop EEG changes following bilirubin infusion and demonstrated minimal or no staining when sacrificed 30 minutes later. For purposes of analysis, we have included only those rats who demonstrated clear differential staining on the ipsilateral side, indicating successful osmotic opening of the blood brain barrier.

Twenty four rats met this criterion. Subjectively, the intensity of staining in all animals appeared to relate to the maximum bilirubin value achieved, although bilirubin extraction and quantification was not attempted. Staining was most intense in the HSA treated animals. Control animals had variable intensity of staining.

Five rats had no EEG change following bilirubin infusion. One HSA primed animal had deep ipsilateral staining in both the base and cortex, with a maximum bilirubin of 71 mg/dl. Four control rats, with maximum bilirubin values of 34, 35, 41, and 50 mg/dl, had

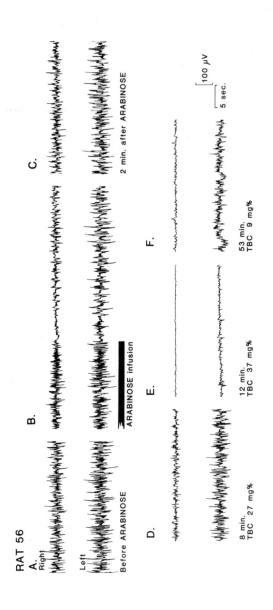

Figure 2 Typical EEG findings. A. Base line B. EEG change following infusion of 0.5 ml 1.6 molal arabinose in the right carotid artery. C. Recovery of EEG two minutes later. D. EEG one minute after the second bilirubin dose (total 10 mg) E. EEG one minute after a third bilirubin infusion (13 mg total dose) showing decreased amplitude on the contralateral side and almost complete loss of activity on the ipsilateral side F. Recovery of the EEG on the contralateral side 42 minutes after administering bilirubin. The right hemisphere was deeply stained, with only faint diffuse yellow coloration in the left hemisphere.

brains with only faint staining at the base of the temporal lobe or olfactory bulb.

Eleven control animals and eight HSA primed rats developed both EEG changes and differential staining of the ipsilateral hemisphere. EEG changes were variable, ranging from a transient decrease in amplitude to complete loss of electrical activity (figure 2, D-E). Most often, the changes would occur during or shortly after a bilirubin infusion, but sometimes appeared two to six minutes later. Recovery of the EEG occured in some animals after 3-5 minutes, and often flattened again 3-10 minutes later. Most often EEG changes occured over both hemispheres, even when staining was clearly unilateral. Differences in time course, character, and magnitude of response indicated that these were related to independent functional abnormalities in each hemisphere.

The bilirubin threshold for EEG changes was markedly different in the control and HSA treated animals. Changes occured at a mean serum bilirubin concentration of 30 mg/dl in the control animals, compared with 55 mg/dl in the HSA primed rats (Table I). Only one treated rat developed EEG changes at a serum bilirubin concentration which was comparable to that of control animals. Total bilirubin loads given the two groups were similar, although several control animals and one treated animal developed EEG changes after only 10 mg bilirubin infusion. The differences in serum bilirubin concentration was therefore due principally to differences in distribution of bilirubin owing to the increased serum binding affinity and/or capacity of the HSA primed animals. However, with disruption of the barrier, albumin with its attached bilirubin had equal access to neurons in both groups of animals. The exposure of neurons to bilirubin, as judged by intensity of staining, was much higher in the HSA treated rats. The exposure to free bilirubin at the time of EEG changes, however, was probably comparable. We measured the apparent unbound bilirubin concentration in the serum of 4 treated and 7 control animals. At comparable total bilirubin concentrations

Table I

SERUM BILIRUBIN LEVELS AT APPEARANCE OF EEG CHANGES

	n	BILIRUBIN CONCENTRATION Mean +/- S.D.	(Range)
HSA Primed	8	54.8 +/- 12.6	(37-72 mg/dl)
Controls	11	30.4 +/- 6.4	(17-38 mg/dl)

t = 5.536, p < .001

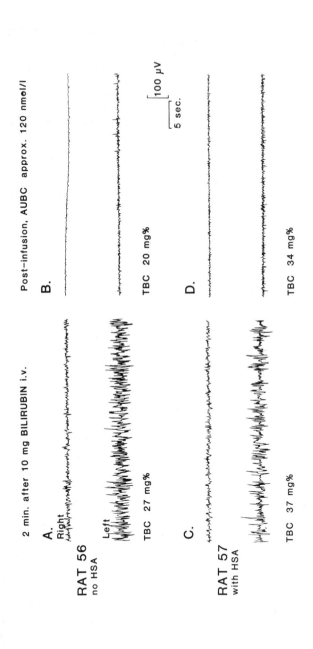

Figure 3 Comparison of serum bilirubin levels and EEG changes in control and HSA treated rats. A and C. Onset of EEG changes after infusion of 10 mg bilirubin. The serum bilirubin concentrations differ greatly. The unbound bilirubin levels were too high to measure accurately in either animal. B and D. EEGs obtained during the decline of serum bilirubin at a time when the concentrations of unbound bilirubin in the animals were nearly identical. Changes in the contralateral side are now apparent. Vital signs remained stable and arterial pH was normal in both animals.

the free bilirubin concentration was higher in control than in
treated animals. These relationships are illustrated in figure 3,
comparing two animals with similar EEG behavior but markedly
different total bilirubin levels.

DISCUSSION

These results indicate that disruption of the blood brain barrier
may potentiate acute neurotoxicity, but only if the serum free
bilirubin is sufficiently elevated. The data do not support Levine's
contention that the bilirubin-albumin complex is toxic, but are
consistent with the large body of evidence which suggests that
bilirubin enters cells unattached to albumin, and that the binding
of bilirubin to albumin prevents its cellular toxicity.[7,8] Opening
of the blood brain barrier to macromolecules gives serum albumin
immediate access to the interstitial space of the brain. The
neuropil is then bathed with a bilirubin-albumin solution, and the
free bilirubin can interact with either albumin or tissue according
to their relative attraction. Under these conditions, albumin
provides a large and relatively static reservoir of bilirubin which
should rapidly equilibrate with alternative binding sites on albumin
or cellular membranes. At some point, the tissue binding will be
sufficient to impair neuronal function, resulting in abnormal
electroencephalographic activity.

When the blood brain barrier is impermeable or only slightly
permeable to albumin, this process would take considerably longer.
Free bilirubin would have to traverse both the capillary endothelium
and the neural tissue to produce toxicity. The rate of this transfer
would depend on four major factors, 1) the free bilirubin
concentration and pH, 2) the dissociation rate from albumin (how
quickly the free bilirubin will be replaced once it is removed), 3)
the transit time through the capillary bed (time available for
equilibrium to occur), and 4) the permeability and surface area of
the capillary endothelium.[9] It is unknown whether the interstitial
concentration of albumin is important as a transport protein to
distribute bilirubin to affected cells

The finding of abnormal EEG's on the unstained contralateral side
and in a few of the "arabinose failures" suggests the possibility
that arabinose can alter permeability of the barrier to bilirubin
itself. In acute toxicity, the yellow staining may represent mostly
interstitial bilirubin bound to albumin rather than cellular
bilirubin accumulation. If the barrier is permeable to bilirubin but
not to albumin, a sudden exposure to a very high free bilirubin load
could produce acute toxicity with minimal staining. This concept is
supported by several clinical and laboratory experiences. Perl
et al[10] reported that infusion of bilirubin in newborn rabbits
produced convulsions and death within hours, yet the brains showed
no evidence of staining. We have previously produced bilirubin

encephalopathy in newborn monkeys following perinatal asphyxia by
maintaining a bilirubin level of 20-30 mg/dl for 6-10 hours.[11] EEG's
were monitored in two of these animals, showing minimal changes
until they received an intravenous infusion of sulfisoxazole,
200 mg/kg. This resulted in apnea, a rapid drop in total bilirubin
concentration and an immediate flattening of the EEG.

The extent to which the yellow staining of kernicterus represents
interstitial bilirubin attached to albumin or neuronal bilirubin
deposition is not clear. Turkel and colleagues[3] demonstrated that
many kernicteric premature babies have spongy changes in brain
consistent with interstitial edema, but few changes in neurons that
could be attributed to bilirubin toxidcity. This would be consistent
with transport of bilirubin-albumin across a disrupted blood brain
barrier. In contrast, Ahdab-Barmada[12] reported a similarly high
incidence of kernicterus, but found that most prematures had typical
findings, both in respect to distribution of lesions and
histological findings.

With respect to the human condition, our observations must not be
over-interpreted. The distribution of staining, while involving
basal ganglia, was diffuse, largely cortical, and not very
characteristic of kernicterus in newborn infants. Osmotic opening of
the barrier, with disruption of capillary endothelial tight
junctions is unlikely to be the mechanism of altered barrier in
newborn infants. However, this study does demonstrate the principle
that both blood brain barrier transport and free bilirubin may be
important in the pathogenesis of bilirubin toxicity. In humans the
distribution of kernicterus is similar to the distribution of
cerebral blood flow, which is linked to metabolic activity. These
associations are probably not coincidental. Cells with higher
metabolic rates may be more susceptible to bilirubin, a metabolic
poison, especially if there is an underlying additive insult such as
hypoxia. Alternatively, the higher blood flow could simply
facilitate the movement of free bilirubin across the capillary
endothelial barrier in these areas.

REFERENCES

1. R. L. Levine, W. R. Fredericks, and S. I. Rapoport, Entry of
      bilirubin into the brain due to opening of the blood brain
      barrier, Pediatrics 69:255 (1982).
2. D. A. Ritter, J. D. Kenny, J. Norton, and A. J Rudolph, A pro-
      spective study of free bilirubin and other risk factors in
      the development of kernicterus in premature infants,
      Pediatrics 69:260 (1982).
3. S. B. Turkel, C. A. Miller, M. E. Guttenberg, D. R. Moynes, and
      J. E. Hodgman, A clinical pathologic reappraisal of
      kernicterus, Pediatrics 69:267 (1982).

4. S. I. Rapoport, W. R. Fredericks, K. Ohno, et al, Quantitative aspects of reversible osmotic opening of the blood-brain barrier, Am J Physiol 238:R421 (1980).
5. J. F. Lucey, Bilirubin and brain damage - A real mess, Pediatrics 69:381, (1982).
6. J. Jacobsen and R. P. Wennberg, Determination of unbound bilirubin in the serum of newborns, Clin Chem 20:783 (1974).
7. W. B. Karp, Biochemical alterations in neonatal hyperbili- rubinemia and bilirubin encephalopathy: a review, Pediatrics 64:361 (1979).
8. R. P. Wennberg, C. E. Ahlfors, and L. F. Rasmussen, The patho- chemistry of kernicterus, Early Human Develop 3/4:353 (1979).
9. W. M. Pardridge, Transport of protein-bound hormones into tissues in vivo, Endocrine Revs 2:103 (1981).
10. H. Perl, A. Nijjar, H. Ebara, et al, Bilirubin toxicity without CNS staining, Pediatr Res 15:303A, (1982).
11. R. P. Wennberg, The pathogenesis of kernicterus: factors influencing the distribution of bilirubin with albumin and tissue, in: "Metabolism and Chemistry of Bilirubin and Related Tetrapyrroles,"- A. F. Bakken and J. Fog, eds., Pediatric Research Institute, Oslo, Norway (1975).
12. M. Ahdab-Barmada, Neonatal kernicterus: Neuropathologic diagnosis, J Neuropath In press.

DISTRIBUTION OF BILIRUBIN BETWEEN SERUM AND CEREBROSPINAL FLUID
IN NEWBORN INFANTS

P. Meisel, D. Jährig, I. Weinke and K. Jährig

Department of Pediatrics
Ernst-Moritz-Arndt University
DDR - 22 Greifswald, G.D.R.

INTRODUCTION

An increased bilirubin (BR) concentration in the cerebrospinal fluid (CSF) is found in newborns either in hyperbilirubinemia or after extravasation of blood into CSF and/or increasing CSF protein concentration. We have hypothesized that the BR concentration of CSF may reflect the pigment level in the brain. Therefore, the estimation of the relationship between circulating bilirubin and its CSF level should offer the possibility to gain some insight into the pathogenesis of BR encephalopathy[1]. Moreover, more subtle indication criteria are necessary to decide whether phototherapy or exchange transfusion is advisable for the treatment of jaundiced infants.

MATERIAL AND METHODS

CSF was obtained from a total of 52 newborn infants by lumbar puncture for diagnostic reasons or post mortem. At the same time a venous blood sample was taken. The infants were divided into two groups: i) "bilirubinemia", including all cases of hyperbilirubinemia and infants presumably without CNS affection (prematurity, RDS, malformations); ii) "CNS affection", including all cases of intracranial hemorrhages and infants suffering from meningitis, sepsis, and congenital toxoplasmosis. Total BR in serum and CSF was determined by standard laboratory methods, CSF-BR was additionally assayed according to van Roy et al.[2], with separation of diazotized dipyrroles by thin layer chromatography. Estimation of BR unbound to albumin (free BR) was performed by the peroxidase technique[3], albumin was estimated by bromocresol green binding[4] .

45

The neurodevelopmental outcome of 19 children of the bilirubinemia group was followed during the first and second years of life
according to the "Functional Developmental Score"[5] and the schedule
of the "Neurodevelopmental Examination"[6].

RESULTS AND DISCUSSION

Although the groups with bilirubinemia and CNS affections were
separated with regard to clinical diagnosis only, significant
differences are obvious in birth weight, blood pH, serum total BR,
BR/albumin ratio, albumin concentration, CSF-BR, albumin and total
protein. However, no significant differences were found in the
serum level of free BR, as well as in the toxic potential of BR[7].
After hemorrhages the CSF-BR content is related to the CSF protein
level only and BR concentration greater than expected are to be
measured due to local BR formation. Thus, CSF specimens obtained
after intracranial bleeding are non-relevant with respect to the
relationship between blood and brain BR levels and the following
examinations were restricted to the bilirubinemia group only.

In Fig. 1 the relationship between the measured CSF-BR level
and the "expected BR" is shown indicating that BR is bound to
albumin in both blood and CSF. Consequently, the CSF-BR level tends
to be lower than expected from the equation

$$BR_{CSF} = BR_{serum} \cdot r \text{ (albumin)}$$

Using the ratios $BR_{CSF}/BR_{serum} = r$ (BR), and $albumin_{CSF}/$
$albumin_{serum} = r$ (albumin) as parameters of the blood brain barrier,
both values are in good agreement in each individual CSB specimen.
However, the BR ratio tends to be lower than the albumin ratio in
the regression analysis: $r(BR) = 0.71 \cdot r(albumin) + 0.003$ (p 0.01).
It is suggested that these differences are due to dilution of the
flowing CSF and/or a transport system which returns BR back into
the circulation, or induces BR binding to tissue constituents.

The CSF-BR levels measured are dependent on the free BR concentration in serum: CSF-BR (umol/l) = 0.16·free BR (nmol/l) +
0.65 (r= 0.87), a finding supporting the free BR concept. This
relationship is indicated in Fig. 2 together with the individual
CSF-BR concentrations of infants examined later for neurodevelopmental outcome. Obviously, the results enabled us to separate the
subjects into two groups. One, the low risk group, with free BR
below 20 nmol/l and low CSF-BR levels in the neonatal period, later
showed predominantly normal psychomotor development.

The other, the high risk group, with free BR above 20 nmol/l
(a value provisionally considered as a risk limit[9]) and high CSF-BR
levels, included a high portion of children with depressed mental

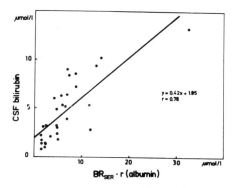

Fig. 1.   The BR concentration measured in CSF related to the
          expected BR level calculated (see text)

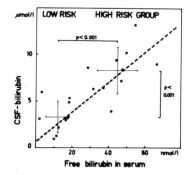

Fig. 2.   Dependence of CSF-BR concentration on serum free BR in
          infants followed for later neurodevelopmental outcome.
          The broken line indicates the least square fit of the
          total of CSF-BR determinations in bilirubinemia group.

or motor development. Exchange transfusions were necessary only in
subjects of the high risk group. No additional risk factors (APGAR
scores, prematurity, etc.) were present as compared with the low
risk group. Three subjects of the high risk group showed considerable
discrepancies between their developmental and chronological age,
with striking abnormalities in perception, active speech, and com=
prehension. It may be speculated that disturbances in these cate=
gories are probably related to BR exposure during neonatal life.

Except for one case, all the children of the high risk group
were neurologically abnormal or retarded. Assuming that the handi=
caps would be, at least partially, a result of increased BR expo=
sure, the exception demonstrates that critical high BR levels during
the neonatal period are essential but not sufficient conditions in

Table 1. Discrimination between the low risk and high risk groups
as a consequence of BR exposure of the CNS as assessed
by the relationship shown in Fig. 2

	CNS-exposure by BR		significance
	low risk	high risk	
Number of subjects	9	10	—
small f. gest. age	1	1	
appr. f. gest. age	8	9	n. s.
five min. APGAR	6–10	7–10	n. s.
5th day			
serum total BR, μmol/l	175.9	339.7	p< 0.01
	± 115.5	± 84.0	
serum BR/albumin	0.37	0.62	p< 0.002
	± 0.24	±0.18	
serum free BR, nmol/l	12.1	44.7	p< 0.001
	± 6.3	±11.2	
CSF total BR, μmol/l	3.3	8.3	p< 0.001
	± 1.7	±2.5	
Number of cases with			
phototherapy	4	7	p< 0.05
exchange transfusion	0	6	
psychomotor appr. developed	7	1	p< 0.05
psychomotor retardation	2	9	

in the etiology of BR encephalopathy. On the other hand, an infant
suffering from Crigler-Najjar syndrome type I, depending on daily
phototherapy, exhibited completely normal neurodevelopmental appearance up to now (age 3 years), in spite of a long lasting exposure
to serum total BR levels above 20 mg/dl. Accordingly, during the
neonatal period dangerous levels of free BR in serum or total BR
in CSF could not be measured. Finally, in one child of the low risk
group assessed as retarded and affected by multiple malformations,
causes of encephalopathy other than hyperbilirubinemia may be present.

In conclusion, the results suggest that the BR level in the
CSF may be related to the pigment concentration in the brain. The
relationship between free BR in serum and total BR in CSF may be
of significance in later neurodevelopmental outcome with regard
to BR encephalopathy, as it includes both the BR chemistry in the
blood and the state of the blood brain barrier[10].

REFERENCES

1. P. Meisel, D. Jähring, I. Weinke, and K. Jähring, Bilirubin in
      CSF of newborns, Kinderärztliche Praxis 49:633 (1981);
      50:370 (1982); 51:70 (1983).
2. F. P. van Roy, J. A. T. P. Meuwissen, F. de Meuter, and K. P. M.
      Heirwegh, Determination of bilirubin in liver homogenates
      and serum with diazotized p-iodoaniline, Clin. Chim. Acta
      31:109 (1971).

3. J. Jacobsen and R. P. Wenneberg, Determination of unbound
    bilirubin in the serum of newborns, Clin. Chem. 20:783 (1974).
4. D. P. Lehane, A. L. Levy, and A. S. Erglis, Colorimetric quan-
    titation of albumin in microliter volumes of serum, Ann.
    Clin. Lab. Sci. 8:122 (1979).
5. T. Hellbrügge, D. Menara, R. Schamberger, and S. Stünkel,
    Funktionelle Entwicklungsdiagnostik im 2. Lebensjahr,
    Fortschr. Med. 89:558 (1971).
6. V. Vojta, Frühdiagnose und Frühtherapie der cerebralen Bewegun-
    gsstörungen im Kindesalter, Z. Orthop. 110:450 (1972).
7. R. Brodersen, Binding of bilirubin to albumin-implications for
    prevention of bilirubin encephalopathy, Crit. Rev. Clin.
    Lab. Sci. 11:305 (1979).
8. K. G. Kjellin, The binding of xanthochromic compounds in the
    cerebrospinal fluid, J. Neurol. Sci. 9:597 (1969).
9. R. P. Wennberg, M. Lau, and L. F. Rasmussen, Clinical signifi-
    cance of unbound bilirubin. Pediat. Res. 10:434 (1976).
10. J. F. Lucey, Bilirubin and brain damage - a real mess,
    Pediatrics 69:381 (1982).

THE CHEMICAL NATURE OF FETAL ALBUMIN

Rolf Brodersen and Christian Jacobsen

Institute of Medical Biochemistry
University of Aarhus
DK-8000 Aarhus C

Henning Iversen and Frank Lundquist

Department of Biochemistry
University of Copenhagen
Blegdamsvej 3c
DK-2200 Copenhagen N

INTRODUCTION

Several observers have reported that serum albumin from the human fetus and newborn infants has a decreased capability for binding bilirubin and certain drugs, when compared with serum albumin from healthy adults,[1] (and references therein). Decreased binding is also seen in pregnant women.[2] The chemical nature of the binding defect has remained unknown.

NEGATIVE RESULTS

Ligands

Reversible binding of the following ligands to albumin in the blood stream could not explain the decreased binding of bilirubin:

Fatty acids (short-, medium- and long-chain as well as branched, saturated acids; oleic acid; polyunsaturated C_{18}-C_{22} acids).

Bile acids.

Other nutrients and metabolites such as cholesterol, cortisol, tryptophan, tyrosine, thyroxine, orotate, citrate, malate, fumarate, lactate, hydroxybutyrate, oxaloacetate, pyruvate, acetone, urea, urate, creatinine, peptides.[3]

Food additives and environmental poisons such as benzoate, hippurate, parabenes, sorbate, oxalate, hydrocarbons.

Calcium, copper and chloride ions.

Chemical Derivations

Covalent changes in the albumin molecule with the following reactants did not result in significantly decreased binding of bilirubin:

Glucose, reacting with lysyl side chains.

Urea, thiourea, cyanate, thiocyanate, reacting with lysyl side chains.

Carbon dioxide, reacting with lysyl side chains.

Sulfhydryl compounds, reacting with the free -SH group and causing "scrambling" of the S-S bond structure.

Oxygen, reacting predominantly with histidine side chains in the presence of unsaturated fatty acids.

Aspirin acetylating one lysyl side chain.

Amino Acid Composition

Differences in amino acid composition of fetal and adult albumin could not explain the difference of bilirubin binding.

POSITIVE FINDINGS

Fetal albumin was isolated from umbilical cord serum by gel chromatography on Sephacryl S-300. Adult albumin was similarly isolated from healthy, non-pregnant adults.

Fetal albumin showed decreased binding of bilirubin, warfarin, sulfamethizole and MADDS (monoacetyl-
-diaminodiphenyl sulfone, a ligand binding competitively with bilirubin). Reserve albumin equivalent[4] for binding of MADDS varied from 50 to 80 percent of that of adult albumin. Binding of diazepam was equal for the two albumin preparations.

Isoelectric focusing showed a main peak with isoelectric point at pH 5.0 for fetal albumin, and 5.6 for the adult protein.

Treatment with charcoal in acid solution, pH 3, changed the fetal albumin to adult type with respect to binding of MADDS and isoelectric focusing pattern.

Fetal albumin (reserve albumin for binding of MADDS in this sample was 77 percent of the adult value) showed a content of acetaldehyde about 2 nmol/mg albumin, when analysed after acid treatment, by gas chromatography. To one volume of the albumin solution (10 mg/ml) was added one volume of 1 M perchloric acid. After incubation in tightly sealed glass tubes 30 min. at 37°C the mixture was chilled in ice and centrifuged. Acetaldehyde was determined in the gas phase by gas chromatography after incubation for 15 min. at 65°C of the protein-free supernatant.

Adult albumin had a significantly lower content of acetaldehyde, 0.1 nmol/mg protein.

Adult albumin, 600 µM, in phosphate buffer solution with acetaldehyde, 10 mM (pH 7.4, 24 h at 37°), formed a product with decreased binding of bilirubin, unchanged binding of diazepam and low isoelectric point.

CONCLUSION AND DISCUSSION

The above observations suggest that the decreased binding of ligands to fetal albumin may be explained by the presence of acetaldehyde, adducted to the protein.

Donohue et al.[5] have described reversible as well as permanent fixation of acetaldehyde to serum albumin. The primary product is a Schiff's base formed with lysyl side chains. One lysyl, lys-240, is essential for binding of bilirubin to human serum albumin.[6]

Acetaldehyde may hypothetically be formed in the fetus by several known processes, breakdown of threonin, hydrolysis of hydroxyethyl-thiaminpyrophosphate, breakdown of deoxyribose-5-phosphate, and by transformation of methyltetrose-1-phosphate to dihydroxyacetone phosphate. The latter process is interesting as a possible source of acetaldehyde since the enzyme involved, muscle aldolase, is present in the fetal liver where it is replaced later in life by another aldolase.

ACKNOWLEDGEMENTS

The authors wish to thank Signe Andersen, Nina Jørgensen, Birthe Lindgaard and Anne-Marie Bundsgaard for technical assistance.

REFERENCES

1. N. Gitzelmann-Cumarasamy, R. Gitzelmann, K.J. Wilson, and C.C. Kuenzle, Fetal and adult albumins are indistinguishable by immunological and physicochemical criteria, Proc. Natl. Acad. Sci. USA 76:2960 (1979).
2. G. Järnerot, S. Andersen, E. Esbjørner, B. Sandström, and R. Brodersen, Albumin reserve for binding of bilirubin in maternal and cord serum under treatment with sulfasalazine, Scand. J. Gastroent. 16:1049 (1981).
3. A. Robertson and R. Brodersen, The effect of lactate, pyruvate, acetone, acetoacetate and β-hydroxybutyrate on albumin binding of bilirubin, J. Pediatr. 102:433 (1983).
4. R. Brodersen, S. Andersen, C. Jacobsen, O. Sønderskov, F. Ebbesen, W.J. Cashore, and S. Larsen, Determination of reserve albumin-equivalent for ligand binding, probing two distinct binding functions of the protein, Anal. Biochem. 121:395 (1982).
5. T.M. Donohue, jr., D.J. Tuma, and M.F. Sorrell, Acetaldehyde adducts with protein: Binding of [^{14}C]acetaldehyde to serum albumin, Arch. Biochem. Biophys. 220:239 (1983).
6. C. Jacobsen, Lysine residue 240 of human serum albumin is involved in high affinity binding of bilirubin, Biochem. J. 171:453 (1978).

ESTIMATION OF RESERVE ALBUMIN EQUIVALENT

CONCENTRATION FOR BINDING OF BILIRUBIN

Rolf Brodersen

Institute of Medical Biochemistry
University of Aarhus
DK-8000   Aarhus C, Denmark

INTRODUCTION

Let us consider a hypothetical case, a prematurely born infant is admitted to an intensive care unit with respiratory distress and jaundice and having received treatment with a sulfonamide. On clinical grounds this infant is thought to be in danger of kernicterus. Is it possible, by studying blood chemistry, to assess the risk in quantitative terms? And can we evaluate the success of therapy, exchange transfusion and light, and tell when the risk is over on the basis of blood tests? These questions have often been asked but have never been finally answered.

It is quite clear that blood chemistry cannot give the full answer. Tissue factors such as the blood-brain barrier and the activity of bilirubin oxidase in the nerve cells are probably important. What we may hope for is that we can measure one factor, the *plasma bilirubin toxicity*. I personally believe that this is an important factor and that, if it can be measured, its use in the clinic will contribute to the understanding of the mechanism of bilirubin encephalopathy and to the improvement of therapeutic results in individual cases.

MEASURING PLASMA BILIRUBIN TOXICITY

The most obvious way of assessing plasma bilirubin
toxicity would be to measure the concentration of free
bilirubin or, to be more specific, to measure the concentration of non protein-bound bilirubin IX-α(Z,Z),
excluding conjugates and other isomers. This is not
possible with present means.

It has accordingly been suggested that we could
measure the total concentration of bilirubin and the
amount of albumin available for binding of bilirubin.
If we have a binding equilibrium of bilirubin, albumin,
and the complex of both, and if we know the binding constant, we could calculate the concentration of free
bilirubin and thus the plasma bilirubin toxicity. This
would be just as good as being able to measure free
bilirubin directly. Let us look at the binding equilibria in the blood plasma of our patient.

Albumin, P, can bind one molecule of bilirubin,
forming the complex PB. This complex can bind a second
bilirubin and possibly even a third. The sulfonamide,
which has been given to the patient, also binds to
albumin, stepwise forming complexes, PS, PS_2 etc. Each
of these can again bind one or two bilirubin, forming
ternary complexes, which can also be formed from binding
the sulfonamide to bilirubin-albumin. We have investigated this whole pattern of equilibria in detail and
have found that considerable amounts of several of the
species are present.

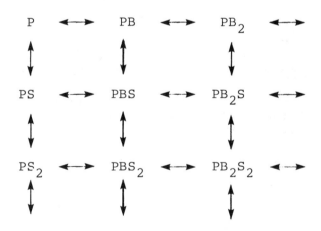

What do we now mean if we talk about the amount of albumin available for binding of bilirubin? It is obvious that this cannot be defined if we have multiple binding of two ligands. It has no clear meaning to talk of the available amount of albumin or the residual binding capacity. This is further underlined if it is taken into account that binding of bilirubin and drugs to albumin is generally non-saturating. Albumin binding curves do not have a level of saturation, as we know it from binding of oxygen to hemoglobin; the curves show a continuous upward trend.

It is therefore not meaningful to talk of *bilirubin binding capacity*. This cannot be defined nor can it be measured.

RESERVE ALBUMIN EQUIVALENT FOR BINDING OF BILIRUBIN

In order to circumvent this difficulty we have had to define another parameter, the reserve albumin equivalent for binding of a ligand, e.g. bilirubin. This is defined as the concentration of a standard albumin preparation which has to be present in pure solution with bilirubin in order to bind the bilirubin equally tight as it is bound in the plasma sample.[1] This is thermodynamically a well-defined entity. It cannot be measured in plasma, however.

We have to use another ligand, a deputy for bilirubin, a substance which is bound to albumin, as far as possible in pure competition with bilirubin and being displaced from binding by the same substances and to the same degree. After an intensive search among many compounds we have found that these criteria are fulfilled to a reasonable degree by a substance, mono-acetyl--diamino-diphenyl sulfone, MADDS.

THE MADDS METHOD

A minute amount of ^{14}C-labelled MADDS in concentrated buffer is added to the plasma sample. Fifteen volumes of plasma are used to one volume of buffered MADDS in order to avoid diluting the sample. The volume used is 25 µl infant plasma. A similar volume of the same plasma sample is mixed with buffer alone, without MADDS. The two mixtures are placed on either side of a dialysis membrane and the *rate* of dialysis of MADDS from

one into the other is measured. The time needed for this
is 10 minutes.

The rate of dialysis depends upon how tight MADDS
is bound to albumin in the sample; the tighter the binding, the slower the dialysis.

A standard curve is prepared, using pure solutions
of a standard albumin instead of plasma. The dialysis
rate is measured as a function of the albumin concentration. The rate measured in the sample is then plotted on
the standard curve and the reserve albumin concentration
is obtained.

This is the reserve albumin concentration, or to be
correct, the reserve albumin equivalent concentration
for binding of MADDS. It is reasonable to use this
figure for practical purposes for the reserve albumin
concentration for binding of bilirubin. The error introduced by using MADDS as a deputy for bilirubin is probably small in most cases although it is admitted that in
principle it is difficult to be sure of this since no
reference method is available for correct determinations
using bilirubin.

It should be understood that this method is not an
equilibrium dialysis. In equilibrium the concentration
of MADDS would be equal on both sides of the dialysis
membrane since the same sample is present on both sides,
and such a determination would not tell us anything of
the bilirubin binding character of the plasma. It is also
clear that dialysis against an equal volume of buffer
would result in removing some of the sulfonamide, thus
causing an error in the determination.

CRITERIA FOR CORRECT DETERMINATIONS
OF BILIRUBIN BINDING

An ideal method for measuring binding of bilirubin
in a plasma sample should fulfill the following criteria:

A.   Dilution of the sample is avoided.

B.   Determination is carried out at $37^{o}C$ and at the
pH of the patient's plasma.

C.   Addition of large amounts of dyes or use of
Sephadex is avoided since this would shift the equilibria to be studied.

D. Titration of a so-called bilirubin binding capacity by adding bilirubin is avoided, partly because this entity cannot be defined nor measured, partly because bilirubin would displace the sulfonamide thus giving a falsely high "capacity".

E. It should be tested by clinical experience whether the technique gives meaningful results, i.e. 1) low reserve albumin in groups of low-icteric infants with clinically known risk of bilirubin encephalopathy, 2) increased reserve albumin after exchange transfusion, albumin infusion, or phototherapy, and 3) low reserve albumin after giving bilirubin displacing drugs.

F. Ideally, binding of bilirubin should be studied directly. Errors introduced by use of a deputy ligand should be investigated.

G. The technique should be easy and not require special manual skill.

None of the available methods fulfill all these criteria. The MADDS technique, as used with the present apparatus, cannot measure reserve albumin at the pH of the patient's plasma since contact with the air is unavoidable. The pH is fixed near 7.4 by adding a buffer. Also, certain errors will be encountered because of the use of a deputy ligand instead of bilirubin. We are at present studying this point further. Finally, the technique is manually difficult and can be mastered only in advanced laboratories. Otherwise the above criteria are met, including E1)-3), as demonstrated by generous cooperation of Cashore in Providence and Ebbesen in Copenhagen.[2-10]

UTILITY OF RESERVE ALBUMIN DETERMINATIONS

The determinations are useful for calculation of the free concentration of bilirubin dianion[1] or other ligands in binding equilibrium with albumin as well as for studies of cobinding of two ligands, such as bilirubin and a displacing drug.

On the further presumption that bilirubin in kernicterus is deposited in the brain as the insoluble acid in a thermodynamically reversible process, the measurements can be utilized for estimation of the actual bilirubin toxicity of plasma, expressed as an index of plasma bilirubin toxicity

$$I = \log \frac{B}{p} - 2 \text{ pH} + 15.5$$

when B is the unconjugated plasma bilirubin concentration, p is reserve albumin equivalent concentration and
15.5 is a constant, theoretically calculated from the
solubility and acidity of bilirubin.

REFERENCES

1. R. Brodersen, S. Andersen, C. Jacobsen, O.
    Sønderskov, F. Ebbesen, W.J. Cashore, and S.
    Larsen, Determination of reserve albumin-equiv-
    alent for ligand-binding, probing two distinct
    binding functions of the protein, Anal. Biochem.
    121:395 (1982).
2. W.J. Cashore, W. Oh, and R. Brodersen, Reserve al-
    bumin and bilirubin toxicity index in infant
    serum, Acta Pædiatr. Scand. 72:415 (1983).
3. F. Ebbesen, Effect of exchange transfusion on serum
    reserve albumin for binding of bilirubin and index
    of serum bilirubin toxicity, Acta Pædiatr. Scand.
    70:643 (1981).
4. F. Ebbesen, The relationship between serum bilirubin
    and reserve albumin for binding of bilirubin
    during phototherapy of preterm infants, Acta
    Pædiatr. Scand. 70:405 (1981).
5. F. Ebbesen, Bilirubin, reserve albumin for binding
    of bilirubin and pH in plasma during phototherapy
    (ordinary and double light) of term newborn in-
    fants, Acta Pædiatr. Scand. 70:223 (1981).
6. F. Ebbesen and R. Brodersen, Albumin administration
    combined with phototherapy in treatment of
    hyperbilirubinemia in low-birth-weight infants,
    Acta Pædiatr. Scand. 70:649 (1981).
7. F. Ebbesen and R. Brodersen, Comparison between two
    preparations of human serum albumin in treatment
    of neonatal hyperbilirubinemia, Acta Pædiatr.
    Scand. 71:85 (1982).
8. W.J. Cashore, M. Funato, G. Peter, and W. Oh, Bili-
    rubin displacement from albumin by beta-lactam
    antibiotics, Pediatr. Res. 16/4:122A (1982).
9. R. Brodersen and F. Ebbesen, Bilirubin displacing
    effect of ampicillin, indomethacin, chlorproma-
    zine, gentamicin, and parabens in vitro and in
    newborn infants, J. Pharm. Sci. 72:248 (1983).
10. F. Ebbesen and R. Brodersen, Risk of bilirubin acid
    precipitation in preterm infants with respiratory

distress syndrome: Consideration of blood/brain
bilirubin transfer equilibrium, <u>Early</u> <u>Hum.</u>
<u>Develop.</u> 6:341 (1982).

POSTNATAL CHANGES IN THE ABILITY OF PLASMA ALBUMIN TO BIND

BILIRUBIN

F. Ebbesen[*] and J. Nyboe[§]

The Departments of [*]Neonatology and [§]Statistics
Rigshospitalet, Copenhagen, Denmark

INTRODUCTION

The ability of plasma albumin to bind bilirubin during the
first 8 days of life was investigated in healthy infants and the
binding ability was related to gestational age, birth weight and sex.
The study included 407 singleborn, newborn infants, who fulfilled
the following criteria: the infant was judged clinically well from
the birth, had received no blood products or medication other than
phytomenadion, did not require phototherapy, direct Coombs' test
was negative, and Apgar score was seven or more 5 min. after birth.

METHODS

The plasma concentrations of unconjugated bilirubin, reserve
albumin for bilirubin-binding, and total albumin were determined
once in each infant during the first 8 days of life. The reserve
albumin concentration for bilirubin-binding was determined by the
^{14}C -MADDS method.[1] MADDS (monoacetyldiaminodiphenyl sulphone) is
a deputy ligand for bilirubin.

The average birth weight of the infants studied was 2,930 g
(range 1,200-4,700 g) and the average gestational age was 269 days.
(range 205-307 days). There were 212 females and 193 males. The
average bilirubin concentration was 40 μmol/l for infants a few
hours old, and rose to a maximal average of 200 μmol/l for infants
3-4 days old, whereafter it decreased slowly in older infants. The
trends in the reserve albumin concentration were more or less opposite to those of the bilirubin concentration. The average reserve
albumin concentration was 180 μmol/l among infants a few hours old,
and it declined to a minimum level (average 115 μmol/l) among

63

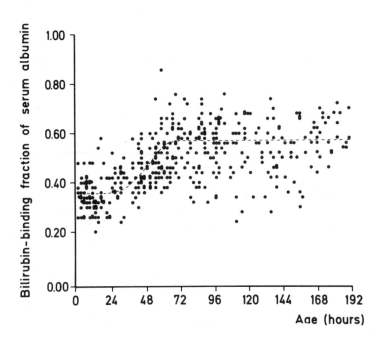

Fig. 1. The bilirubin-binding fraction of plasma albumin plotted against postnatal age. The curve represents smoothed mean values.

Table 1. The bilirubin-binding fraction of plasma albumin in relation to gestational age and birth weight in two age groups.

	AGE GROUP			
	0 - 24 HOURS		60 - 192 HOURS	
	NUMBER OF INFANTS	MEAN OF BINDING FRACTION	NUMBER OF INFANTS	MEAN OF BINDING FRACTION
GESTATIONAL AGE (DAYS)				
LESS THAN	10	0.362	20	0.442
240 - 259	19	0.368	26	0.481
260 - 274	12	0.328	68	0.574
275 - 284	20	0.370	78	0.573
285 OR MORE	20	0.355	38	0.594
BIRTH WEIGHT (G)				
LESS THAN 2000	21	0.356	21	0.433
2000 - 2290	16	0.380	23	0.504
2300 - 2990	16	0.368	58	0.540
3000 - 3490	10	0.347	63	0.606
3500 OR MORE	18	0.340	65	0.576

infants 24-72 h old, whereafter it rose again in older infants. The
average total albumin concentration was almost the same for infants
of all ages up to 8 days (580, μmol/l). The average total albumin
concentration was almost the same for infants of all ages up to 8
days (580 μmol/l). The fraction of albumin capable of binding bilirubin was calculated as the sum of the concentrations of the concentrations of unconjugated bilirubin and reserve albumin, divided by
the total albumin concentration.

RESULTS

In Fig. 1 the bilirubin-binding fractions of plasma albumin
were plotted against the postnatal age of the infants. No trend in
the fraction was discrenible during the first 24 h after birth, the
mean fraction being 0.36. Thereafter, the binding fraction increased
with age until about 60 h after birth, and from this point there
was no apparent change up to the end of the 8th day of life. In
the following, we consider the two levels of bilirubin-binding
fraction of plasma albumin: the primary level in infants 0-24 h
old, and the secondary level in infants 60-192 h old. The intermediate data of infants 24-60 h old are used to obtain details of
the transition from the primary to the secondary level. Apparently,
the secondary level depended on the maturity of infants, as expressed by their birth weight or gestational age, whereas this was not
the case for the primary level. This is indicated in Table 1, which
shows means of the bilirubin-binding fraction of albumin in the
two age groups, again divided into 5 birth weight groups and 5
groups of gestational age. No relation was apparent between the
bilirubin-binding fraction and birth-weight or gestational age among
the 0-24 h old infants, while among the 60-192 h old infants the
binding fraction increased with increasing birth weight up to at
least 3,000 g and with increasing gestational age up to 275 days,
when the mean binding fraction was about 0.58.

These apparent trends have been futher studied by means of
regression analysis using sex, postnatal age, and birth weight/ge-
stational age as describing variables. As the relation between the
binding fraction and birth weight was not linear for 60-192 h old
infants, a separate analysis was made for infants with birth weight
less than 3,000 g and birth weight of 3,000 g or more, assuming
linearity within each group. Similar assumptions have been made for
gestational age less than 275 days and 275 days or more.

None of the regression coefficients for postnatal age and sex
were significantly different from zero (thus supporting our use
of the term "level" of bilirubin-binding fraction of albumin within
the two age groups). For the 0-24 h old infants there was no significant relation between the binding fraction and birth weight or

gestational age, whereas the 60-192 h old infants displayed a
binding fraction which was positively correlated with birth weight
up to 3,000 g and with gestational age up to 275 days. These rela-
tions were highly significant.

DISCUSSION

The risk of bilirubin encephalopathy in newborn infants may
depend on many factors including the plasma concentration of unconjugated bilirubin, the albumin concentration, the ability of
albumin to bind bilirubin, the plasma pH, the permeability of the
blood-brain barrier, and the activity of bilirubin oxidase present
in the mitochondria of the central nervous system cells. In this
study, we have investigated the postnatal changes of the ability
of plasma albumin to bind bilirubin.

Kapitulnik et al.[2] observed that the bilirubin-binding capacity of albumin was greater in sera from term infants aged 3 to 8
days than in cord sera,whereas Cashore et al.[3] found that the capacity remained unchanged during the initial ten days of life, both
in healthy preterm and term infants, but the capacity was lower in
preterm than in term infants. Our main findings indicate that during
the initial 24 h of life the fraction of albumin available for
binding of bilirubin was stable, i.e. the ability of albumin to
bind bilirubin was constant. This ability was low - only a little
more than a third of the albumin could bind bilirubin - and the
binding ability was independent of the maturity of the infant. From
about the 24th h to about the 60th h of life, the bilirubin-binding
fraction increased. From the 60th h to the 8th day of life, the
fraction remained stable. This new level prevailing after 60 h of
age was related to the maturity of the infant. The level increased
with increasing birth weight up to 3,000 g and with increasing
gestational age up to 275 days, where its average approached 0.58.
This level was below that found in healthy adults,[4] indicating that
a further improvement of the binding ability of albumin occurs after
the first week of life. Kapitulnik et al.[2] found that the "adult"
level is reached at about 5 months of age.

The fact that bilirubin encephalopathy is most often seen for
very preterm infants together with our observation that there is
very little increase of the bilirubin - binding fraction of albumin
among the very preterm infants may indicate that the binding ability of albumin plays a major role in the development of bilirubin
encephalopathy. On the other hand, the lower resistance to bilirubin encephalopathy among boys than among girls cannot be explained
ned by differences in the ability of albumin to bind bilirubin,
since we found this ability to be identical in the two sexes. The
low bilirubin-binding ability of albumin in newborn infants and its
increase after the first day of life may be explained by either
changes in the albumin structure or the presence of competing ligand.

REFERENCES

1. R. Brodersen, S. Andersen, and C. Jacobsen, Determination of
    reserve albumin for ligand-binding, probing two distinct
    binding functions of the protein, Anal. Biochem. 121:395(1982)
2. J. Kapitulnik, R. Horner-Mibashan, S. H. Blondheim, N. A.
    Kaufmann, and A. Russel, Increase in bilirubin-binding affi-
    nity of serum with age of infant, J. Pediatr. 86:442 (1975).
3. W. J. Cashore, A. Horwich, J. Laterra, and W. Oh, Effect of
    postnatal age and clinical status of newborn infants on
    bilirubin-binding capacity, Biol. Neonat. 32:304 (1977).
4. F. Ebbesen, Effect of exchange transfusion on serum reserve
    albumin for binding of bilirubin and index of serum bilirubin
    toxicity, Acta Paediatr. Scand. 70:643 (1981).

INTERACTIONS OF BILIRUBIN AND DRUGS

William J. Cashore and Masahisa Funato

Department of Pediatrics
Brown University Program in Medicine and
Women and Infants Hospital of RI
Providence, Rhode Island, U.S.A.

INTRODUCTION

Many drugs given to mothers and their newborns are bound to albumin. After 25 years of experience in the United States, sulfisoxazole still remains as the only drug clearly associated with an epidemic of kernicterus in newborn infants; however, several other drugs that are often used and most of the newer drugs being developed for possible use in the perinatal period have not been adequately tested for their effects on bilirubin binding, distribution, and metabolism. As the routine use of multiple drugs increases in high-risk newborns, it is appropriate to review the methods available for testing bilirubin-drug interactions. In this presentation we shall review several methods potentially useful for studying bilirubin displacement from albumin by drugs, using examples from our own laboratory.

We shall demonstrate that:
1. Different in vitro methods may give different results and conclusions concerning bilirubin - drug interactions; so that
2. Multiple methods are needed to study the effects of drugs on bilirubin binding;
3. In vivo study of effects on bilirubin binding is possible for some drugs.

Finally, while the effects of phototherapy on bilirubin-drug interactions are beyond the scope of the data presented here, possible interactions between drugs and bilirubin photoproducts, or between bilirubin and light-induced changes in the drugs themselves, need to be considered when phototherapy is an additional variable in the treatment of infants receiving drugs.

MATERIALS AND METHODS

In all studies, we used standard colorimetric methods[2,3] for
measurement of serum bilirubin and albumin and the method of
Jacobsen and Wennberg[4] for estimation of free bilirubin or
apparent free bilirubin. Sephadex gel filtration was performed by
the method of Schiff et al[5], salicylate saturation index by the
method of Odell et al[6], and MADDS (mono-acetyl diamino diphenyl
sulfone) dialysis by the method of Brodersen[7] with equipment
kindly donated by Dr. Brodersen. Whole blood fluorometry for
bilirubin binding was performed by the method of Lamola et al[8],
with equipment provided by Bell Laboratories and by Aviv
Biomedical, Inc. Sephadex, peroxidase, and salicylate techniques
were performed at 23-24°C and MADDS dialysis and whole blood
fluorometry at 37°C. In vitro studies requiring sample dilution
with buffer were performed at pH 7.4. Study conditions
substantially different from those listed above will be described
below with the results of the particular studies. All methods were
standardized with both model serum (Fraction V Albumin, 2.5 - 5.0%)
and adult blood prior to studies on infant specimens. Studies
requiring blood samples from newborn infants were performed with
approval of the Research and Human Rights Committee of our hospital
and with informed consent by the parents.

EXAMPLES OF BILIRUBIN DISPLACEMENT BY DRUGS

It is possible to demonstrate bilirubin-drug interactions by
spectral changes. Addition of Salicylic acid, 25 mmol/l, to a

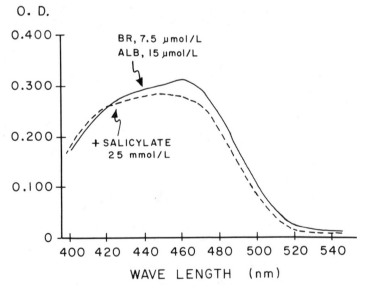

Fig. 1: Change in the spectrum of bilirubin bound to albumin when
salicylate, 25mmol/L, is added.

model serum with a ratio of 0.5 moles of BR per mole of albumin
produces a shift in the spectral curve of the bilirubin-albumin
complex with a decrease in optical density at 460nm; Odell
confirmed that this shift was caused by dislacement of bilirubin
from albumin and speculated that salicylate, which has a lower
affinity constant for albumin than bilirubin, was displacing
bilirubin from one of its secondary, or lower affinity sites on the
protein.

Another way to demonstrate the same effect is to capture
bilirubin on a Sephadex gel column and measure the amount of
bilirubin displaced by the drug. In this example, it appears that
salicylate can displace BR from its primary or high-affinity site,
because the recovery curve of bilirubin is shifted to the left
before the bilirubin concentration reaches one mole of bilirubin
per mole of albumin. This aspect of the binding relationship

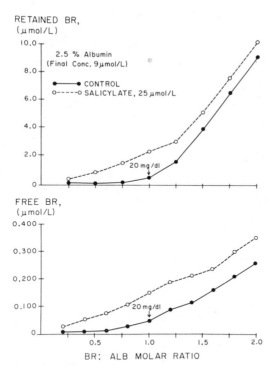

Fig. 2: Displacement of bilirubin by addition of salicylate
(0----0) to a bilirubin-albumin solution. The y-axis shows
bilirubin retained by Sephadex G-25 columns in the upper panel and
free bilirubin estimated by peroxidase oxidation in the lower
panel.

between bilirubin, albumin, and salicylate is better shown by the
more sensitive peroxidase method. When albumin is titrated with
bilirubin in the presence of excess salicylate, the drug increases
the oxidizable or free fraction of bilirubin at all bilirubin
concentrations, even far below a bilirubin:albumin ratio of one.

Since the plasma bilirubin:albumin molar ratio is usually less
than one in jaundiced newborns, important displacers of bilirubin
should be drugs which are strongly bound and compete for the
primary, or higher affinity, bilirubin binding site (unless
bilirubin is equally bound among 2 or more sites, which seems
unlikely from bilirubin-albumin binding kinetic studies). In model
serum, sulfisoxazole as well as salicylate appears to compete for
the primary bilirubin binding site, since addition of sulfisoxazole
to a bilirubin-albumin solution causes a straight linear increase
in free bilirubin even at bilirubin-to-albumin and drug-to-albumin
ratios less than one. However, the diuretic furosemide shows a
different pattern of bilirubin displacement. Furosemide added to
model serum does not displace bilirubin until the drug:albumin
ratio is 2:1 or greater, but is a moderately strong displacer at
higher concentrations, with an overall curvilinear displacement
effect. We infer from this finding that one or more high-affinity
sites for binding furosemide are non-competitive for bilirubin. A
well-known and more striking case is that of the fatty acids, such
as oleate. In an albumin solution of 9.5 umol/l and
bilirubin:albumin ratio 0.75, oleate concentrations less than 40
umol/l do not displace bilirubin; thereafter, oleate is a stong
displacer with a high affinity for bilirubin binding sites. As
with most other studies of bilirubin displacement by fatty acids, a
fatty acid:albumin ratio of 4 or greater is needed before
significant bilirubin displacement occurs. Clinically, high
circulating concentrations of drugs with multiple non-competitive
binding sites would be needed before bilirubin displacement by such
drugs became a major concern.

Different methods of testing drugs for displacement of
bilirubin may occasionally give divergent results. For example,
cefoperazone, a beta-lactam antibiotic, appears to be a weak
displacer of bilirubin when studied by Sephadex column elution,[10]
peroxidase oxidation, and dialysis of MADDS. However, in the
spectrum of the bilirubin-albumin complex, cefoperazone shows no
recognizable displacement effect and actually produces a slight
increase in the optical peak at 460nm. A specific effect of
cefoperazone on the spectrum of bound bilirubin, or competition
between cefoperazone and bilirubin at a different albumin site than
that for salicylate, may explain the discrepancy between methods.

For drugs of similar structure and function, the extent to
which the drug is protein-bound may correlate with its ability to

displace bilirubin. This is the case for ampicillin, moxalactam, and cefoperazone (none of which produce a decrease in the spectral peak at 460 nm.) Ampicillin, which is 15% albumin-bound, does not decrease reserve albumin binding or increase free bilirubin even at very high drug-to-albumin ratios. Moxalactam, 38% bound, is a weak displacer of bilirubin, with an affinity constant, K_D, $5x10^3$ Mol^{-1}. Cefoperazone, 70% bound with a K_D of $9x10^3$ Mol^{-1}, is a stronger displacer than moxalactam. In the same in vitro system which showed no changes in bilirubin binding with ampicillin, 0.5 mmol/L concentrations of moxalactam and cefoperazone decreased reserve albumin by 13% and 33% and increased unbound bilirubin by 3-fold and 5.5-fold, respectively. In the same system, 0.5 mmol/L of sulfisoxazole, with a K_D of $3x10^4$ Mol^{-1}, was a stronger displacer than moxalactam or cefoperazone and produced a 60% decrease in reserve albumin and an 11-fold increase in unbound bilirubin.

In Vivo Studies of Bilirubin Displacement: Animal Studies.

    Most drugs may be evaluated for potential bilirubin displacement by in vitro screening techniques, such as those described above. Under some circumstances, in vivo evaluation of bilirubin displacement by drugs is possible. First, animal models may be used. In adult rats weighing 175-250 gm, we achieved stable plasma bilirubin levels by continuous intravenous infusion of bilirubin at 20-25 mg/kg/hr for 3 hrs. The control animals and those receiving drugs were studied simultaneously in pairs. After 60 mins., plasma bilirubin levels of 10-15 mg/dl were identical in control and study animals. One of each pair was then given 50 mg/kg of sulfisoxazole as a single intravenous bolus dose and 50 mg/kg intraperitoneally. Plasma bilirubin level remained stable in the control rats, but in the rats given sulfisoxazole plasma bilirubin fell significantly while brain bilirubin at the end of the experiment was found to be increased. Free bilirubin concentration increased only transiently after the intravenous dose of the antibiotic; for most of the observation period, free bilirubin remained in equilibrium with the bound bilirubin in the plasma and was not significantly greater than control levels[11]. These findings confirm earlier observations by Øie and Levy that drug-induced increases in free bilirubin may be only transient, as the bilirubin displaced by the drug redistributes to multiple equilibrium sites within the body, including the brain. While massive, quantitative displacement of bilirubin by drug may cause a measurable decrease in plasma total bilirubin, measurement of free bilirubin or apparent free bilirubin in neonatal plasma "after the fact" of drug administration may fail to identify the displacement and redistribution of bilirubin. An additional conclusion to be drawn from these findings is that drug-induced redistribution of bilirubin may be very rapid, especially if the blood-brain barrier is permeable to free bilirubin.

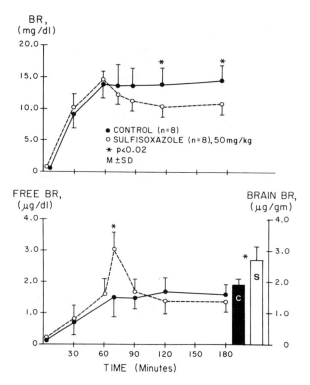

Fig. 3: Total bilirubin (upper panel), free bilirubin (lower panel), and brain bilirubin (bar graphs) in 8 pairs of rats given saline (●———●) or sulfisoxazole (O----O).

In Vivo Studies in Newborns

If an administered drug persists for some time in the circulation as the albumin-bound form, a decrease in reserve binding may identify the tendency of the drug to displace bilirubin. In such cases, a trace amount of a "deputy" ligand, analogous in its binding properties to bilirubin, such as ^{14}C-MADDS, may be used with undiluted and virtually unmodified serum or plasma to measure changes in reserve albumin induced by the drug, and to make an indirect estimate of the drug's potential to displace bilirubin in vivo. This indirect approach avoids the ethical problem of testing potentially displacing drugs in jaundiced infants, since the drug's effect on reserve albumin measured in this way will be the same, whether the newborn is jaundiced or not. We have used this approach for clinical studies of the effect on reserve albumin of the diuretic furosemide and the antibiotic cefoperazone given to newborns with minimal to no jaundice.[10,12]

Eight infants weighing from 980-1680 gms were given furosemide, 1 mg/kg i.v., by order of their physicians for treatment of pulmonary edema or congestive heart failure. With parental permission, a blood sample was taken immediately before the diuretic was given; furosemide, 1 mg/kg diluted in 1 ml of 5% glucose and water, was then given over 4-5 minutes by slow intravenous injection; a second blood sample was then obtained 5-7 minutes after completion of the injection. Pre- and post- dosing samples were analyzed for total and direct bilirubin, albumin, and reserve albumin (MADDS dialysis technique). There were no significant differences in bilirubin, albumin, or reserve albumin before and after the diuretic. When we calculated the maximum possible concentration achievable with a 1 mg/kg dose of furosemide, using the estimated plasma volume as its immediate volume of distribution, the estimated plasma concentration of drug and the drug-to-albumin ratio were below the concentration required to displace bilirubin or decrease reserve albumin in in vitro studies of the same drug - an observation confirmed by our in vivo results. Since furosemide is rapidly distributed to its sites of action and is not appreciably recirculated either as the unchanged drug or as an active metabolite, any effect on bilirubin binding caused by this drug should be immediate and transitory. As early as 5-10 minutes after administration, furosemide given at 1 mg/kg appeared to have little or no effect on reserve albumin in the newborn.

SERUM BILIRUBIN, ALBUMIN, AND RESERVE

ALBUMIN BEFORE AND AFTER FUROSEMIDE,

1mg/kg, IN 8 INFANTS (MEAN$\pm$S.D.)

	BILI-RUBIN μmol/L	ALBUMIN μmol/L	RESERVE ALBUMIN μmol/L
BEFORE	70$\pm$33	406$\pm$43	55$\pm$26
AFTER	72$\pm$34	406$\pm$58	52$\pm$23
p VALUE	n.s.	n.s.	n.s.

The antibiotic cefoperazone has a half-life of 5-7 hours and in the usual clinical situation would be given repeatedly at regular intervals to maintain therapeutic blood levels for several days. Our preliminary screening of this drug identified it as a potential displacer of bilirubin. In a clinical trial of cefoperazone for neonatal sepsis, we obtained pre- and post-injection serum samples from 5 infants given single doses of 50 mg/kg of cefoperazone. The five infants showed a significant (-29%) decrease in reserve albumin from 67±10 to 47±8 umol/l at 30 minutes after cefoperazone injection, in association with blood levels of 144±16ug/ml (216±24umol/l) of the drug. In vitro screening of cefoperazone predicted that a drug level of 250umol/l would cause a 25% decrease in reserve albumin, a finding confirmed by this in vivo study.

CONCLUSIONS

Evaluation of the bilirubin-displacing properties of albumin-bound drugs should be a routine part of the evaluation of any new drug before it is used clinically in newborn infants. However, the complexity of bilirubin-drug interactions makes it advisable to use multiple methods to study these interactions.

For most drugs, documentation of bilirubin displacement by capture of increased bilirubin on Sephadex or by an increase in the fraction of oxidizable "free" bilirubin are useful preliminary screening tests. Drugs which appear to displace bilirubin when screened in this way should be further tested for:
1)   The affinity of the drug for albumin;
2)   The number of binding sites for the drug;
3)   Whether the primary binding site for bilirubin is also the primary site for the drug; and
4)   The amount of bilirubin displaced by a therapeutic concentration of the drug (best evaluated in an undiluted assay system).
5)   Whenever practically possible and ethically acceptable, in vivo evaluation should be done in newborns receiving the drug.
Finally,
6)   If there is a valid choice between 2 drugs of equal effectiveness, one of which is strongly bound to albumin while the other is not, the less strongly bound drug should usually be chosen.

Studies to date of a large number of compounds suggest that only a few have practical clinical importance as displacers of bilirubin. However, as increasing numbers of new drugs are given to high risk infants, and as new uses are found for older drugs in the nursery, some way of estimating the potential of a drug to displace bilirubin from albumin is still necessary.

REFERENCES

1. R. C. Harris, J. F. Lucey, and J. R. Maclean, Kernicterus in
    premature infants associated with low concentrations of bili-
    rubin in plasma, Pediatrics, 21:875 (1958).
2. R. J. Martinek, Improved micromethod for determination of serum
    bilirubin, Clin. Chem. Acta, 13:161 (1966).
3. B. T. Doumas, T. Watson, and II. G. Biggs, Albumin standards
    and the measurement of serum albumin with bromcresol green,
    Clin. Chem. Acta, 31:87 (1971).
4. J. Jacobsen and R. P. Wenneberg, Determination of unbound bili-
    rubin in the serum of newborns, Clin. Chem., 20:783 (1974).
5. D. Schiff, G. Chan, and L. Stern, Sephadex G-25 quantitative
    estimation of free bilirubin potential in jaundiced newborn
    infants' sera, A guide to the prevention of kernicterus,
    J. Lab. Clin. Med., 80:455 (1972).
6. G. B. Odell, S. N. Cohen, and P. C. Kelly, Studies in kernicte-
    rus. II. The determination of the saturation of serum albu-
    min with bilirubin, J. Pediatr., 74:214 (1969).
7. R. Brodersen, S. Andersen, C. Jacobsen, et al., Determination
    of reserve albumin equivalent for ligand binding, probing
    two distinct binding functions of the protein, Analytical
    Biochem., 121:395 (1982).
8. W. J. Cashore, W. Oh, W. E. Blumberg, J. Eisinger, and A. A.
    Lamola, Rapid fluorometric assay of bilirubin and bilirubin
    binding capacity in blood of jaundiced neonates: comparisons
    with other methods, Pediatrics, 66:411 (1980).
9. R. Brodersen, Competitive binding of bilirubin and drugs to
    human serum albumin studied by enzymatic oxidation, J. Clin.
    Invest., 54:1353 (1974).
10. W. J. Cashore, M. Funato, G. Peter, and W. Oh, Displacement of
    bilirubin from albumin by two Cephalosporins, Ped. Res., 16:
    122A (1982) (abstract).
11. S. Øie and G. Levy, Effect of sulfisoxazole on pharmacokinetics
    of free and plasma protein bound bilirubin in experimental
    unconjugated hyperbilirubinemia, J. Pharmaceut. Sci., 68:6
    (1979).
12. W. J. Cashore, R. Brodersen, and W. Oh, In vitro and in vivo
    effects of furosemide on bilirubin binding to albumin,
    Develop. Pharmacol. and Therapeut., (1983) (in press).

ESTIMATION AND CLINICAL SIGNIFICANCE OF BILIRUBIN BINDING STATUS

Timos Valaes

Department of Pediatrics, Tufts-New England Medical
Center Hospital
171 Harrison Avenue, Boston, MA 02111

The association between hyperbilirubinemia and neurotoxicity was established by epidemiologic data in the early fifties[1,2] and was strengthened by the successful prevention of kernicterus following control of hyperbilirubinemia by exchange transfusion and phototherapy. The purists have argued that in the absence of randomized clinical trials a causal relationship was never proven. The difficulty in deciding when an epidemiologically established association should be considered proof of a causal relationship is well known from the story of tobacco smoking and lung cancer. In both associations the distinction between legitimate doubts and unreasonable demands for the perfect proof is difficult to make. An additional problem is the lack of a generally accepted pathogenetic mechanism for bilirubin*(BR) neurotoxicity[3], which invites the search for alternative explanations.

In this review we will examine the theoretical and practical reasons that limit our ability to answer the question: "how much of what kind of bilirubin is toxic and to whom?"[4] We will also examine the epidemiologic evidence supporting a causal relationship between BR concentration and BR toxicity. This may be considered redundant in a conference on phototherapy. Afterall, the rationale for phototherapy rests on the assumption that decreasing the BR level reduces the risk of BR toxicity. Recently expressed doubts on the validity of the concept of BR toxicity and the recycling of old alternative theories for kernicterus make it clear that such a review is needed.

---

*Throughout this text unless otherwise specified unconjugated (indirect) bilirubin is referred simply as bilirubin.

The order of the review is seemingly reversed. In the first part
we assume as proven the association that we examine in the second
part. It was felt that this order will be helpful in evaluating
the epidemiologic data.

BASIC CONCEPTS OF BILIRUBIN BINDING AND TOXICITY.

Bilirubin binding to the high affinity site of albumin is
expressed by the equation:

$$Ka = \frac{[Bilirubin-Albumin]}{[Bilirubin] [Albumin]}$$

Where:
Ka=Affinity Constant. [Bilirubin-Albumin]=Concentration of BR
bound to Albumin (BBR). [Bilirubin]=Concentration of unbound,
"free" BR (UBR). [Albumin]=Concentration of albumin with empty
sites to bind BR - Reserve BR binding Capacity-(RBRBC).
This equation indicates that an increase in total BR (which, in
practical terms, is equal to the concentration of BBR) or a
decrease in albumin concentration leads to elevation of UBR and that
provided Ka is known, the level of UBR can be predicted by the molar
ratio: BR/Albumin. The existence of low affinity binding sites in
the albumin, other plasma proteins and in the red cells and the
fact that a variable proportion of the albumin is not available for
binding BR at the primary site, particularly in newborns (presence
of competitors? non-binding variety-fetal albumin?)[5] make such a
prediction often inaccurate. These reservations not withstanding
one should be able, given a large and homogeneous study population,
to demonstrate correlations between BR concentration and UBR or
"loosely bound BR" (UBR plus BR bound to low affinity sites) or
RBRBC. The correlation should become tighter if the BR/Albumin
molar ratio, or its easily available substitute: BR(mg/dl)/Total
plasma protein(gm/dl) is used. Furthermore, in the same population
an association between plasma BR concentration and neurotoxicity
will be apparent irrespective of which is the actual "toxic species"
of BR. Similarly, the demonstration of a relationship between the
results of any of the BR binding assays and neurotoxicity does not
necessarily prove that the "BR species" measured by the assay is
the important one for the toxic effect. To define the "toxic
species" we need situations where the usual relationship between
the various BR binding parameters has been perturbed, as for
instance in the Gantrisin experience[6,7], which, of course, cannot
be recreated. These theoretical considerations have not been
examined systematically in clinical material, but the evidence
available so far is consistent with these concepts. For instance,
all the assays of BR binding, irrespective of which "BR species"
the assay is measuring, gave almost identical results for BRBC
when similar groups of patients were compared (Fig. 1). Agreement
between several BR binding tests was also obtained when the same
samples[11-14] or the same problem (effect of maturity, clinical
status[8-13], exchange transfusion[5-7,15-17]) was examined by various

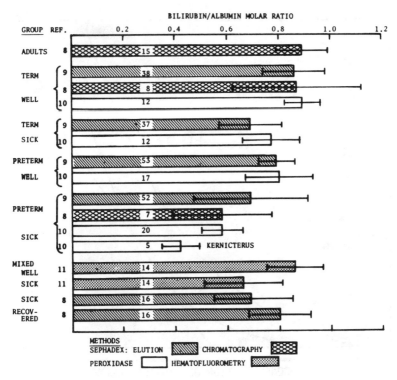

Fig. 1.   Estimation of bilirubin binding capacity in various groups
          and by four different methods. All values expressed as
          mean ± 1SD. Numbers inside bars=number of subjects studied.

methods.   These results are reassuring in regard to the methodology
of the various BR binding assays but cannot help define the "toxic
species".   Without a satisfactory pathogenetic mechanism and no
empirical method to decide on the "toxic species" we cannot, a
priori, select the assay most likely to predict BR toxicity on the
basis of the BR binding parameter measured.   Nevertheless, as
already pointed out, this may be more of a conceptual than a practical problem.   The inter-relationship between the various BR
binding parameters makes it possible, for practical purposes, to
ignore this objection.   In any event, the basic concepts are independent of which is the toxic substance.   There is no good reason
to expect that BR will be different from any other endogenous or
exogenous toxic substance.   Intragroup and intergroup variability
in the dose (level)-effect relationship should be expected.   Factors
as maturity, age, concurrent disturbances, length of exposure, etc..
are likely to effect this relationship.   Three theoretical situations are presented in Fig. 2.   We have no information to determine
which of the lines best represents the risk of BR toxicity for any
of the clinical groups.   The issue is of considerable practical

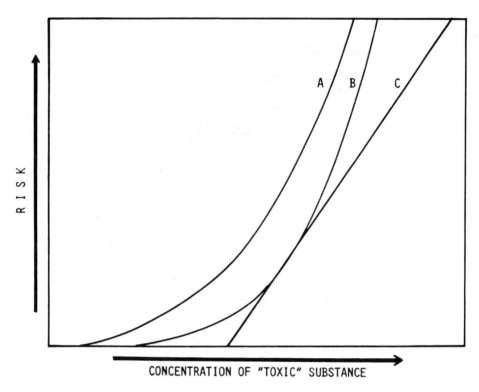

Fig. 2. Three theoretical lines expressing the relationship between
         concentration of a toxic substance and the risk of toxic
         effects.

importance. Since BR neurotoxicity can be prevented but cannot be
reversed, criteria for intervention should be of very high sensitivity while the degree of specificity required should be a function
of the risk of intervention itself. Obviously, there is no difficulty in picking up a critical level, if line C represents the
level-risk relationship. In contrast, the situation depicted by
either line B or A makes it very difficult to decide on a critical
level for intervention and unless we are able to eliminate hyperbilirubinemia altogether failures in preventing neurotoxicity will
be inevitable. There is an obvious question: Was the success of
the past and the failures of the present due to a population
represented predominantly by line C in the past and by lines either
B or A at present? This is another of the questions for which
there is no available answer. The factors that determine the position or the shape of the level-risk line, which of course expresses
the susceptibility of the CNS to BR-induced damage, are of great
importance but they do not affect the basic concept that the risk
is related to the level of the "toxic species". Epidemiological

or experimental studies of these factors will be possible only after the "toxic species" has been determined and reliable assays of its level are available.

EPIDEMIOLOGY OF BILIRUBIN TOXICITY: "CLASSICAL" versus "POST NEONATAL INTENSIVE CARE" KERNICTERUS.

The current interest in BR toxicity is the result of a resurgence of the problem of nuclear BR staining in many Neonatal Intensive Care Units (NICU). Aggressive policies of intervention even at much lower BR levels than those used in the past, were of no avail. In separating the epidemiologic data into "classical" and "NICU kernicterus" we are not distinguishing studies only according to their chronologies but also in reference to the clinical material, thus pursuing the answer to the question of "who" is susceptible to BR toxicity. Six criteria that have been accepted as useful in assigning etiologic significance to epidemiologic associations[18] will be used to examine the association of BR to kernicterus in these two populations of patients.

I. Consistency: The association of "classical kernicterus" with high unconjugated BR levels was independent of the cause of hyperbilirubinemia (isoimmune hemolytic disease, hereditary, spherocytosis, red-cell enzyme defects, DIC, immaturity, infections, inborn errors of metabolism--Crigler-Najjar Syn.,etc...), age and sex (in Crigler-Najjar Syn.[19] and with fulminant viral hepatitis[20] kernicterus was seen even in adolescents), or the presence of other conditions or abnormalities as hypoxia, acidosis, hypoglycemia. In contrast, "NICU kernicterus" was restricted to sick, mainly preterm, infants dying from a variety of complications with hyperbilirubinemia apparently the least important of their problems[21-27].

II. Strength of association: In the series of "classical kernicterus" (provided measurements of BR were reliable) levels of unconjugated BR in the 40-45mg/dl range resulted almost always in kernicterus. In the series of "NICU kernicterus" there was no apparent relation with BR levels and only a weak association with decreased BR binding[27]. Nevertheless, it should be pointed out that vigorous control of hyperbilirubinemia is part of modern neonatal intensive care.

III. Gradient (Dose-response): In all the studies of "classical kernicterus" whether in patients with hemolytic disease[1,2] or in preterm[28-33] infants the risk of kernicterus increased with the level of BR. The level of BR at which the risk started was not the same in all the series. Series that reported a very high incidence of marked hyperbilirubinemia also reported higher limits of safety[29,30,32,33], suggesting that this conclusion resulted from the known difficulties with the standardization of BR measurements. There has been only one and extremely significant exemption to the rule that the risk of kernicterus increased with the BR level. Preterm infants allocated to Gantrisin prophylaxis had not only remarkably higher rate of kernicterus but also lower peak BR levels than the group given oxytetracycline[6,7]. The shifting of emphasis from plasma BR levels to BR binding dates from this pivotal observation. All the studies on "NICU kernicterus" are of the case-control type and cannot provide data for calculating the risk in relation to BR levels or to BR binding status.

IV. Temporal sequence: In "classical kernicterus", whether in infants with hemolytic disease or in preterm otherwise well infants, an acute neurological syndrome manifested itself during the phase of increasing BR levels. Those with the most severe symptoms died, the age at death being related to the rate of increase in BR concentration, i.e., earlier in isoimmune hemolytic disease, later in preterm infants or in the Crigler-Najjar syn. An occasional infant was discovered to have nuclear BR staining at autopsy or survived to develop athetoid cerebral palsy without a recognizable acute neurological syndrome. All the reports of "NICU kernicterus" stress the absence of a recognizable neurological syndrome. Death was always adequately explained by other complications of immaturity and there was no clustering of the deaths around the time of peak BR levels[21-27]. Moreover, follow-up studies from several centers have not reported an increase in athetoid cerebral palsy at the same period that unsuspected nuclear BR staining was seen at autopsy.

V. Specificity: For "classical kernicterus" the only common denominator present in all the conditions and diseases that could lead to kernicterus was a high unconjugated BR level. Conversely, no other disease or noxious agent is known to produce a similar clinicopathological picture. The only common feature of the infants with "NICU kernicterus" was that they were sick, predominately preterm infants who died, inspite of modern intensive care, from overwhelming complications and after repeated efforts to resuscitate. No clinical or laboratory predictors of this type of "kernicterus" could be identified[23-25]. The gross pathological picture seems to be identical in both "classical and NICU kernicterus" but the identity and specificity of the microscopic picture of "NICU kernicterus" is disputed[34,35].

VI. Epidemiological sense: The incidence of "classical kernicterus" in various populations paralleled the incidence of marked hyperbilirubinemia irrespective of its cause (Rhesus HDN, G-6-PD deficiency, etc..). In the same populations, control of hyperbilirubinemia by exchange transfusion or phototherapy or eradication of the cause, as with "Rhogam", coincided with a fall or disappearance of kernicterus. In Contrast, the incidence of "NICU kernicterus" is increasing inspite of stricter control of hyperbilirubinemia[24,25,36].

We examined the existence of a causal relationship between

kernicterus and BR levels by applying the same epidemiologic criteria and we arrived at the conclusion that while "classical kernicterus" fulfills all the criteria "NICU kernicterus" meets none. There are three possible explanations for these results: (a) Inappropriate use of epidemiologic methods. (b) "Classical and NICU kernicterus" have different pathogenetic mechanisms and therefore should be considered different entities. (c) Combination of (a) and (b).

There are important methodologic differences between the old studies of "classical kernicterus" all of which were of the cohort type, and the recent studies of "NICU kernicterus" all of which were of the case-control type. In the cohort studies, a series of patients were followed prospectively and the small number that developed kernicterus was compared with the rest. In the case-control studies, after the group with autopsy-proven nuclear BR staining was identified, a control group was chosen from those without staining at autopsy. It was felt that the population of survivors could not provide the controls as it could include infants with unsuspected BR toxicity. The limitations of the case-control

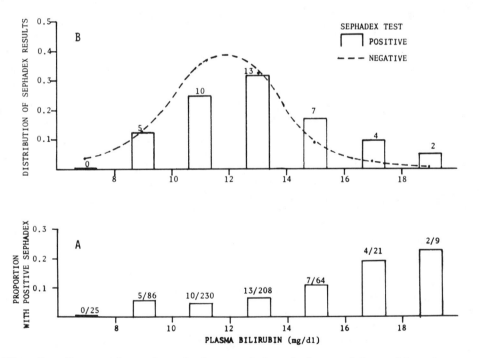

Fig. 3.   Proportion of sephadex positive infants (plate A) and
          distribution of sephadex positive and negative infants
          (plate B) in relation to maximum plasma bilirubin
          concentration.

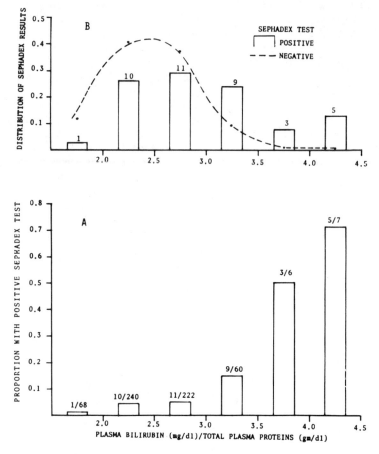

Fig. 4.   Proportion of sephadex positive infants (plate A) and
          distribution of sephadex positive and negative infants
          (plate B) in relation to maximum value of the ratio:
          plasma bilirubin to total plasma proteins.

studies are a favorite subject for epidemiologists. Their theoretical objections are well known. I will use a concrete example to
demonstrate that opposite conclusions can be reached from the same
material depending on which epidemiologic method is used. We use
sephadex column chromatography to assess the BR binding status in
sick preterm infants and the results of the test are the basis of
the clinical management[37]. For the purpose of this discussion, it
is immaterial whether it is accepted or not that the results of the
test correlate well with the risk of BR toxicity[38,39]. In Figs. 3
and 4 we examined the relation between BR concentration or the
ratio:BR/Total plasma proteins and positive sephadex test. Graphs A
demonstrate that as the BR level or the ratio values increased the

proportion of babies with a positive sephadex also increased, the relation being much more impressive with the BR/Total plasma proteins values, as predicted by the BR binding equation. This is an example of a cohort type of study and the conclusions are the same as those of studies proving that the risk of kernicterus increased with the BR levels[1,2,23]. In graphs B, the same sephadex positive infants are plotted according to their BR level or BR/Total plasma proteins ratio. The positive infants have a normal distribution with a small shifting to the right from the distribution of the sephadex negative infants. The relation between BR levels and the probability of obtaining a positive sephadex test disappeared. In statistical parlance this is called: "Numerators in search of denominators". In the case-control studies we don't have the denominators, i.e., the total population at risk. A control group is selected to substitute for the population at risk. Whether we will be able to demonstrate the small difference in distribution between the positive and negative infants depends on the sample size drawn from the two populations and the perfection of the matching of the two groups in relation to the factors (apart from the BR levels) that influence the outcome. All the studies of "NICU kernicterus" were of insufficient statistical power because of small numbers (5-30 cases). In addition, the patients were managed according to strict criteria and almost none was allowed to develop BR levels over 14-15mg/dl. If we had followed the same criteria, we would have been unable to demonstrate the relationship between BR levels and positive sephadex test. To simulate the case-control studies we selected a control group of sephadex negative infants matched for sex, gestational age, birth weight, and date of birth with the 41 cases of positive sephadex. As expected, the degree of overlap of individual values (Fig. 5) is more striking than the fact that there is a statistically significant difference in the mean values. When we reduced the number of cases and controls to 20 (by including only half the cases from each gestational age group) the difference was no longer statistically significant. Obviously if we had, as a result of a management protocol, no infants with high BR levels, the overlap of the values between positive and negative infants would have been perfect. This example makes it obvious that the methodology used in the studies of "NICU kernicterus" was totally inappropriate and their conclusions that "kernicterus" is not related to BR levels should not be accepted. A similar criticism should be applied to the other conclusions that there are no clinical predictors of "NICU kernicterus"[23-25]. It could easily be anticipated that there was no possibility of finding a difference since both cases and controls were infants that died from the same conditions and under the same circumstances. The decision not to use the cohort method cannot be justified on the basis that only autopsy can prove the absence of BR toxicity. In preterm infants a case-fatality rate for kernicterus of 70-75% was well documented in the past. It is unlikely that this has changed. Thus a cohort study will not be invalidated by the small number of infants with undiagnosed BR

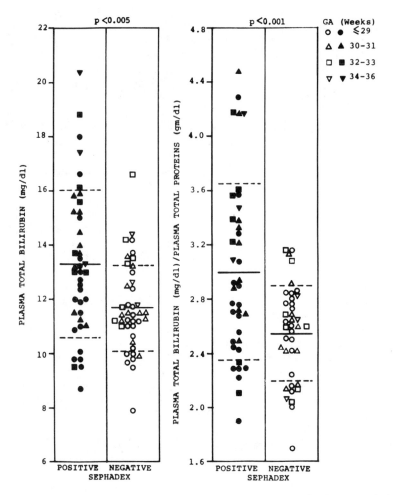

Fig. 5.   Comparison of individual values of sephadex positive
          infants and matched sephadex negative controls.
          ———— mean, ----- 1SD.

toxicity, particularly if follow up is included in the study.

    The above methodologic objections, although sufficient to
explain the confusion regarding "NICU kernicterus", are probably
only part of the story. Of the triad included in the term "kernicterus": (a) acute neurological syndrome, (b) selective nuclear BR
staining for the patients that die, and (c) athetoid cerebral palsy
for the patients that survive, "NICU kernicterus" comprises only
(b). A legitimate questions is raised: Are the two conditions the
same and should the term kernicterus be applied to both conditions?

In order not to prejudice the answer to this question we should use the term "BR encephalopathy" for the complete clinicopathological picture, as described in "classical kernicterus", and the term "Nuclear BR Staining" for the gross pathologic picture shared by both "classical and NICU kernicterus". We would like to propose that two, partly separate, mechanisms can lead to nuclear BR staining. The epidemiologic evidence for this is the old Gantrisin experience[6,7] and the temporal association between the introduction of the NICU techniques and the resurgence of the problem of "kernicterus"[37]. The theory is also supported by important experimental data [40-44]. In the mechanism operating in "classical kernicterus" UBR diffusely enters the brain. At certain levels the metabolism of only a few nuclear masses is interferred with and subcellular changes are produced. This results in the selective opening of the blood-brain barrier and massive entrance of BR bound to albumin. It is only at this stage that BR staining becomes obvious and irreversible neuronal damage occurs. This mechanism represents true BR toxicity as the UBR precipitates the sequence of events that lead to neuronal death. In the second mechanism, which we believe is compatible with at least a proportion of the current cases of nuclear BR staining, other insults interfere with the cellular metabolism and affect the blood-brain barrier of the same nuclear masses with subsequent entrance of BR bound to albumin. The final pathologic picture is the same but in these cases BR is an innocent bystander. This type of nuclear BR staining obviously cannot be prevented by focusing on BR or BR binding. If the theory is correct, we are faced with an impossible situation: Nuclear BR staining cannot be considered the ultimate proof of BR toxicity. In the absence of a firm end-point how are we to assess laboratory methods and management protocols for the prevention of BR toxicity in the current population of NICU?

CONCLUSIONS

The sorry state of the art regarding BR toxicity is not due to the fact that the BR binding methods have not lived up to our expectations. Our expectations were both simplistic and impossible. Simplistic, because we were looking for a magic number valid for everyone despite all that is known about toxic effects. Impossible, because without the informative material and specific end-points and with the wrong epidemiologic methods we tried to answer the questions in a reverse order: "how much" before "which species". The predicament we find ourselves in should not be used as license to continue with the old management protocols. In the face of uncertainties we can still choose between alternative protocols using the clinical decision analysis process. Data for such an analysis are provided in the table. We applied to our population--managed by albumin infusion supplemented by exchange transfusion on the basis of the sephadex results[37]--the criteria for exchange transfusion based on BR levels, birth weight and clinical condition[45]. Both methods of

Comparison of Two Criteria for Intervention in
the Same Population of Jaundiced Sick Preterm Infants

CRITERIA	Gestational Age Groups				TOTAL
	≤29	30-31	32-33	34-36	
Sephadex - BR criteria*-	40 (49%)	55 (70.5%)	140 (92%)	301 (96%)	545 (85%)
Sephadex - BR criteria +	31 (31%)	12 (15%)	5 (3.3%)	9 (2.9%)	57 (8.9%)
Sephadex + BR criteria -	1 (1%)	3 (3.8%)	3 (2%)	2 (0.6%)	9 (1.4%)
Sephadex + BR criteria +	19 (19%)	8 (10.2%)	4 (2.6%)	1 (0.3%)	32 (5%)
Exchange Transfused**	9 (9%)	1 (1.3%)	3 (2%)	1 (0.3%)	14 (2.2%)
Total	100	78	152	313	643

*As per Ref. 40.
**On the basis of positive Sephadex not reversed by
   albumin (1gm/kg) infusion.

management were successful in preventing nuclear BR staining in the
respective populations of sick preterm infants. The difference
between 89 cases that ought to be exchanged using the BR criteria
and the 14 we actually exchanged by our protocol means that the two
methods result in quite different risk to benefit ratios. The good
correlation between sephadex and several other BR binding methods
allows us to predict that similar results will be obtained if
management protocols based on these methods were to be used.

REFERENCES

1. D.Y-Y. Hsia, F.H. Allen Jr., S.S. Gellis and L.K. Diamond,
    Erythroblastosis Fetalis VIII. Studies of serum bilirubin in
    relation to kernicterus, N.Engl.J.Med. 247:668 (1952).
2. P.L. Mollison and M. Cutbush, Haemolytic disease of the new-
    born, in: "Recent Advances in Paediatrics", D. Gairdner, ed.,
    Churchill, London, p. 110 (1954).
3. W.B. Karp, Biochemical alterations in neonatal hyperbilirubin-
    emia and bilirubin encephalopathy: A review. Pediatrics 64:
    361 (1979).
4. A.K. Brown and A.F. McDonagh, Phototherapy for neonatal hyper-
    bilirubinemia: Efficacy, mechanism and toxicity, Adv.Pediatr.
    27:341 (1980).
5. F. Ebbesen, Effect of exchange transfusion on serum reserve
    albumin for binding of bilirubin and index of serum bilirubin
    toxicity, Acta Paediatr.Scand. 70:643 (1981).
6. W.A. Silverman, D.H. Anderson, W.A. Blanc and D.N. Crozier, A
    difference in mortality rate and incidence of kernicterus
    among premature infants allotted to two prophylactic anti-
    bacterial regimens, Pediatrics 18:614 (1956).

7. R.C. Harris, J.F. Lucey and J.R. MacLean, Kernicterus in pre-
    mature infants associated with low concentrations of bili-
    rubin in the plasma, Pediatrics 21:875 (1958).

8. T. Valaes and M. Hyte, Effect of exchange transfusion on bili-
    rubin binding, Pediatrics 59:881 (1977).

9. W.J. Cashore, A. Horwich, J. Laterra and W. Oh, The effect of
    postnatal age and clinical status of newborn infants on bili-
    rubin binding capacity, Biol. Neonate 32:304 (1977).

10. W.J. Cashore, Free bilirubin concentrations and bilirubin-
    binding affinity in term and preterm infants, J.Pediatr. 96:
    521 (1980).

11. W.J. Cashore, W. Oh, W.E. Blumberg, J. Eisinger and A.A. Lamola,
    Rapid fluorometric assay of bilirubin and bilirubin binding
    capacity of jaundiced neonates: Comparison with other methods,
    Pediatrics 66:411 (1980).

12. W.J. Cashore, P.J.P. Monin and W. Oh, Serum bilirubin binding
    capacity and free bilirubin concentrations: A comparison
    between sephadex G-25 filtration and peroxidase oxidation
    techniques, Pediatr. Res. 12:195 (1978).

13. A.K. Brown, J. Eisinger, W.E. Blumberg, J. Flores, G. Boyle,
    and A.A. Lamola, A rapid fluorometric method for determining
    bilirubin levels and binding in the blood of neonates: Compari-
    sons with a diazo method and with 2-(4'Hydroxybenzene)
    azobenzoic acid dye binding, Pediatrics 65:767 (1980).

14. R. Wells, K. Hammond, A.A. Lamola and W.E. Blumberg, Relation-
    ships of bilirubin binding parameters, Clin.Chem. 28:432(1982).

15. A.D. Arkans and G. Cassady, Estimation of unbound serum bili-
    rubin by the peroxidase method: Effect of exchange transfusion
    on unbound bilirubin and serum bindings, J.Pediatr.92:1001
    (1978).

16. R.C. Banagale, Effect of exchange transfusion on bilirubin
    binding parameters as measured by bilirubin hematofluorometer,
    Pediatr.Res. 17:303A (1983).

17. E. Cepeda and S. Shankaran, Exchange transfusions and bilirubin
    binding, Pediatr.Res. 17:306A (1983).

18. Report of the Advisory Committee to the Surgeon General on
    Smoking and Health, PHS Publ. No. 1103 (1964).

19. A.W. Wolkoff, J.R. Chowdbury, L.A. Gartner, A.L. Rose, L.
    Biempica, D.R. Giblm, D. Fink, and I.M. Arias. Crigler-
    Najjar syndrome (type I) in an adult male, Gastroenterology
    76:840 (1979).

20. K.C. Ho, R. Hodach, R. Varma V. Thorsteinson, T. Hess and
    D. Dale, Kernicterus and central pontine myelinolysis in a
    14 yr. old boy with fulminating viral hepatitis, Ann.Neurol.
    8:633 (1980).

21. L.M. Gartner, R.N. Snyder, R.S. Chabon and J. Bernstein,
    Kernicterus: High incidence in premature infants with low
    serum bilirubin concentrations, Pediatrics 45:906 (1970).

22. M.A. Perlman, L.M. Gartner, K. Lee, A.I. Eidelman, R. Morecki
    and D.S. Haroupian, The association of kernicterus with

bacterial infection in the newborn, Pediatrics 65:26 (1980).

23. S.B. Turkel, M.E. Guttenberg, D.R. Moynes and J.E. Hodgman,
     Lack of identifiable risk factors for kernicterus, Pediatrics
     66:502 (1980).

24. M.H. Kim, J.J. Yoon, J. Sher and A.H. Brown, Lack of predictive
     indices in kernicterus: A comparison of clinical and patho-
     logical factors in infants with or without kernicterus.
     Pediatrics 66:852 (1980).

25. D.A. Ritter, J.D. Kenny, J. Norton and A.J. Rudolph, A pro-
     spective study of free bilirubin and other risk factors in
     the development of kernicterus in premature infants, Pediatrics
     69:260 (1982).

26. D.R. Pledger, J.M. Scott and A. Belfield, Kernicterus at low
     levels of serum bilirubin: The impact of bilirubin albumin-
     binding capacity, Biol. Neonate 41:38 (1982).

27. W.J. Cashore and W. Oh, Unbound bilirubin and kernicterus in
     low-birth weight infants, Pediatrics 69:458 (1982).

28. V.M. Crosse, The incidence of kernicterus not due to haemo-
     lytic disease among premature babies, in:"Kernicterus", A.
     Sass-Kortsak, ed., Univ. of Toronto Press, Toronto (1961).

29. G. Rapmund, J.M. Bowman and R.C. Harris, Bilirubinemia in non-
     erythroblastic premature infants, Am.J.Dis.Child.94:604(1960).

30. C.A. Koch, D.V. Jones, M.S. Dine and E.A. Wagner, Hyperbili-
     rubinemia in premature infants, J.Pediatr. 55:23 (1959).

31. K. Hugh-Jones, J. Slack, K. Simpson, A. Grossman and D.Y-Y
     Hsia, Clinical course of hyperbilirubinemia in premature
     infants, N.Engl.J.Med. 263:1223 (1960).

32. A. Mores, I. Fogasova, E, Minarikova, Relation of hyperbiliru-
     binemia in newborns without isoimmunisation to kernicterus,
     Acta Paediatr.Scand.48:590 (1959).

33. L. Wishingrad, M. Corblatt, T. Takakura, I.M. Rozenfeld, L.D.
     Elegant, A. Kaufman, E. Lassers and R.I. Klein, Studies of
     non-hemolytic hyperbilirubinemia in premature infants. I.
     Prospective randomized selection for exchange transfusion with
     observations on the levels of serum bilirubin with and with-
     out exchange transfusion and neurologic evaluations one year
     after birth, Pediatrics 36:162 (1965).

34. S.B. Turkel, C.A. Miller, M.E. Guttenberg, D.R. Moynes and J.E.
     Hodgman, A clinical pathologic reappraisal of kernicterus,
     Pediatrics 69:267 (1982).

35. M. Ahdab-Barmada, Neonatal kernicterus: Neuropathologic diagno-
     sis, in: "Hyperbilirubinemia In The Newborn". Report of the
     85th Ross Conference, Ross Laboratories, Columbus (1983).

36. A.J. Barson and D.G. Sims, Kernicterus in a special care baby
     unit, Arch.Dis.Childh.55:243 (1980).

37. T. Valaes, M. Hyte, K. Murphy and L. Nielson, The management
     of jaundiced ill preterm infants using the sephadex column
     chromatography bilirubin binding test, in: "Intensive Care
     of the Newborn", L. Stern, B. Salle, and B, Friis-Hansen,
     ed., Masson, New York (1980).

38. J. Kapitulnik, T. Valaes, N.A. Kaufmann and S. Blondheim, Clinical evaluation of sephadex gel filtration in estimation of bilirubin binding on serum in neonatal jaundice, Arch. Dis.Child. 49:886 (1974).

39. T. Valaes, J. Kapitulnik, N.A. Kaufmann and S.K. Blondheim, Experience with sephadex gel filtration in assessing the risk of bilirubin encephalopathy in neonatal jaundice, in: "Bilirubin Metabolism In the Newborn (II)", S.H. Blondheim and D. Bergsman, ed., Birth Defects 12:215 (1976).

40. I. Diamond and R. Schmid, Experimental encephalopathy. The mode of entry of bilirubin^{14}C into the central nervous system, J.Clin.Invest. 45:678 (1966).

41. H.S. Schutta and L. Johnson, Bilirubin encephalopathy in the Gunn rat: A fine structure study of the cerebellar cortex, J.Neuropath.Exp.Neurol. 26:377 (1967).

42. H.S. Schutta, L. Johnson and H.E. Neville, Mitochondrial abnormalities in bilirubin encephalopathy, J.Neuropath.Exper. Neurol. 29:296 (1970).

43. B. Rozdilsky and J. Olszewski, Permeability of cerebral vessels to albumin in hyperbilirubinemia, Neurol. 10:631 (1960).

44. R.L. Levine, W.R. Fredericks and S.I. Rapoport, Entry of bilirubin into the brain due to opening of the blood-brain barrier, Pediatrics 69:255 (1982).

45. M.A. Pearlman, L.M. Gartner, K. Lee, R. Morecki and D.S. Haroupian, Absence of kernicterus in low-birth-weight infants from 1971 through 1976: Comparison with findings in 1966 and 1967, Pediatrics 62:460 (1978).

FACTORS AFFECTING THE TRANSCUTANEOUS MEASUREMENT OF BILIRUBIN:

INFLUENCE OF RACE, GESTATIONAL AGE, PHOTOTHERAPY AND ALBUMIN BINDING CAPACITY

A.K. Brown, M.H. Kim, G. Valencia, P. Nuchpuckdee, and
G. Boyle

Department of Pediatrics, State University of New York-
Downstate Medical Center
Brooklyn, N.Y. 11203

INTRODUCTION

Most previous studies in infants have found surprisingly good correlation between transcutaneous bilirubin indices and serum bilirubin indices and serum bilirubin levels.[1-6] However, exact correlation between such measurements should not be expected since the instrument measures the yellowness of the skin and not the concentration of bilirubin in the blood. Many factors can influence the relationship between these two measurements, including race, gestational age, the rate of bilirubin accumulation as well as the bilirubin binding capacity, and other factors that affect the distribution of bilirubin between the intravascular and extravascular spaces. These influences preclude the use of any objective measurement of skin jaundice as a complete substitution or replacement for the measurement of serum bilirubin under all circumstances. Nevertheless, previous studies have tested the validity of transcutaneous bilirubinometry almost solely by comparing the degree of exact correlation with the serum value.

During the period before marketing of the transcutaneous bilirubinometer we helped to establish guidelines for the interpretation of readings obtained with this device. In our pre-marketing trials of the instrument we demonstrated the usefulness of specific transcutaneous bilirubin indices that could serve as "action levels" for identifying infants who required that serum bilirubin levels be drawn, as well as those infants who might be exempt safely from such a procedure. Subsequently, we have tested the instrument more extensively and would like to present the findings relevant to the determination of "action levels" in our institution.

Since we are aware that many factors may affect the relationship between icterus and serum bilirubin, we determined whether sufficient correlation could be found between transcutaneous measurements of jaundice and serum bilirubin to allow its use as a screening device. We sought to establish objective indices by which infants could be safely selected for, or exempt from, the necessity of determining the serum bilirubin concentration by an invasive procedure. Because of the known influences of skin color, gestational age and use of phototherapy on the degree of jaundice perceptible at a given biliru-bin concentration, the study included black, white, term and preterm infants with and without phototherapy. The degree to which these factors affected the relationship of TcB or jaundice meter readings and serum bilirubin was determined.

MATERIALS AND METHODS

During a 12 month period 291 measurements were taken with the Air Shields Jaundice Meter on 169 newborn infants; simultaneous serum bilirubin determinations were made using the American Optical Biliru-binometer. (We shall use the terms transcutaneous bilirubinometer (TcB) and electronic jaundice meter interchangeably). The Air Shields jaundice meter is a noninvasive hand-held instrument which employs fiber optic techniques to illuminate the skin and subcutaneous tissue, and then spectrophotometrically analyzes the intensity of the yellow color of the skin. There is a digital display of the index of that intensity of color. We studied 169 infants; 33 white (22 term and 11 preterm), and 136 black (79 term and 57 preterm); 291 determinations were made. Subsequently, 53 infants in the study received photothe-rapy, and data collected during this treatment were analyzed separa-tely. Since the jaundice meter readings may be influenced by the darkness of skin color, black infants were further subdivided into light (48 infants), medium (56 infants) and dark (32 infants) groups.

The jaundice meter readings were taken from both forehead and sternum; the mean of three serial measurements was recorded. In some of the infants receiving phototherapy, a round light reflecting patch (2.5 cm in diameter) was placed on the infant's sternum and the rea-dings were done on the area of skin beneath the patch, unexposed to phototherapy. Linear regression analyses were performed.

In addition to these studies, in a group of 30 term and preterm infants not receiving phototherapy, simultaneous information was obtained using the Bilirubin Hematofluorometer.[7] With this instru-ment, albumin-bound bilirubin (B), total bilirubin (T), and reserve bilirubin binding (R) are measured. From these measurements additio-nal information may be derived. For example, B+R measures total bili-rubin binding capacity of the albumin; B/R correlates with unbound bilirubin. From these simultaneous studies we sought to examine the relationships between these factors and the degree of jaundice as measured transcutaneously. It was hoped that such studies would give insight into the factors that determine the distribution of the bilirubin between the vascular compartment and the other tissues of the body.

RESULTS

Correlation between Jaundice Meter Readings (Transcutaneous Bilirubin Meter of TcB) Indices and Serum Bilirubin Concentrations.

a) Term Infants: for white infants receiving no phototherapy there was good correlation between jaundice meter readings and serum bilirubin values, as shown in fig. 1A (r=0.87, slope 1.04, intercept 9.43). Among light black infants, the correlation was quite good (r=0.81, slope 0.86 and intercept 10.3; see fig. 1B). Among medium black infants the correlation between jaundice meter readings and serum bilirubin values was good, as shown in fig. 1C (r=0.82, slope 0.95, intercept 11.8), but in the dark black infants the correlation was not as good (r=0.7, slope 0.59) and the intercept was higher (14.1), as shown in fig. 1D.

b) Preterm Infants: as shown in fig. 2 (A-D), among white and black preterm infants receiving no phototherapy, the correlation coefficients between jaundice meter readings and serum bilirubin values were comparable to those for term infants.

c) Variation in the baseline readings with race and gestational age: the intercepts of the baseline jaundice meter readings for term infants ranged from 9.4 in white term infants to 14.1 in dark black term infants. Baseline TcB values were higher in preterm infants than in term infants of the same race except in the dark black infants.

Use of the Electronic Jaundice Meter To Identify Infants with Significant Bilirubinemia: Action Point for all Infants (Black or White) in the First Week of life.

We sought a simple action point for the group of infants that would screen for those infants with a serum bilirubin concentration equal to or greater than 10 mg/dl. This is the general level at which all infants, term or preterm, should be reassessed to determine the cause of such "hyperbilirubinemia". It is at this point that the clinician should determine whether there is a possible clinical explanation, such as breast feeding, infant of a diabetic mother, or, more seriously, a missed hemolytic disease or infection. Also, if treatment is to be used to control hyperbilirubinemia, phototherapy has proven to be more effective in controlling bilirubinemia at this, rather than at higher, levels. As shown in table 2, no infant with a TcB index less than 19 had a serum bilirubin concentration greater than 10 mg/dl; thus there were no false negatives. The negative

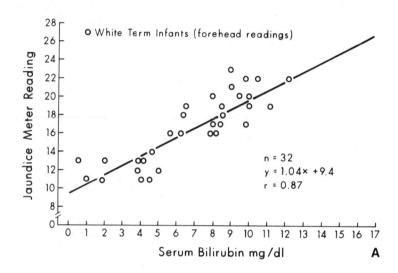

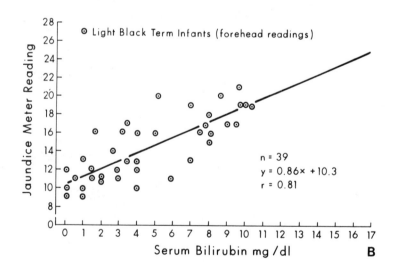

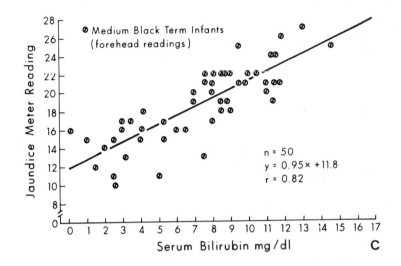

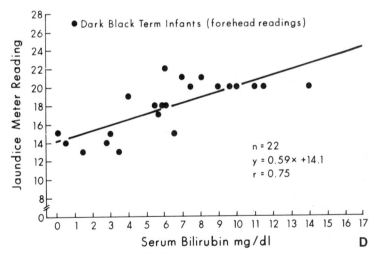

Fig. 1, A-D. Comparison of Jaundice Meter (Transcutaneous Bilirubin Meter) readings and serum bilirubin concentrations in term infants of different race and/or skin color.

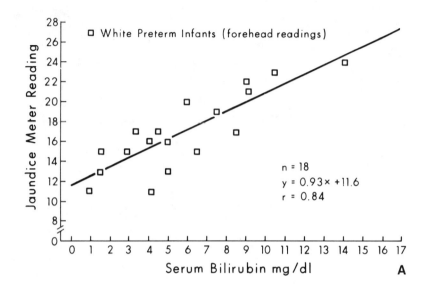

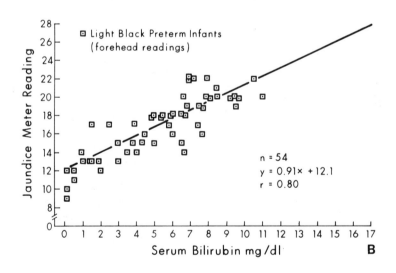

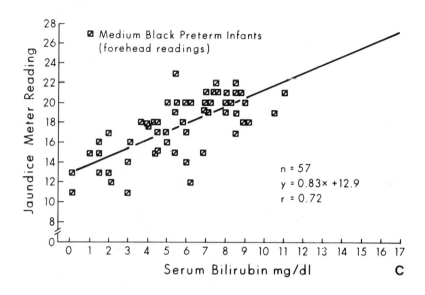

C

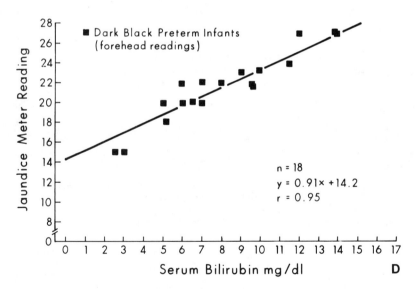

D

Fig. 2, A-D. Comparison of Jaundice Meter readings and serum bilirubin concentrations in preterm infants of different
races and/or skin color.

Table 1. Variation of baseline jaundice meter readings with skin
          color and gestational age.

Color	Term	Preterm
White	9.4	11.6
Light Black	10.3	12.1
Medium Black	11.6	12.9
Dark Black	14.6	14.2

predictive value was 100%. As expected, there were 30% false positives, but false positives are less serious than false negatives.
Screening at the action point of 19 then would identify all infants
with bilirubin levels of > 10 mg/dl, and spare a majority of infants
with bilirubin levels under 10 mg/dl an invasive procedure to determine whether or not their serum bilirubin level was in a zone that
required further attention (table 2).

It was of interest that more preterm than term infants had
moderately high TcB readings at low bilirubin levels, as might be
expected since preterm infants whether black or white had higher
baseline TcB readings. Among both black and white infants, preterm
infants had significantly more false positive readings than did term
infants (56 of 147 preterm vs. 36 of 144 term infants, p < 0.025).
Since preterm infants are more susceptible to bilirubin toxicity,
an error in this direction is not necessarily bad, since it leads
to an increased number of evaluations in these infants.

Influence of Phototherapy

Correlation between TcB readings and serum bilirubin values
were not good in any group of infants treated with phototherapy when
jaundice meter readings were taken from either the forehead or the
sternum (r=0.55, fig. 3). When readings were taken from areas that
had been covered ("patched") during phototherapy, the correlation
between serum bilirubin and jaundice meter readings was quite good
(r=0.89, slope 0.96 and intercept 9.2). These studies were done only
in the white infants (fig. 4).

Comparison of Jaundice Meter Readings and Visual Detection of Jaundice in the Neonate

In 24 of 169 infants, jaundice had not been seen by the nursery
personnel prior to the jaundice meter reading. Simultaneous serum
bilirubin concentrations in these infants ranged from 6 to 14 mg/dl;
17 of the 24 infants had serum bilirubin concentrations of 8 mg/dl

Table 2.   Predictive value of TcB index. All races and all gestational ages.

| TcB Index | Bilirubin | | Total |
	>10 mg/dl	10 mg/dl<	
>19	35 (12%)	88 (30%)	123
	True Pos (a)	False Pos (b)	
<19	0	168 (58%)	168
	False Neg (c)	True Neg (d)	
Total	35	256	291

Negative Predictive value = 100% d/(c+d)
Positive Predictive value = 28.5% a/(a+b)
Sensitivity = a/(a+c)
Specificity = d/(b+d)

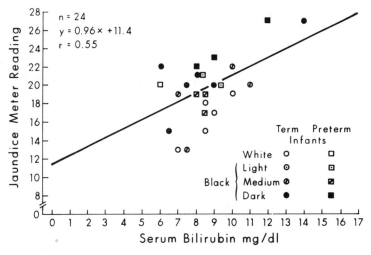

Fig. 3.   Influence of phototherapy on the relationship between skin bilirubin (Jaundice Meter readings) and serum bilirubin concentrations in term and preterm infants.

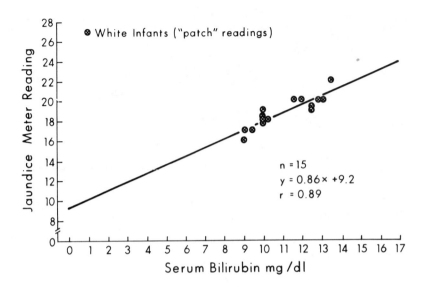

Fig. 4.   Relationship between Jaundice Meter readings in unexposed
          areas of skin ("patch") and serum bilirubin during photo-
          therapy.

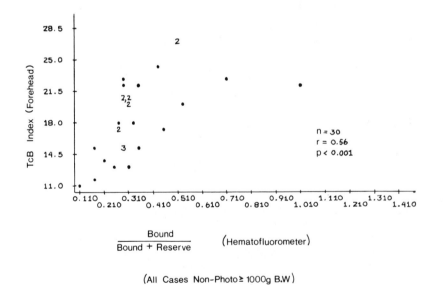

Fig. 5.   Relationship between skin bilirubin (TcB index) and satura-
          tion of the albumin binding capacity, B/B+R. (B= albumin
          bound bilirubin; R= albumin reserve bilirubin binding capa-
          city.)

Table 3.

CORRELATION OF TcB INDEX WITH HEMATOFLUOROMETER DATA
POPULATION: INFANTS $\geq$1000 g.; N = 30
NON - PHOTOTHERAPY

Bound Bilirubin (B)	r=0.77; p <0.0001
Total Bilirubin (T)	r=0.75; p <0.001
$\dfrac{\text{Bound Bilirubin}}{\text{Bound + Reserve}} \quad \dfrac{B}{B+R}$	r=0.56; p <0.001
Reserve Albumin Binding Capacity (R)	r=0.38; p <0.05 (Inverse)
TOtal Bilirubin - Bound (T-B)	N.S.

Table 4.

RELATIONSHIP OF BILIRUBIN RESERVE BINDING CAPACITY
AND SATURATION INDEX TO BIRTH WEIGHT

Birth Wt. (g)	n	Bound Bilirubin(B)* (mg/dl)	Reserve(R)* (mg/dl)	Saturation Index 10 x (B/R)
1000-2000	13	mean 6.43 range (2.4-9.6)	12.33	9.0
2001-2500	5	mean 7.68 range (4.6-13.3)	15.8	4.7
2501	12	mean 7.20 range (3.3-13.2)	18.08	4.0

*Using Bell Labs
Hematofluorometer

Table 4.

ALBUMIN BINDING CAPACITY
COMPARISON OF SICK AND WELL PRE-TERM INFANTS
(BIRTH WEIGHT <2000 g.)

	Sick n=14	Well n=18	
Reserve Binding	8.3+3.8	12.6+6.3	p<0.001
Albumin Binding Capacity (B+R)	13.7+3.1	19.4+5.6	p<0.0005
Bilirubin mg/dl (AO)	7.2+2.7	6.1+2.8	p<0.1 N.S.

or more. All had jaundice meter reading from 13 to 27, and 16 of the infants had readings of 19 or greater. In the two very dark black infants in whom jaundice had not been detected, the jaundice meter readings were both 27, and the corresponding serum bilirubin concentrations were 12 mg/dl and 14 mg/dl during the third day of life.

Comparison of Jaundice Meter Readings (TcB Index) and Hematofluorometer Bilirubin, Bilirubin Binding and Reserve

Table 3 displays the general relationship between the TcB index and the values for unconjugated bilirubin, bilirubin binding capacity and reserve bilirubin binding obtained simultaneously using the Bilirubin Hematofluorometer. The TcB index correlated very well to the albumin bound (B) and total (T) unconjugated bilirubin in whole blood. Correlation was good for B/B+R, a value that indicates the degree to which the total binding sites on the serum albumin are saturated. There was an inverse relationship between the reserve albumin binding capacity and the TcB index; as the reserve (R) binding sites decreased, the TcB index rose. The difference between the total bilirubin and the bound bilirubin (T-B) is thought to represent the amount of bilirubin bound to red blood cell sites, as well as to sites other than the prime bilirubin binding sites on albumin. This value did not correlate with the TcB index in these studies.

The value of the albumin saturation index (B/R) x 10, which has been found to correspond to the unbound bilirubin, did correlate with the TcB index, indicating that as the "unbound" bilirubin rises, the TcB index increases. This was true of the relationship between the TcB index and the ratio of albumin-bound bilirubin (B) to the total albumin-binding capacity (B+R) (fig. 5).

In this study, as in our previous studies,[8] the reserve as well as the total bilirubin binding capacity of low birth weight infants (< 2000 g) was found to be less than that of larger infants (> 2000 g) at comparable bilirubin levels (table 4). These values were also low (table 5) in sick infants compared to those that were well (p = < 0.001).

DISCUSSION

The usefulness of transcutaneous bilirubin measurements should be gauged against the problem of assessing the serum bilirubin concentration. While micromethods are available for assessing serum bilirubin, none can be performed without using an invasive technique for sampling the infant's blood. Because of this, determination of bilirubin on the first day of life or at the time of discharge from the hospital is not performed routinely. There is marked variation in both the skill and accuracy with which neonatal jaundice is appraised, yet it is this initial observation which determines the next important step in appraisal and management, that is the decision to perform an invasive procedure to determine serum bilirubin concentration.

In our study, correlation between jaundice meter readings and serum bilirubin concentration were good in both white and black infants. However, the correlation in very dark black infants was not as good as in light or medium black infants. Correlation between the TcB index and serum bilirubin concentration in infants under phototherapy was poor, but when these indices were read using areas of skin protected from light by a patch, the correlation was quite good, but we do not know how long after phototherapy such relationships hold. Baseline TcB readings were influenced by skin pigmentation and gestational age; the darker the skin pigment, the higher the baseline reading. It is of interest that baseline readings are higher in preterm than in term infants in both black and white populations. This may relate to the decreased bilirubin binding capacity of the preterm infant or to variations in the nature of the immature skin itself.

Despite the lack of exact correlation with serum bilirubin concentration, TcB readings correspond well to ranges of serum bilirubin concentrations; this gave ample objective indication for the development of action points, allowing the use of the electronic jaundice meter as means of identifying infants with degrees of jaundice. Further investigation including serum bilirubin determinations and use of the TcB action point to identify infants who may be safely exempt from such an invasive procedure is stimulated. In the entire group of infants, regardless of race or gestational age, TcB indices of less than 19 (in infants not receiving phototherapy) identified infants with serum bilirubin levels of less than 10 mg/dl. The electronic jaundice meter can be used upon to screen for significant degrees of hyperbilirubinemia at the time of discharge from the hospital, and for follow-up of hyperbilirubinemia. Comparison of TcB indices with the visual perception of jaundice by nursery personnel indicated that the jaundice meter is more reliable. We suggest that each nursery using such an instrument develop its own correlative data and selective action points. Since serum bilirubin is not measured by the jaundice meter, the TcB index should not replace serum bilirubin determinations; however, the indices clearly identify infants with potentially dangerous levels of serum bilirubin. Such infants should then have a serum bilirubin determination done.

The finding that the TcB index rises as both the saturation of albumin bindings sites (i.e. B/B+R) and the unbound bilirubin (B/R x 10) increase, may explain in part why TcB indices are in general higher in preterm than in term infants at comparable bilirubin levels. These findings also hold promise that further study of the TcB index in conjunction with measurements of unbound bilirubin, reserve binding capacity, and other factors such as pH, may help elucidate phenomena which influence bilirubin distribution and movement from the vascular bed into the tissues.

REFERENCES

1. I. Yamanouchi, Y. Yamauchi, and I. Iagarashi, Transcutaneous bilirubinometry: Preliminary studies of noninvasive transcutaneous bilirubin meter in the Okayama National Hospital, Pediatr. 65:195 (1978).

2. T. Hegyi, I. N. Hiatt, and L. Indyk, Transcutaneous Bilirubinometry. I. Correlations in term infants, Pediatr. 98:195 (1980).

3. R. R. Engel, B. B. Henis, and R. E. Engel, Effect of race and other variables on transcutaneous bilirubinometry, Pediatr. Res. 15:531 (1981).

4. K. Vangyanichyakorn, S. Sun, and A. Abubaker, Transcutaneous bilirubinometry in black and Hispanic infants, Pediatr. Res. 15:653 (1981).

5. R. E. Hanneman, R. L. Schreiner, and D. P. Dewitt, Evaluation of the Minolta bilirubin meter as a screening device in white and black infants, Pediatr. 69:107 (1982).

6. W. J. Maisels and S. Conrad, Transcutaneous bilirubin measurements in full-term infants, Pediatr. 70:464 (1982).

7. A. A. Lamola, J. Eisinger, and W. E. Blumberg, Fluorometric
    study of the partition of bilirubin among blood components:
    basis for the rapid microassays of bilirubin and bilirubin
    binding capacity in whole blood, Anal. Biochem. 100:25 (1980).
8. A. K. Brown, J. Eisinger, W. E. Blumberg, J. Flores, G. Boyle
    and A. A. Lamola, A rapid fluorometric method for determining
    bilirubin levels and binding in the blood of neonates: com-
    parisons with a diazo method and with 2-(4'-hydroxybenzene)
    azobenzoic acid dye binding, Pediatr. 65:767 (1980).

RECENT ADVANCES IN THE CHEMISTRY OF BILE PIGMENTS

Raymond Bonnett

Department of Chemistry
Queen Mary College
London E1 4NS, U.K.

INTRODUCTION

The bile pigments have long been familiar as products of haem catabolism in the animal kingdom. In recent years their importance in the plant world - notably as biliproteins, such as phycoerythrin, phycocyanin, and phytochrome - has become increasingly evident. In a very real sense the name "bile pigment" is inappropriate for these substances, and it is perhaps more fitting to use the terms "linear tetrapyrrole" or "bilindione" to refer to the series as a whole. The term bilin is now formally assigned[1] to the unsubstituted parent (1), and the naturally occurring derivatives so far known are all dihydroxy derivatives of this, essentially in the bis lactam, bilindione, tautomeric form. The commonest oxidation levels are the bilindione or verdin system (2) and the 10,23-dihydrobilindione or rubin system (3).

In the present paper attention is directed in a comparative way to the chemistry of (2) and (3), as represented by the type molecules biliverdin IXα (4) and bilirubin IXα (5). Certain model systems are also considered, particularly octaethylbilindione, the 2,3,7,8,12,13,17,18-octaethyl derivative of (2).

(1) Bilin (22H shown by convention)

111

(2) Bilindione (formally 21H,24H-bilin-1,19-dione)
or verdin system

(3) 10,23-Dihydrobilindione or rubin system

(4) Biliverdin (IXα)
(P = −CH₂ CH₂ CO₂ H)

(5) Bilirubin (IXα)

STRUCTURAL CONSIDERATIONS

The chemical structures of these substances were established
in the sense of atom connectivities by the Fischer school, using
the methods of chemical degradation and total synthesis.[2] This
work left two questions unresolved - the configuration at bridge
double bonds, and the conformation of the molecule as a whole.
It is interesting to note that for many years the configurational
problem was not really recognised, and in the older liteature (and
even today) both E and Z configurations tend to be represented
indiscriminately.

In recent years these questions have been answered for the
solid state by X-ray crystal structure analysis. The structure of

biliverdin itself has not yet been obtained: repeated attempts
in our laboratories to grow suitable crystals have so far been
unsuccessful, and the attempted analysis of the model system,
octaethylbilindione, has given only a partial solution.[3]   However,
the structure of biliverdin dimethyl ester has been solved,[4] as
have the structures of bilirubin,[5,6,7] its diisopropylammonium
salt,[8] and mesobilirubin.[9]

The biliverdin dimethyl ester molecule has the syn-Z geometry
at the meso bridges, and adopts a helical conformation in the
crystal. The rubins, on the other hand, each have two approximately
planar regions (comprising the pyrromethenone units i.e. rings A +
B and rings C + D) with an interplanar angle of 96°-104°.   The C-5
and C-10 bridges both have the syn-Z geometry. This arrangement
generates, with the aid of a system of six hydrogen bonds, a
molecular shape referred to as the ridge-tile conformation.[5]   The
six intramoleculear hydrogen bonds involve all the polar residues
in the molecule, and the low solubility of bilirubin in water may
be rationalised in terms of this feature.   It seems likely that
hydrogen bonding also occurs in the biliverdin free acid structure:
but, because of the double bond at the C-10 bridge it cannot be the
same as the arrangement in bilirubin, and intermolecular hydrogen
bonding is probably important here.

Table 1. Bond lengths for carbon-carbon bonds at meso bridges
          (Å, rounded to two decimal places)

	Ref.	C-4—C-5	C-5—C-6	C-10—C-11 C-11—C-12	C-14—C-15	C-15—C-16
Biliverdin dimethyl ester	4	1.36	1.48	1.37 1.385	1.42	1.35
Bilirubin[a]	6	1.30	1.45	1.51		
Bilirubin .CHCl$_3$.MeOH	7	1.37	1.42	1.47 1.49	1.40	1.37
Bilirubin diisopropyl ammonium salt[a]	8	1.35	1.43	1.50		
Mesobilirubin	9	1.32	1.49	1.54 1.58	1.45	1.34

[a]Average values for the two pyrromethenone units

Overall, the X-ray work has confirmed the bis-lactam formulation which previously rested largely on infra-red evidence. A consideration of bond lengths at the meso bridges (Table 1) shows the considerable degree of bond localisation at the C-4 - C-5 and C-15 - C-16 bonds: although the system is to some extent delocalised, these bonds have a high degree of double bond character, and can sustain geometrical isomerism. This has become an important feature in the photochemistry of the linear tetrapyrroles. The situation at the C-10 bridge in the verdin structure is not so clear cut, and extensive delocalisation evidently occurs over the pyrromethene unit (rings B and C).

METAL COMPLEXES

Metal complexes of bile pigments have been known for a considerable number of years - Kuster[10] referred to silver and zinc derivatives of bilirubin in 1912 - but their structures and chemistry are still not well understood. More recent work has shown that metal complexes of bilirubin are generally unstable[11] but nonetheless a number of such substances (e.g. Sm III[12] and Zn II[13]) have been studied. Metal complexes of verdins have also been prepared,[14] and have been shown to be subject to a ready one-electron oxidation to give rather stable π-cation radicals.[15]

We have recently prepared the nickel and difluoroboron complexes of the model verdin system octaethylbilindione, and carried out X-ray crystal structural determinations on both complexes.[16] Both compounds are 1:1 complexes. The nickel complex has a helical "macrocyclic" conformation, as shown in Figure 1. Of particular interest is the observation that such complexes show ligand radical character.[17] This may be ascribed to the oxidation of the ligand during the preparation of the complexes.

With boron trifluoride, octaethylbilindione forms a series of interconvertible boron complexes which were originally prepared at Queen Mary College by Dr. McDonagh in 1970. One of these has been obtained crystalline: it has a quite different conformation when compared with the nickel complex, and its structure is shown in Figure 2. The pyrromethene unit (rings B and C) is coordinated to the boron atom, and the bond lengths at the C-10 bridge indicate a markedly delocalised system (C-10 - C-11 = 1.37Å; C-9 - C-10 = 1.37Å) in this region. However the A and D rings are turned away from the boron atom, and although the "double" bonds at the C-5 and C-15 bridges have the Z configuration, the arrangement about the "single" bonds is anti.

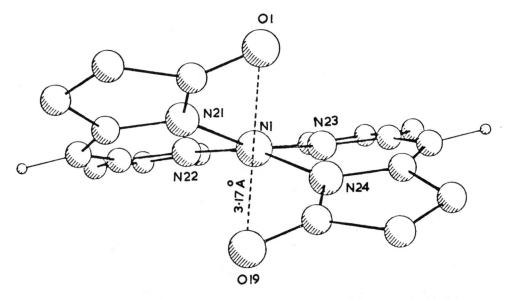

Figure 1 Helical conformation of nickel complex of octaethylbilindione.   The ethyl substituents are omitted for clarity.[16]

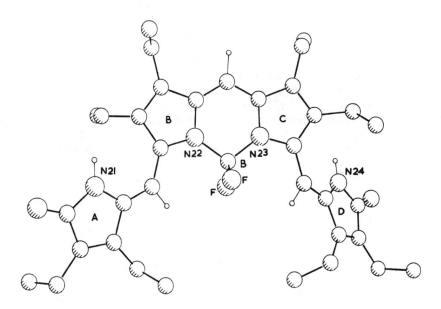

Figure 2.   Extended conformation of the difluoroboron
complex of octaethylbilindione.[16]

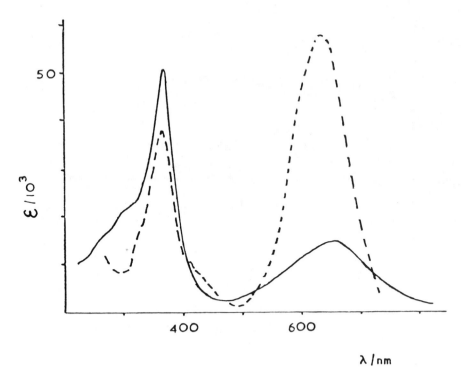

Figure 3.   Electronic spectra in chloroform of octaethylbilin-
            dione (————) and its difluoroboron complex (------)

A particularly interesting feature of the difluoroboron
complex is its electronic spectrum, which, since the boron atom
can be regarded as neutral from the point of view of electronic
transitions, can be compared with that of the parent verdin, octaethylbilindione. Figure 3 shows the comparison. Octaethylbilindione has a typical verdin spectrum – a strong absorption at about
380 nm, and a weaker one at about 650 nm. In the boron complex
the visible band is the more intense, a result which accords with
predictions made some years ago[18] for verdin systems in such an
extended arrangement as is shown by this particular structure.

MESO REACTIVITY

The addition of alcohols to the double bonds at the 5 and 15
bridges of the verdins under oxidative conditions has been known
for some time.[19] Recently two X-ray crystal analyses of such
dialkoxy derivatives have appeared.[20,21]

Substitution reactions have been observed at C-5 and C-15
(deuteriation, nitration).[21] The deuteriation may be followed by

[1]H nmr spectroscopy as is shown in Figure 4 for octaethylbilindione in [2]H-trifluoroacetic acid. These are formally electrophilic sub-stitutions. At C-10, on the other hand, nucleophilic attack occurs. This may lead to an overall addition, as with sodium borohydride[22] and nucleophiles such as alcohols, thiols and amines, to generate the rubin system. Falk has shown that in many cases this process is readily reversed.[23] With cyanide in dimethylsulphoxide/LiBr a formal (oxidative) nucleophilic substitution is observed to give the 10-cyanoverdin, the electronic spectrum of which shows a marked bathochromic shift of the visible band (λ_{max}(CHCl$_3$) 380, 680 sh, and 726 nm).[24]

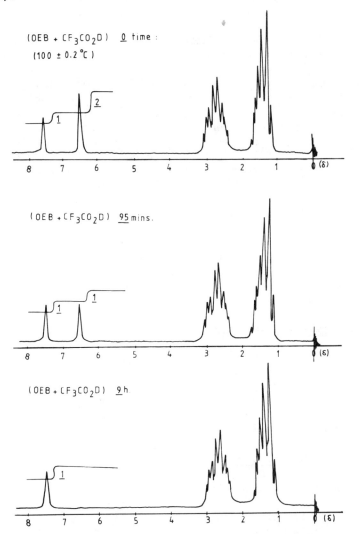

Figure 4. Deuteriation of octaethylbilindione (OEB) at C-5 and C-15 in CF$_3$CO$_2$[2]H, followed by nmr spectroscopy

CLEAVAGE AT THE C-10 BRIDGE

There are two long established reactions which cleave linear tetrapyrroles at the C-10 bridge. Fusion with resorcinol (the Schumm reaction) was employed by the Fischer school in degradative work on these pigments: it is a complex reaction, and is seldom used. The van den Bergh reaction (the diazo reaction), in which a diazonium ion attacks at C-9 (and C-11) is well established in clinical chemistry as the basis of an analytical method for bilirubin. Scheer has recently reexamined this reaction, and has shown that the initial products are an azo derivative of a pyrromethenone (purple) and an alkoxymethylpyrromethenone (yellow).[25]

Two other cleavage reactions merit comment. The first is the acid-catalysed pyrrole exchange reactions by which bilirubin IXα is converted into an equilibrium mixture of the starting material and the isomeric bilirubins IIIα and XIIIα. Originally encountered during the acid-catalysed dehydrogenation of bilirubin,[26],[27] it has been developed as a preparative method.[28],[29] The second cleavage reaction is of the verdin system with thiobarbituric acid, a reaction which is plausibly initiated by nucleophilic attack at C-10 (see above), followed by participation of the thiobarbituric moiety in the cleavage of the rubinoid C-10 bridge so generated.[30]

PHOTOCHEMISTRY

Finally, I propose to look in outline at the photochemistry of bile pigments, concentrating on the familiar verdin and rubin systems, and so create a link with the main topic of this meeting. Three areas have received attention – photoaddition, photo-oxidation, and photoisomerisation.

Photoaddition

The photoaddition of nucleophilic species occurs slowly at the vinyl groups (and particularly the _exo_ vinyl group) and has been studied by Manitto and his colleagues.[31],[32] The photoaddition proceeds in the Markovnikov sense. A thermal addition of this sort (with mercaptoacetic acid) has been developed to provide a useful route to bilirubin XIIIα.[33]

Photo-oxidation (Photo-oxygenation)

This has been extensively studied. It is currently thought to play a minor role in jaundice phototherapy. Since photoisomerisation (see below) occurs the more readily, it seems likely that the photoisomers are also subject to photo-oxidation. The reaction has been studied in a variety of solvents.[34] In ammoniacal methanol the photo-oxidation proceeds with cleavage at the _meso_ bridges to give maleimides (methylvinylmaleimide from rings A and D, haematinic acid imide from rings B and C), and three methanol-propentdyopent adducts.[35] The latter are derived from rings A + B and C + D: the stereochemistry of these propentdyopent adducts is at present unknown.

There is a great deal of evidence that singlet oxygen is involved in this reaction. It has been generally presumed that bilirubin is the sensitiser, although the actual sensitiser may well be one of the photoisomers (see below). Bilirubin certainly reacts very rapidly with singlet oxygen to give a similar distribution of products to those found in the photo-oxidation.

Photoisomerisation

The postulate that the photoinitiated geometrical isomerisation of C-4 and/or C-15 double bonds of bilirubin would lead to an isomer which would be more soluble in water followed hard on the heels of the X-ray crystal analysis of bilirubin,[6] and the observed photo-isomerisation of a model pyrromethenone.[36] The latter result was highly relevant because bilirubin contains two slightly dissimilar pyrromethenone chromophores.

Irradiation of bilirubin in a variety of solvents and in the absence of air gives a mixture of products. In dimethylsulphoxide or ammoniacal methanol irradiation with a tungsten filament (500 watts) or a clinical "blue" light source (λ_{max} ca. 440 nm, 100 watts) gives rubinoid products which are more polar than is bilirubin and which have been called photobilirubin I (two components, A and B) and photobilirubin II (the more polar, again two components, A and B). Photobilirubin I readily reverts to bilirubin,[37] and initial attempts to isolate solid photobilirubin I and to study its properties at room temperature[38] are now realised to have given misleading results. Photobilirubin II is somewhat more robust than is photobilirubin I, but is still a sensitive compound: a few milligrams can be isolated and examined, but it gradually decomposes when kept at room temperature. On further irradiation it is partly unchanged, but some bilirubin is detected and a new compound, photobilirubin III, is also formed.[39]

In recent studies by McDonagh and Lightner on the one hand, and Falk and his colleagues on the other, the substances which are referred to here as photobilirubin IA/B have been shown to be a mixture of the 4E,15Z and 4Z,15E isomers of bilirubin, which can be effectively analysed by hplc. The conclusions have rested primarily on nmr correlations, particularly with the photoisomers of symmetrically substituted systems (bilirubin IIIα and bilirubin XIIIα).[40] An elegant chemical correlation has also been achieved. The photoisomers of bilirubin, after enrichment by extraction into methanol at low temperature, have been dehydrogenated with

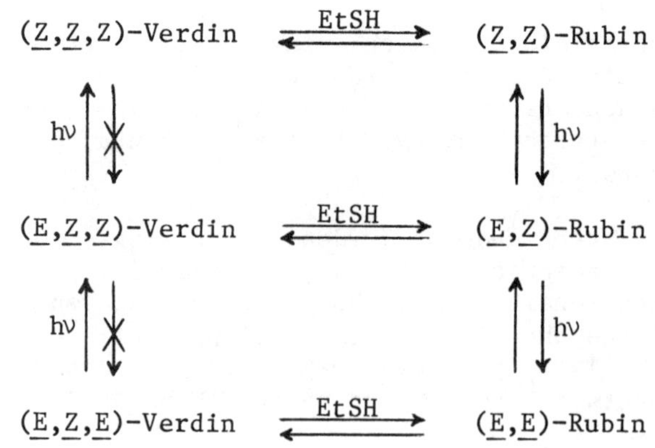

(Z̲,Z̲,Z)-Verdin $\xrightarrow{\text{EtSH}}$ (Z̲,Z̲)-Rubin

hν ⇅ ⤬   ⇅ hν

(E̲,Z̲,Z)-Verdin $\xrightarrow{\text{EtSH}}$ (E̲,Z̲)-Rubin

hν ⇅ ⤬   ⇅ hν

(E̲,Z̲,E̲)-Verdin $\xrightarrow{\text{EtSH}}$ (E̲,E̲)-Rubin

Figure 5. Proposed scheme for the photoisomerisation
of the verdin system in the presence of a
nucleophile, after Falk.[23]

chloranil to the known E̲Z̲Z̲- and Z̲Z̲E̲-biliverdin isomers (as their
dimethyl esters).[41] These verdin isomers are more robust: they
are prepared by irradiation of biliverdin IXα in the presence of a
nucleophile (e.g. ethanethiol) which adds reversibly (see above)
to give a rubin system.[23] It is the latter that photoisomerises:
the verdin system resists direct photoisomerisation. The various
equilibria are summarised in Figure 5.

A product formulated as the E̲,E̲-bilirubin has also been
observed as a minor product of the photoreaction.[40] Photobilirubin II was originally regarded as the E̲,E̲-bilirubin.[38] However,
subsequent nmr studies at high field have indicated that the endovinyl group has disappeared, and, since the substance appears to
be isomeric with bilirubin, an intramolecular cyclisation must have
occurred. Two structures (6, 7) fit the nmr data,[39] and each has
subsequently been favoured (7)[42] or supported (6)[43]. In fact the
infrared evidence argues against the δ-lactone structure (7), and
we have adopted the seven-membered carbocyclic ring formulation (6).
This appears to be the first cycloderivative of bilirubin to be
recognised.

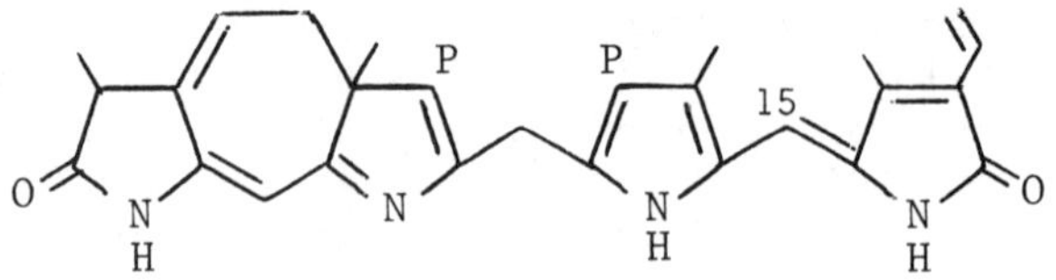

(6)

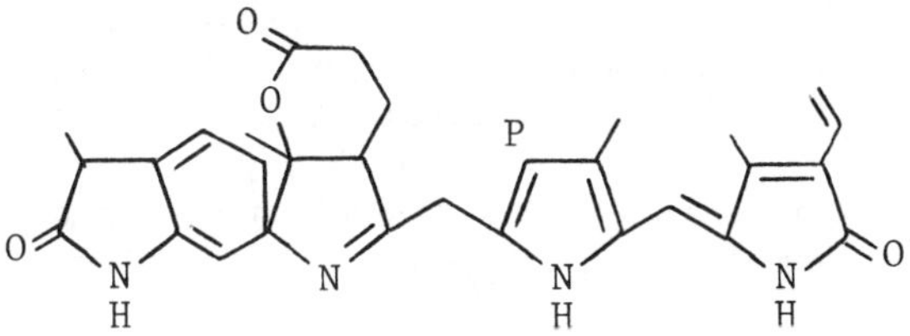

(7)

Photobilirubin III is more polar than is photobilirubin II. On keeping it reverts to photobilirubin II, and is therefore formulated as the 15E isomer of photobilirubin II (i.e. 6, with the E configuration at C-15).[39]

Because a number of workers have been engaged in this field, trivial names have multiplied. On the whole, if we have to use trivial names here (and perhaps we do) I prefer the Stoll/Ostrow names which are simple and descriptive, even though these workers were not able to isolate the (EZ)- and (ZE)-bilirubins in a pure state. We must bear in mind that no one has published satisfactory elemental analyses on any of the rubin photoisomers as yet. These are difficult compounds.

In Figure 6 a correlation is provided between the trivial names and current structure assignments which may be found helpful.

Structure (as denoted by a systematic name)	Trivial Names
(4E,15Z)-Bilirubin[b]	Photobilirubin IA (IB)[a] Peak 3[c]
(4Z,15E)-Bilirubin[b]	Photobilirubin IB (IA)[a] Peak 3[c]
(4E,15E)-Bilirubin[b]	
3²,7-Cyclo(15E)-bilirubin (two pairs of enantiomers 2S,7S; 2R,7R & 2S,7R; 2R,7S)	Photobilirubin IIA and IIB Lumibilirubin and isolumibilirubin Peak 2 ("unknown pigment")[c]
3²,7-Cyclo-(15Z)-bilirubin (two pairs of enantiomers as before)	Photobilirubin III (A & B)[a]

Figure 6. Correlation for names used by different workers. (a: Stoll and Ostrow, used here. b: McDonagh and Lightner. c: Onishi)

The photochemistry of linear tetrapyrroles is very active at present, and not just in the bilirubin area. In closing let me call attention to the plant bilindiones that I mentioned in passing at the outset. The way in which algal biliproteins act as accessory pigments in photosynthesis and the mechanism by which phytochrome undergoes a photochemical rearrangement which triggers off morphological change in plants, are two topics which have their own followers, and they may seem far removed from clinical matters which we are relating to at this meeting. But these, too, are photochemical changes involving linear tetrapyrrole chromophores, and we should, I think, be well advised to keep an eye on what is happening in another part of the forest.

I would like to acknowledge the contributions made by my colleagues and coworkers in our published work referred to below. The support of the Medical Research Council and the Science and Engineering Research Council is acknowledged.

REFERENCES

1. IUPAC/IUB Joint Commission on Biochemical Nomenclature, Nomenclature of Tetrapyrroles, Pure Appl. Chem. 51: 2251 (1979) and there, section TP6.
2. H. Fischer and H. Plieninger, Synthesis of biliverdin and bilirubin, Hoppe-Seyler's Z. Physiol. Chem. 274:231 (1942) and references therein.
3. E.F. Meyer and G. Pepe, Interactive graphics with the aid of force field calculations, Amer. Cryst. Assoc. Abstr. Ser. 2: 93 (1979).
4. W.S. Sheldrick, Crystal and molecular structure of biliverdin dimethyl ester, J. Chem. Soc., Perkin Trans. 2, 1457 (1976).
5. R. Bonnett, J.E. Davies, and M.B. Hursthouse, Structure of bilirubin, Nature (London) 262: 326 (1976).
6. R. Bonnett, J.E. Davies, M.B. Hursthouse, and G.M. Sheldrick, The structure of bilirubin, Proc. Roy. Soc. London B202: 249 (1978).
7. G. LeBas, A. Allegret, Y. Mauguen, C. de Rango, and M. Bailly, The structure of triclinic bilirubin chloroform-methanol solvate, Acta Cryst. B36: 3007 (1980).
8. A. Mugnoli, P. Manitto, and D. Monti, Structure of di-isopropyl-ammonium bilirubinate, Nature (London) 273: 568 (1978).
9. W. Becher and W.S. Sheldrick, The crystal structure of meso-bilirubin IXα - bis(chloroform), Acta Cryst.,B34: 1298 (1978).
10. W. Kuster and P. Deihle, Bilirubin and haemin, Hoppe Seyler's Z. Physiol Chem. 82: 463 (1912).
11. R.A. Velapoldi and O. Menis, Formation and stabilities of free bilirubin and bilirubin complexes with transition and rare earth elements, Clin. Chem. 17: 1165 (1971).

12. C.C. Kuenzle, R.R. Pelloni, and M.M. Weibel, A proposed novel structure for the metal chelates of bilirubin, Biochem. J. 130: 1147 (1972).
13. D.W. Hutchinson, B. Johnson, and A.J. Knell, Metal complexes of bilirubin in aprotic solvents, Biochem. J. 133: 399 (1973).
14. For review see J. Subramanian and J.-H. Fuhrhop, Metal complexes of open-chain tetrapyrrole pigments, in: "The Porphyrins, Vol. 2", D. Dolphin, ed., Academic Press, New York (1978).
15. C. Krauss and H. Scheer, Long-lived π-cation radicals of bilindionato zinc complexes, Tetrahedron Letters 3553 (1979).
16. J.V. Bonfiglio, R. Bonnett, D.G. Buckley, D. Hamzetash, M.B. Hursthouse, K.M.A. Malik, A.F. McDonagh, and Jill Trotter, Syntheses and X-ray analyses of boron and nickel complexes of octaethyl-21H,24H-bilin-1,19-dione, Tetrahedron, in press.
17. J. Subramanian, J.-H. Fuhrhop, A. Salek, and A. Gossauer, Esr studies of metal complexes and π-radicals of biliverdin derivatives, J. Mag. Res. 15: 19 (1974).
18. M.J. Burke, D.C. Pratt, and A. Moscowitz, Low-temperature absorption and circular dichroism studies of phytochrome, Biochemistry 11: 4025 (1972).
19. H. von Dobeneck, U. Sommer, E. Brunner, E. Lippacher, and F. Schnierle, Classification of tripyrrenes: addition to the double bone of methylenepyrrolinones, Justus Liebig's Ann. Chem. 1934 (1973).
20. D.L. Cullen, N. van Opdenbosch, E.F. Meyer, K.M. Smith, and F. Eivazi, Crystal and molecular structure of a 4,5-dimethoxybilindione derived from etiobiliverdin IVγ, J. Chem. Soc., Perkin Trans. 2, 307 (1982).
21. J.V. Bonfiglio, R. Bonnett, D.G. Buckley, D. Hamzetash, M.B. Hursthouse, K.M.A. Malik, S.C. Naithani, and J. Trotter, Substitution and addition reactions of octaethyl-21H,24H-bilin-1,19-dione, a model verdin system, J. Chem. Soc., Perkin Trans. 1, 1291 (1982).
22. M.S. Stoll and C.H. Gray, The preparation and characterisation of bile pigments, Biochem. J. 163: 59 (1977).
23. H. Falk, N. Muller, and T. Schlederer, A regioselective reversible addition to bilatrienes-abc, Monatsch. Chem. 11: 159 (1980).
24. H. Falk and T. Schlederer, A formal nucleophilic substitution of biliatrienes-abc, Monatsch. Chem. 109: 1013 (1978).
25. W. Kufer and H. Scheer, The diazo reaction of bilirubin: structure of the yellow products, Tetrahedron, in press (1983).
26. R. Bonnett and A.F. McDonagh, The isomeric heterogeneity of biliverdin dimethyl ester derived from bilirubin, J. Chem. Soc., Chem. Commun. 238 (1970).

27. R. Bonnett, D.G. Buckley, D. Hamzetash, and A.F. McDonagh, Pyrrole exchange reactions in the bilirubin series, Isr. J.Chem. in press (1983).

28. A.F. McDonagh and F. Assisi, Direct evidence for the acid-catalysed isomeric scrambling of bilirubin IXα, J. Chem. Soc., Chem. Comm. 117 (1972).

29. A.F. McDonagh, "Bile pigments: bilatrienes and 5,15-biladienes" in: "The Porphyrins", Vol. 6, D. Dolphin ed., Academic Press, New York, 1979 and there p. 455.

30. P. Manitto and D. Monti, Reactions of biliverdins with thiobarbituric acid. A novel fragmentation reaction of bilin-1,19-(21H,22H)-diones, J. Chem. Soc., Chem. Commun. 178 (1980).

31. P. Manitto, Photochemistry of bilirubin, Experientia 27: 1147 (1971).

32. P. Manitto and D. Monti, Photoaddition of sulphydryl groups to bilirubin in vitro, Experientia 28: 379 (1972).

33. D. Monti and P. Manitto, A simple procedure for preparing bilirubin XIIIα, Synth. Commun. 11: 811 (1981).

34. For a review see D.A. Lightner, The photoreactivity of bilirubin and related pyrroles, Photochem. Photobiol. 26: 427 (1977).

35. R. Bonnett and J.C.M. Stewart, Photo-oxidation of bilirubin in hydroxylic solvents, J. Chem. Soc., Perkin Trans. 1, 224 (1975).

36. H. Falk, K. Grubmayer, U. Herzig, and O. Hofer, The configuration of the isomeric 3,4-dimethyl-5-(1H)-2,2'-pyrromethenones, Tetrahedron Lett. 559 (1975).

37. A.F. McDonagh, D.A. Lightner, and T.A. Wooldridge, Geometric isomerisation of bilirubin IXα and its dimethyl ester, J. Chem. Soc., Chem. Commun. 110 (1979).

38. M.S. Stoll, E.A. Zenone, J.D. Ostrow, and J.E. Zarembo, Preparation and properties of bilirubin photoisomers, Biochem. J. 183: 139 (1979).

39. M.S. Stoll, N. Vicker, C.H. Gray, and R. Bonnett, Concerning the structure of photobilirubin II, Biochem. J. 201: 179 (1982).

40. A.F. McDonagh, L.A. Palma, F.R. Trull, and D.A. Lightner, Phototherapy for neonatal jaundice. Configurational isomers of bilirubin, J. Am. Chem. Soc. 104: 6865 (1982).

41. H. Falk, N. Muller, M. Ratzenhofer, and K. Winsauer, The structure of 'photobilirubin', Monatsh. Chem. 113: 1421 (1982).

42. S. Onishi, S. Itoh, K. Isobe, H. Togari, H. Kitoh, and Y. Nishimura, Mechanism of development of bronze baby syndrome in neonates treated with phototherapy, Pediatrics 69: 273 (1982).

43. A.F. McDonagh, L.A. Palma, and D.A. Lightner, Phototherapy for neonatal jaundice. Stereospecific and regioselective photoisomerisation of bilirubin bound to human serum albumin and NMR characterisation of intramolecularly cyclised photoproducts, J. Am. Chem. Soc. 104: 6867 (1982).

SOLUTION CONFORMATIONS, PHOTOPHYSICS, AND PHOTOCHEMISTRY

OF BILIRUBIN AND BILIVERDIN DIMETHYL ESTERS

Kurt Schaffner

Max-Planck-Institut für Strahlenchemie
Stiftstrasse 34 - 36
D-4330 Mülheim a. d. Ruhr, West Germany

INTRODUCTION

This review will focus on the results of the investigations into the solution conformation, the photophysics and photochemistry of BRE, BVE, and related linear open-chain tetrapyrroles,* which have been carried out in

BR (R = CO$_2$H) Bilirubin (IXα)
BRE (R = CO$_2$CH$_3$) Bilirubin dimethyl ester (IXα)

BVE (R = CO$_2$CH$_3$) Biliverdin dimethyl ester (IXα)

---

*Abbreviations: D(UV)/D(Vis), ratio of dipole strengths of absorption and fluorescence excitation bands; OAS, optoacoustic spectroscopy; CD, circular dichroism; PP, picosecond pump-probe; RT, room temperature; SPT, single-photon timing; MTHF, 2-methyltetrahydrofuran; see also formula captions.

Mülheim under the competent direction of Professor Silvia
E. Braslavsky and Dr. Alfred R. Holzwarth (cf. ref 1 for a
more extensive review of this and the literature work).
The linear pigments are extended chromophores of unusual
conformational flexibility in both the electronic ground
and excited states. In principal, various configurational,
conformational and tautomeric forms are possible, and in-
terconversions of these forms can include E-Z photo-
isomerizations of the C=C bonds and rotations around the
C-C bonds of the bridges, as well as intra- and intermolecular proton transfer processes. Some of these processes
will link species which are almost isoenergetic and have
overlapping spectra. These species often possess significantly different excited state properties, with thermally
reversible photochemical changes. Direct experimental detection is thus often difficult, and reversible photochemical processes may appear as "energy wasting" channels
difficult to distinguish from direct radiationless
deactivation of the excited state to the ground state.

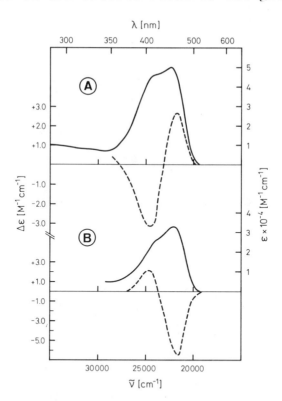

Fig. 1. RT absorption (——) and solvent-induced CD (---)
        spectra of BRE in ethyl (S)-(-)-lactate (A) and
        (R,R)-(-)-butane-2,3-diol (B) (2).

BILIRUBIN AND BILIRUBIN DIMETHYL ESTER

Spectroscopy of BRE in Solution. Coexistence of Different Forms

A combination of absorption, luminescence, solvent-induced CD and NMR studies has shown that BRE in very dilute solution can adopt at least two (families of) diffe-

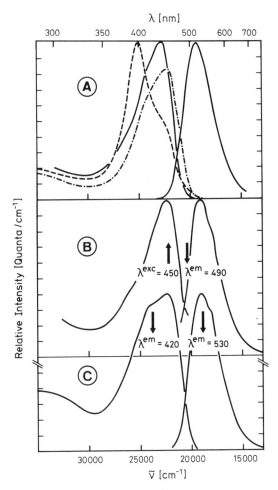

Fig. 2. Corrected RT fluorescence and fluorescence excitation spectra of BRE in MTHF (A) and ethyl lactate (B, C). In (A) the spectra are independent of λ(exc) and λ(em) and in (B) and (C) they arise from different components when λ(exc) and λ(em) are varied. The RT absorption spectra in EtOH (---) and MTHF (—·—) are also given.

rent forms, depending on solvent and temperature (see, e.
g., Figs. 1 and 2) (2). BR and its dianion behave in a
qualitatively similar way. At RT one species has an absorption maximum at 448 nm (Fig. 2A: in EtOH; = "450 nm"
species), the other at 397 nm (in MTHF; = "395 nm" species). The fluorescence lifetime in EtOH at 77 K is 1.9 ns
for the "450 nm" and 11.9 ns for the "395 nm" component.
At RT the relative lifetimes are reversed, and the "395
nm" species has an about tenfold lower emission quantum
yield and a correspondingly shorter lifetime than the
"450 nm" species.

The Nature of the Coexisting Ground-State Forms. Iso-
phorcarubin Dimethyl Ester

For an evaluation of the nature of the two forms of
BRE in dilute solutions it is best to first consider analogous results obtained for IPRE (Chart 1) (3). IPRE possesses a more rigid tetrapyrrole backbone than the parent
BRE, and the fusion of the central rings B and C forces
the two pyrromethenone moieties into a stretched alignment
with the nitrogens in anti position. This rigidity provi-

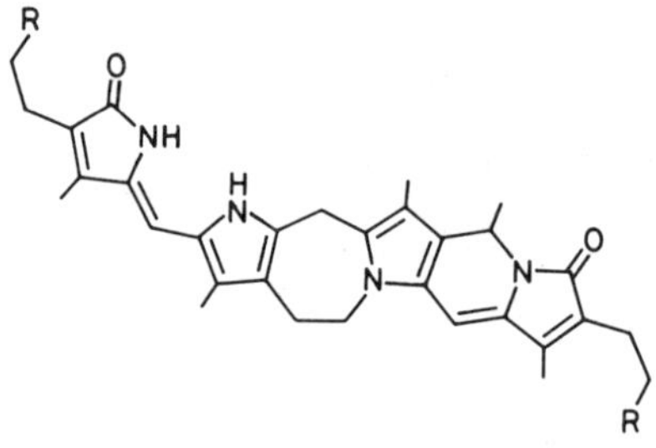

IPRE   Isophorcarubin dimethyl ester

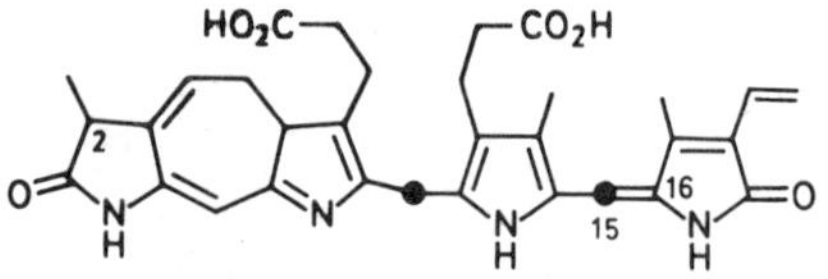

(E)- and (Z)-LR   Lumirubins
(E)- and (Z)-ILR   Isolumirubins (C2 epimers)

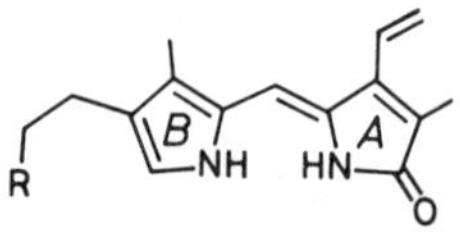

1

R = CO₂CH₃

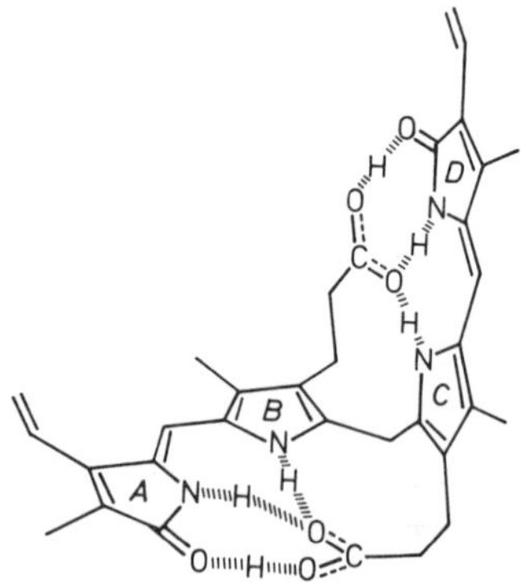

Chart 1. Constitution of IPRE, LR, ILR and the parent
         ring A/B model compound 1, as well as the
         "ridge tile" crystal conformation of BR (4).

des some structure to the UV absorption of IPRE even at
RT, whereas the coexistence of several forms of the more
flexible BRE gives rise to broad bands. It is even more
clearly illustrated by the fact that IPRE has the highest
fluorescence quantum yield [0.04 at RT (3)] of all rubins
[cf. BRE: 0.0008, 1: 0.001 (5)] owing to the lack of
conformational mobility of the C/D chromophore. The simi-
larity of the spectral characteristics of BRE and IPRE,
and the negligible contribution at RT of the non-cyclized
pyrromethenone moiety (cf. 1) to the total emission of
IPRE suggest that the major contribution to the heterogeneity in emission comes from different orientations of the
A/B and C/D partial structures with respect to each other.

In accordance with this conclusion the spectral properties of the "395 nm" species of BRE resemble those of
the parent model 1 (5,6). The absorption of the "450 nm"
form, however, cannot be extrapolated from the spectra of
the individual partial chromophores. Rather, it must arise
from electronic coupling of the two subchromophores.

The Photochemistry of BRE

The singlet-excited BR and BRE undergo a rapid Z → E
photoisomerization of either of the C-4 or C-15 double
bonds, and a less efficient photocyclization to LR and ILR
(8-12). The E photoproducts again revert photochemically
and thermally to the all-Z isomers. As a consequence of
the heterogeneous composition of the BRE solutions the
phochemistry is dependent on the irradiation wavelength
(13). The "395 nm" species isomerizes less efficiently
than the "450 nm" form, and the distribution of the photoproducts and their reactivities in secondary phototrans-
formations is different. The following then is a minimum
scheme for the C=C bond isomerizations, not including additional processes such as diagonal ones across the scheme
(e.g., Z,Z-BRE' ⇌ Z,E-BRE'' etc.) which are also
possible provided that the preferences for the reaction
pathways are maintained:

(4Z,15Z)-BRE'("395 nm")   (4Z,15Z)-BRE''("450 nm")

    hν ↑↓ hν   hν ↑↓ hν

(4E,15Z)-BRE'   (4Z,15E)-BRE''

   hν ⟍ hν   hν ⟋ hν

(4E,15E)-BRE

Internal Conversion

Much of the wasting channels for the remainder of the overall quantum efficiency associated with the Z → E iso-merization (i.e., relaxation via k(1) and k(2) of the twisted excited singlet; Fig. 3) is turned into fluores-cence upon cooling or embedding the molecule into a solid matrix (5,8). Rotation modes around the C-C and C=C modes at C-5 and C-15 must therefore be important in the direct deactivation of the first singlet excited state at room temperature. The temperature-dependent fluorescence yield characteristics show that the "450 nm" is the more rigid of the forms. In BR this is attributed to conformational fixation thorugh intramolecular hydrogen bonds, analogous to the crystal "ridge tile" conformation (Chart 1), which slows down the excited-state twisting towards the Z → E isomerization (8,14,15). In BRE the constraints are simi-lar but less important since there are fewer hydrogen bonds involved, and the overall rate of isomerization of BRE is faster (14). The greater flexibility of the "395

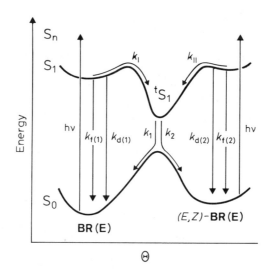

Fig. 3. Potential energy levels and deactivation paths for any given conformer of BR, BRE and their E,Z iso-mers. Θ: twist angle about the C-4 or C-15 double bond; k(d): sums of rate constants for deactiva-tion by C-C rotation and hydrogen bridge-mediated processes; k(f): for fluorescence; k(I,II): for twisting around a C=C bond; k(1,2): for relaxa-tion of twisted singlet to BR(E) and photoisomers, respectively. Not depicted are are the k(d) acti-vation energies and the paths for (I)LR formation.

nm" species is due to the lack of intramolecular hydrogen bonds. It is more readily subjected to rotations around the C-C bonds at C-10 and less so to hydrogen bond-mediated deactivation.

In conclusion we may extend somewhat an earlier diagram (16) of the potential energies of BR and BRE by including rotational and hydrogen bridge-mediated processes deactivating the singlet excited states of any given forms of BR and BRE and their E,Z photoisomers (Fig. 3). Since in a rigid matrix Z → E isomerization is negligible and yet the fluorescence yield does not reach unity, the ratio k(1)/k(2) is assumed close to 1, which implies that the efficiency of twisting is less than unity and different for the two singlet excited states. The remainder is thus available for direct deactivation via the k(d)´s.

BILIVERDIN DIMETHYL ESTER

Spectroscopy of BVE Dimethyl Ester in Solution and in Liposomes. Coexistence of Helically Coiled and Stretched C-10 Isomers

The stationary spectroscopic techniques, which have served for the initial investigation of BVE (5,17-23), have recently been supplemented by time-resolved methods (LIOAS, PP, SPT), which afford a better insight into the relationship between structure and radiationless processes of individual species (24,25). Chart 2 exemplifies the complex situation which is to be anticipated in the case of ground state BVE, even when lactam-lactim tautomerizations and geometrical changes within the A/B and C/D partial structures are a priori excluded.

The distinct thermochromic and solvatochromic properties of the absorption, fluorescence, fluorescence excitation and solvent-induced CD spectra of BVE, at low concentrations, have again been interpreted in terms of helically coiled and stretched forms coexisting in solution. The spectral differences between these forms is best illustrated with BVE incorporated in liposome membranes (Fig. 4). The emission of the initially predominating coiled form changes into that of the stretched species when in liquid-crystalline liposomes, or on sonication or heating above the phase transition temperature when in more rigid gel-type membranes. A similar stretching in solution at RT requires a higher activation energy, in the order of solvent viscosity activation. By comparison, the barriers between the "395 nm" and "450 nm" conformers of BRE are much lower.

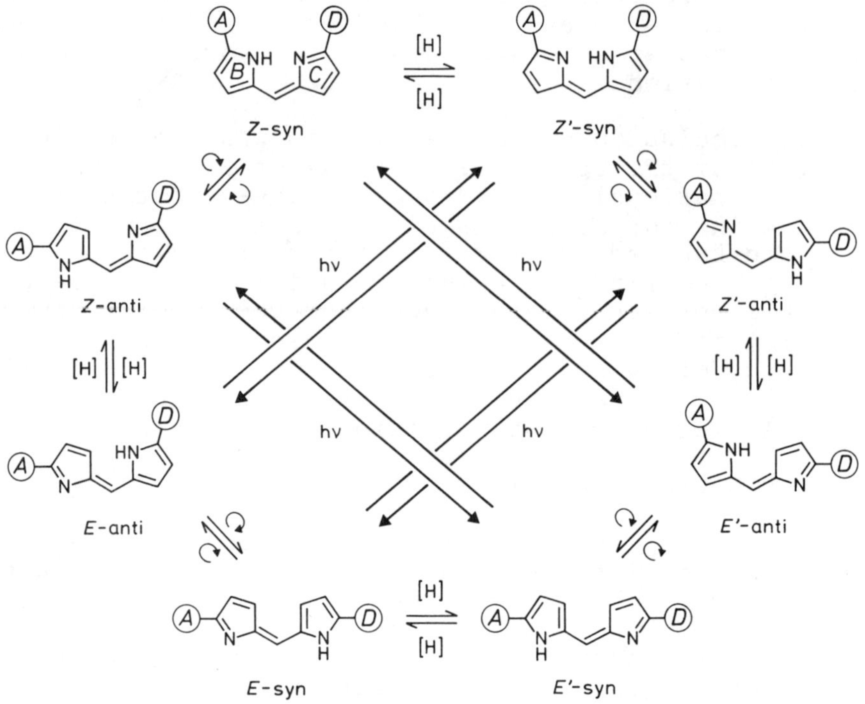

Chart 2. Helically coiled Z-syn and the stretched E-anti, E-syn, and Z-anti C(10)-isomeric forms of an A/D unsymmetrically substituted bilatriene, with interconverting proton transfers between the B/C nitrogens ([H]) and C-C rotation at C-10 in the ground state, and E - Z isomerization of the C-10 double bond in the excited state.

Picosecond Kinetics of Excited State Relaxation in BVE

The detailed study of radiationless deactivation by emission quantum yield determinations and LIOAS has been impaired by the spectral overlaps of the individual BVE forms. These difficulties have been overcome by an investigation (25) which combined picosecond absorption and fluorescence detection using the PP and SPT techniques, respectively. As exemplified in Fig. 5, up to 4 fluorescing species, 2 short-lived (picosecond) and 2 long-lived (nanosecond) ones, are detected.

The remarkably long-lived nanosecond decay components originate from the stretched forms which are attributed an inherently rigid anti conformation preventing

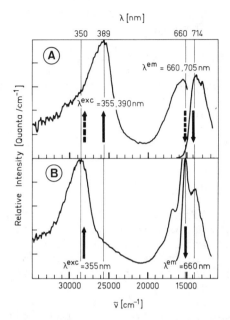

Fig. 4. Corrected fluorescence and excitation spectra at 298 K of BVE in gel-type liposome membranes (dipalmitoyl lecithine); A: helically coiled BVE; B: stretched forms of BVE (22).

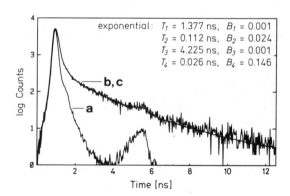

Fig. 5. Semilogarithmic plot of fluorescence decay of BVE in MTHF at RT (SPT); λ(exc) = 580 nm, λ(em) = 650 nm; a: exciting pulse; b: measured decay; c: decay function calculated from the best-fit kinetic parameters; inset: calculated lifetimes T(1)...T(n) and amplitudes B(1)...B(n) of the decay components (25).

ultrarapid radiationless deactivation by proton transfer
between the B/C nitrogens.

The picosecond components are related to either one
or two coiled ground states. Both decay components are
subject to ultrarapid radiationless deactivation induced
by temperature-(or rather, viscosity-)dependent C-C rotations, and the shorter-lived of the two is additionally
deactivated by way of intramolecular proton transfer.

The Photochemistry of BVE. The Conformation-selective
Photocyclization of BVE-IXγ

The photocyclization to PBE (Chart 3) selectively occurs with the stretched 10Z-anti form of BVE-IXγ, in competition to the excited-state twisting at C-10 and relaxa-
tion to the starting material and the E,Z photoisomers
(23). Analogous ring closures across one of the lateral
bridges are not observed, neither in BVE-IXγ as an alternative to the closure in the center nor in BVE where one
vinyl group is adjacent to a lateral bridge. Stretching of
the coiled form is evidently confined to thermal and photochemical transformations within the B/C moiety, while
the Z-syn geometry of the A/B and C/D halves is retained.

Low-temperature irradiation (20) and LIOAS studies
(24) show that BVE at low concentrations (cf. Fig. 6) pho-
toisomerizes to the stretched Z-syn,E-anti,Z-syn species.
Reverting back to BVE on the μs time scale at RT, these
isomers are thermally more labile than E-syn-BVE which is
the stretched species formed on heating or ultrasonica-

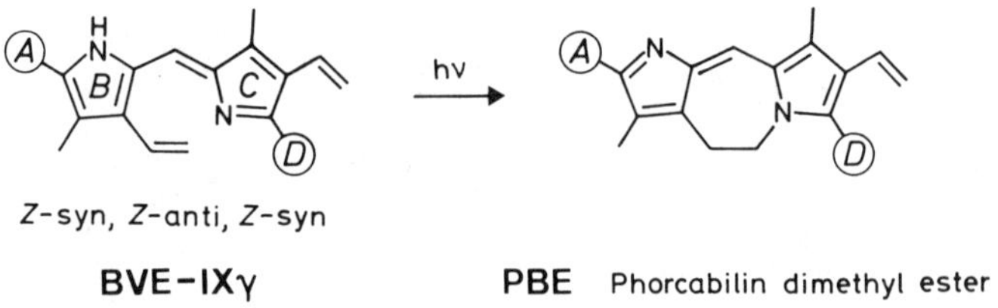

Z-syn, Z-anti, Z-syn

BVE-IXγ   **PBE**   Phorcabilin dimethyl ester

Chart 3. Selective photocyclization of the coiled Z-
         syn,Z-anti,Z-syn-BVE-IXγ to PBE in dimethyl-
         sulfoxide (23). The highest reaction efficiency
         is achieved in the region 575-600 nm where the
         stretched forms absorb. At longer wavelengths,
         where the absorption of the coiled form becomes
         increasingly more important, the efficiency
         sharply declines.

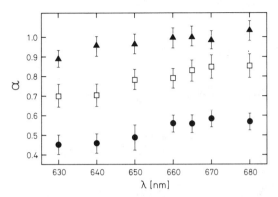

Fig. 6. Concentration dependence of the LIOAS of BVE at RT: "Prompt" heat dissipation fractions α of $\bullet$ = 1.0 10^{-6} M, $\square$ = 2.0 10^{-6} M, and $\blacktriangle$ = 1.3 10^{-5} M BVE in ethanol (24). The $(1-\alpha)$ values in the more dilute solutions ($\bullet$,$\square$) are a measure of the formation of E-anti photoisomers reverting back to BVE on the microsecond time scale.

tion. The photochemical behaviour of BVE and its IXγ isomer suggests that 10E-10Z photoisomerization may play an appreciable role as a radiationless deactivation channel of excited BVE.

This photochemistry is different from the "bilirubin-type photoreactions" of BVE observed when adsorbed on alumina (26) or when in solution in the presence of strong electron donors (27,28), and brought about by nucleophilic attacks at C-10 (5,7,29-30). The resulting rubinoid intermediates undergo photochemical Z → E isomerizations and additions at C-5 and C-15. They have also been recognized as the trace sources of the so-called "blue" or "anomalous" fluorescence of BVE (5,32) and of phytochrome (7,32).

The Formation of Aggregates

The tendency to form aggregates manifests itself in various ways. One is that BRE and BVE form strong adducts of varying stoichiometry with many solvents (21). Another one is shown by the LIOAS results in Fig. 6 (24). The static inhibition of the formation of the Z,E,Z photoisomers at higher concentrations has recently been shown (Fig. 7) to involve dimerization of the stretched E-syn BVE molecules (33).

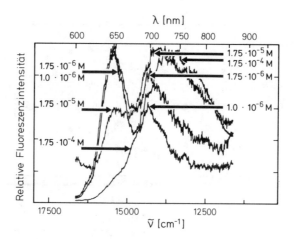

Fig. 7. Concentration dependence of the fluorescence of
BVE at RT in methanol. At the highest concentration, the 735 nm dimer emission of the stretched
E isomer prevails, and on dilution it is replaced
by the 650 nm emission of the corresponding monomer. The fraction of fluorescence from the coiled
all-Z,all-syn monomer at around 700 nm, hidden
under the dimer emission at the highest concentration, has been found to remain unchanged in
this dilution experiment (33).

REFERENCES

1. S. E. Braslavsky, A. R. Holzwarth, and K. Schaffner,
   Solution Conformations, Photophysics, and Photochemistry of Bile Pigments. Bilirubin and Biliverdin
   Dimethyl Esters and Related Linear Tetrapyrroles,
   Angew. Chem. Int. Ed. 21:in press (1983).
2. A. R. Holzwarth, E. Langer, H. Lehner, and K. Schaffner, Absorption, Luminescence, Solvent-induced Circular Dichroism and NMR study of Bilirubin Dimethyl
   Ester: Observation of Different Forms in Solution,
   Photochem. Photobiol. 32:17 (1980).
3. W. Kufer, H. Scheer, and A. R. Holzwarth, Isophorcarubin - A Conformationally restricted and Highly Fluorescent Bilirubin, Isr. J. Chem. 23:in press
   (1983).
4. R. Bonnett, J. E. Davies, M. B. Hursthouse, and G. M.
   Sheldrick, The Structure of Bilirubin, Proc. R.
   Chem. Soc. B 202:249 (1978).
5. A. R. Holzwarth, H. Lehner, S. E. Braslavsky, and K.
   Schaffner, The Fluorescence of Biliverdin Dimethyl
   Ester, Liebigs Ann. Chem. 2002 (1978).

6. H. Falk and F. Neufingerl, Zur anaeroben Photochemie
    von Gallenpigmenten: Die Lumineszenz von Gallenpig-
    ment-Partialstruktursystemen und integralen Farb-
    stoffen, Monatsh. Chem. 110:987 (1979).
7. A. R. Holzwarth, S. E. Braslavsky, S. Culshaw, and K.
    Schaffner, The Blue Anomalous Emission of Large and
    Small Phytochrome, Photochem. Photobiol. 36: 581
    (1982).
8. A. A. Lamola and J. Flores, Effect of Buffer Viscosity
    on the Fluorescence of Bilirubin Bound to Human Se-
    rum Albumin, J. Am. Chem. Soc. 104:2530 (1982).
9. A. A. Lamola, J. Flores, and F. H. Doleiden, Quantum
    Yield and Equilibrium Position of the Configuratio-
    nal Photoisomerization of Bilirubin Bound to Human
    Serum Albumin, Photochem. Photobiol. 35:649 (1982).
10. A. F. McDonagh, L. A. Palma, F. R. Trull, and D. A.
    Lightner, Phototherapy for Neonatal Jaundice. Con-
    figurational Isomers of Bilirubin, J. Am. Chem. Soc.
    104:6865 (1982).
11. A. F. McDonagh, L. A. Palma, and D. A. Lightner, Photo-
    therapy of Neonatal Jaundice. Stereospecific and Re-
    gioselective Photoisomerization of Bilirubin Bound
    to Human Serum Albumin and NMR Characterization of
    Intramolecularly Cyclized Photoproducts, J. Am.
    Chem. Soc. 104:6867 (1982).
12. H. Falk, N. Müller, M. Ratzenhofer, and K. Winsauer,
    The Structure of "Photobilirubin", Monatsh. Chem.
    113:1421 (1982).
13. A. R. Holzwarth and K. Schaffner, Wavelength Dependence
    of Quantum Yields and Product Distribution in the
    Anaerobic Photochemistry of Bilirubin Dimethyl
    Ester, Photochem. Photobiol. 33:635 (1981).
14. A. F. McDonagh, D. A. Lightner, and T. A. Wooldridge,
    Geometric Isomerisation of Bilirubin-IX and its
    Dimethyl Ester, J. Chem. Soc., Chem. Commun. 110
    (1979).
15. G. Favini, D. Pitea, and P. Manitto, Intramolecular
    Energy Map for 3,3'-Dimethylpyrrol-2-yl Methane,
    Nouv. J. Chim. 3:299 (1979).
16. B. I. Greene, A. A. Lamola, and C. V. Shank, Pico-
    second Primary Photoprocesses of Bilirubin Bound to
    Human Serum Albumin, Proc. Natl. Acad. Sci. USA
    78:2008 (1981).
17. H. Lehner, S. E. Braslavsky, and K. Schaffner, Isola-
    tion, Characterization and Solution Conformation of
    Biliverdin Dimethyl Ester and its XIII Isomer,
    Liebigs Ann. Chem. 1990 (1978).

18. H. Lehner, S. E. Braslavsky, and K. Schaffner, Enan-
    tiomerism and Diastereoisomerism of Bishelical Bi-
    latriene Dimers in the Crystal Lattice, Angew.
    Chem., Int. Ed. 17:948 (1978).
19. H. Lehner, W. Riemer, and K. Schaffner, The Intercon-
    version Barrier of the Bilatriene Helix, Liebigs
    Ann. Chem. 1798 (1979).
20. S. E. Braslavsky, A. R. Holzwarth, E. Langer, H.
    Lehner, J. I. Matthews, and K. Schaffner, Conforma-
    tional Heterogeneity and Photochemical Changes of
    Biliverdin Dimethyl Ester in Solution, Isr. J.
    Chem. 20:196 (1980).
21. S. E. Braslavsky, H.-J. Herbert, A. R. Holzwarth, and
    K. Schaffner, Chromatographic Detection of Solvent
    Adducts of Bilinoid Pigments, J. Chromat. 205:85
    (1981).
22. I.-M. Tegmo-Larsson, S. E. Braslavsky, S. Culshaw, R.
    M. Ellul, C. Nicolau, and K. Schaffner, Conforma-
    tion Control by Membrane of Biliverdin Dimethyl
    Ester Incorporated into Lipid Vesicles, J. Am.
    Chem. Soc. 103:7152 (1981); see also I.-M. Tegmo-
    Larsson, S. E. Braslavsky, C. Nicolau, and K.
    Schaffner, Biophys. Struct. Mech., Suppl. 6:112
    (1980).
23. S. E. Braslavsky, H. Al-Ekabi, C. Pétrier, and K.
    Schaffner, Conformation Selectivity of the Photo-
    cyclization of the Biliverdin IXγ and IXδ Dimethyl
    Esters, in preparation.
24. S. E. Braslavsky, R. M. Ellul, R. G. Weiss, H. Al-
    Ekabi, and K. Schaffner, The Photoisomerization of
    Biliverdin Dimethyl Ester in Ethanol Measured by
    Laser-induced Optoacoustic Spectroscopy (LIOAS),
    Tetrahedron 39:in press (1983).
25. A. R. Holzwarth, J. Wendler, K. Schaffner, V.
    Sundström, A. Sandström, and T. Gillbro, Picosecond
    Kinetics of Excited State Relaxation in Biliverdin
    Dimethyl Ester, Isr. J. Chem. 23:in press (1983);
    see also idem, in: "Picosecond Chemistry and Bio-
    logy," T. Doust and M. A. West, eds., Science Re-
    views, Northwood (1983).
26. H. Falk, K. Grubmayr, E. Haslinger, T. Schlederer, and
    K. Thirring, The Diastereomeric (Geometrically Iso-
    meric) Biliverdin Dimethyl Esters - Structure, Con-
    figuration and Conformation, Monatsh. Chem. 109:
    1451 (1978).
27. W. Kufer, E. Cmiel, F. Thümmler, W. Rüdiger, S.
    Schneider, and H. Scheer, Regioselective Photoche-
    mical and Acid Catalyzed Z,E Isomerization of Di-

hydrobilindione as Phytochrome Model, Photochem. Photobiol. 36:603 (1982).

28. C. Krauss, C. Bubenzer, and H. Scheer, Photochemically Assisted Reaction of A-Dihydrobilindione with Nucleophiles as a Model for Phytochrome Interconversion, Photochem. Photobiol. 30:473 (1979).

29. P. Manitto and D. Monti, Addition of Sulphydryl Groups to Biliverdin, Experientia 35:1418 (1979).

30. H. Falk, N. Müller, and T. Schlederer, A Reversible Regioselective Addition to Bilatrienes-abc, Monatsh. Chem. 11:159 (1980).

31. W. Kufer and H. Scheer, Rubins and Rubinoid Addition Products from Phycocyanin, Z. Naturforsch. 37c: 179 (1982).

32. P.-S. Song, Q. Chae, D. A. Lightner, W. R. Briggs, and D. Hopkins, Fluorescence Characteristics of Phytochrome and Biliverdins, J. Am. Chem. Soc. 95:7892 (1973).

33. S. E. Braslavsky, H. Al-Ekabi, A. R. Holzwarth, and K. Schaffner, unpublished results.

PHOTOPHYSICAL PROPERTIES OF BILE PIGMENTS

E.J. Land[*], R.W. Sloper[**] and T.G. Truscott[**]

[*]Paterson Laboratories, The Christie Hospital and Holt
Radium Institute, MANCHESTER, M20 9BX
[**]Dept. of Chemistry, Paisley College, PAISLEY, PA1 2BE

Phototherapy has been successfully used for a number of years
for the treatment of neonatal hyperbilirubinemia.   Although the
major mechanism is now known to involve photoisomerisation[1,2,3,4,5],
other photoprocesses involving bilirubin (BR) may still have
biological relevance.   Thus an understanding of the photophysics
of BR is important for assessing any other possible processes
related to phototherapy.

Photo-excitation of BR leads not only to excited states (BR^*)
which undergo well known processes such as isomerisation and triplet
state production but can also lead to radicals, produced either
directly via photo-oxidation or via an electron transfer process
involving an excited state and some other species (A or B below) -
such processes can be written as, for example:-

$$BR^{2-} \xrightarrow{h\nu} BR^{\cdot -} + e^- \tag{1}$$

$$BR^{2-} + e^- \rightarrow BR^{\cdot 3-} \tag{2}$$

$$BR^{2-*} + A \rightarrow BR^{\cdot -} + A^{\cdot -} \tag{3}$$

$$BR^{2-*} + B \rightarrow BR^{\cdot 3-} + B^{\cdot +} \tag{4}$$

so that a comprehensive study of the processes which may occur
following photo-excitation of BR requires a study of BR radical
ions as well as excited states.

Probably the best combination of techniques available to study
both transient excited states and radical ions are laser flash
photolysis and nano-second pulse radiolysis.   The usual description

141

of excited state generation and photophysical processes of polyatomic
molecules (such as BR) following flash photolysis in terms of a
modified Jablonski diagram are well known; however the pulse
radiolysis induced processes in aqueous solution may not be so well
understood and may be summarised as follows:-

$$H_2O \xrightarrow{\text{\Large$\wedge\wedge\wedge$}} e_{aq}^- + H^{\cdot} + OH^{\cdot} + H_2 + H_2O_2 + H_3O^+ \tag{5}$$

with e^- and $H^{\cdot}$ being reducing species and $OH^{\cdot}$ oxidising. Various
methods exist of generating more or less exclusively reducing or
oxidising environments and in the present work we added tertiary
butanol to remove $OH^{\cdot}$ and to produce a reducing situation (leading
to semi-reduced radical production $BR^{\cdot 3-}$).

$$OH^{\cdot} + (CH_3)_3COH \rightarrow CH_2^{\cdot}(CH_3)_2COH + H_2O \tag{6}$$

To obtain primarily oxidising conditions we removed the electron
with nitrous oxide

$$e_{aq}^- + N_2O + H_2O \rightarrow N_2 + OH^- + OH^{\cdot} \tag{7}$$

and converted $OH^{\cdot}$ radicals into azide radicals which are oxidising
($OH^{\cdot}$ radicals themselves sometimes undergo other processes such as
addition).

$$OH^{\cdot} + N_3^- \rightarrow OH^- + N_3^{\cdot}$$

so that semi-oxidised radicals are formed by the process

$$N_3^{\cdot} + BR^{2-} \rightarrow N_3^- + BR^{\cdot -} \tag{9}$$

PHOTOISOMERISATION

As noted above the major and possibly sole process responsible
for the effectiveness of the phototherapy treatment is a very rapid
cis-trans photoisomerisation via the S_1 state of Z,Z bilirubin.
The process, when monitored by differential absorption spectroscopy,
shows characteristic photoisomer peaks at $\lambda \sim 500$ nm and <350 nm and
a depletion at $\lambda \sim 460$ nm. The photoisomers (ZE, EZ and EE) can be
separated by chromatography and are unstable in the dark at room
temperature.

We have reported a fast-formed permanent (>50 μs) product
following 347 nm laser flash photolysis of BR in solvents such as
methanolic ammonia and benzene[6]. The spectrum of this product
showed similarities with the difference spectrum obtained by
continuous irradiation of BR and assigned to the mixture of isomers
known as "photobilirubin" [1,2,3]. The photoisomers of BR have a
less introverted structure with less hydrogen bonding and might be
expected to be more water soluble than the naturally occurring 5Z,15Z

isomer.   There is much evidence that this increased solubility is
the primary reason for the lowered BR levels achieved by phototherapy
of infants.   No evidence for photoisomerisation was found from 347
or 694 nm laser flash photolysis of biliverdin (BV) in any of the
solvent systems studied[7].

In the blood BR is primarily bound to HSA and laser flash
photolysis[6][8] has been used to study the transient species obtained
from irradiation of the BR-HSA complex in aqueous solution and we
have obtained a quantum yield of photoisomerisation (Φ_{isom}) of ~ 0.2.
A similar value has been obtained[9] using a fluorescence technique.

TRIPLET STATE

We have used laser flash photolysis with 347 nm excitation to
estimate the triplet quantum yield (Φ_T) in various solvent systems
and typical values are <0.005 in chloroform with varying amounts of
triethylamine (0-20%), various detergents and methanolic ammonia.
In benzene we obtain a Φ_T of ~ 0.01 and a similar value has been
reported in this solvent using a technique based upon enhancing the
BR intersystem crossing by high oxygen concentrations[10].

Clearly in such solvent systems intersystem crossing is an
inefficient process, nevertheless S_1 to T_1 crossover must occur to
some extent to account for the reported self-sensitised photooxidation process of BR[11],[12].   However it can be shown that $\Phi_{isom}/$
$\Phi_{ox} \gg 100$ where Φ_{ox} is the quantum yield of self-sensitised photooxidation.

RADICALS

Laser excitation, at 265 nm, of Ar flushed alkaline aqueous
solutions of BR, BV and xanthobilirubinic acid (XBR) yielded the
characteristic e_{aq} absorption at 720 nm which disappeared upon N_2O
saturation.   Transient spectra measured after flash photolysis of
N_2O-saturated samples of the same solutions containing added tBuOH,
are fairly similar to those of the semi-oxidised radicals.   Neither
the decay of these species, which were long-lived ($t_{\frac{1}{2}} \gg 100$ μs) nor
their spectra were affected by O_2, indicating in the case of BR the
absence of the triplet state.   A similar conclusion cannot be
reached for BV since its triplet is not quenched by O_2.   Furthermore, no clear evidence for BR photoisomerisation was seen.

Transient yields for all three systems showed a linear
dependence on laser excitation intensity implying that photo-
ionisation was a monophotonic process (some biphotonic photo-
ionisation was detected for XBR at high laser intensities).   The
quantum yields of photo-ionisation (Φ_I) for BR, BV and XBR were
estimated as 0.08 ± 0.02; 0.03 ± 0.01 and 0.13 ± 0.03 respectively.

For BR and BV the effect of variation of pH was studied within
the range pH 10-14.   The results show an increased Φ_I at pH > 12,
suggestive of further deprotonation of the BR and BV dianions.
Although it is not possible to determine pK_a values from these data,
the approximate limits of pK_a > 14 for BR and pK_a > 13 for BV can be
assessed.

Although monophotonic photo-ionisation of BR has been observed
in this 265 nm laser study, it was not observed in 347 nm laser
studies of similar solutions so that this process seems unlikely to
present a possible hazard in neonatal jaundice phototherapy,
particularly if effectively filtered lamps are used.

However 347 nm laser flash excitation of BR in highly purified
chloroform did lead to a transient (in addition to those from photoisomers $\lambda_{max} \sim 500$ nm) with $\lambda_{max} \sim 550$ nm which was not due to a
triplet because it was not quenched by oxygen.   We suggest that
this longer wavelength species is due to the presence of radicals.
Since the solvated electron is not observed in halogenated hydrocarbons, it is not immediately clear whether the radicals resulted
from photo-ionisation or from a photo-dissociation or abstraction
reaction.   The fact that xanthobilirubinic acid (a model compound
representing half of a BR molecule) showed no equivalent absorption
even though its photo-ionisation yield from 265 nm excitation in
aqueous solution was rather higher than that of BR, strongly
suggests that the radicals observed here resulted from a process
other than photo-ionisation.

These data, together with those from 265 nm excitation of BR in
aqueous solutions, correlate quite well with the observations of a
wavelength and solvent dependence of BR photoreactivity under
anaerobic conditions[13].   Thus the increased reactivity following
280 nm excitation can be explained by the present observation of
photo-ionisation and the increased reactivity in chloroform
correlated with our observation of radicals in that solvent.

ELECTRON TRANSFER REACTIONS

In order to determine whether the semi-oxidised BR radical,
resulting from photo-ionisation, can react with serum proteins, a
preliminary pulse radiolysis study of its reaction in alkaline
solution (pH 11) with tryptophan (TrpH) has been made.   Included,
for the sake of completeness, have been the reaction of the semi-
reduced radical with TrpH and the reactions of TrpH radicals with
BR.   Semi-oxidised and semi-reduced radicals were produced by
reaction with N_3^- and e_{aq}^- respectively, as described above.   In each
case, the mixture contained a suitable excess of the compound whose
radical was to be produced, based on a knowledge of the relative
reaction rates. $BR^{\cdot -}$ and $BR^{\cdot 3 -}$ were monitored at 590 nm, where
interference from TrpH radicals is minimal, and Trp radicals were

monitored at 540 nm, where the $(BR^{\bullet})^{-}/(BR)^{2-}$ system is approximately isosbestic, and at 350 nm.

In these experiments, only the transfer between the deprotonated semi-oxidised $Trp^{\bullet}$ radical (the NH_3^{+} group is also deprotonated at this pH) and BR was observed.

$$Trp^{\bullet} + BR^{2-} + H_2O \quad \rightarrow \quad TrpH + BR^{\bullet-} + OH^{-} \qquad (10)$$

with a second-order rate constant of $4.3 \times 10^8 \ M^{-1}s^{-1}$.

We have also attempted to observe electron transfer reactions occurring after $N_3^{\bullet}$ oxidation of the BR-HSA complex.   Generating $N_3^{\bullet}$ via pulse radiolysis as described above we studied mixtures of BR and HSA and observed mainly TrpH oxidation with no indication of any electron transfer process involving BR.   However a radical transformation involving TrpH and tyrosine (TyrOH) residues similar to that previously reported with a number of peptides and proteins was readily observed[14],[15],[16],[17].

$$Trp^{\bullet} + TyrOH \quad \rightarrow \quad TrpH + TyrO^{\bullet} \qquad (11)$$

From studies of the $Trp^{\bullet}$ decay at 510 or 540 nm and $TyrO^{\bullet}$ build-up at 405 nm, the reaction was found to proceed with $k = 3.8 \times 10^3 \ s^{-1}$ with HSA alone and with $k = 1.6 \times 10^3 \ s^{-1}$ with the BR-HSA complex. The reduced electron transfer rate which occurred upon complexation can be interpreted in terms of a conformational change in the protein.   HSA has only one TrpH residue but three possible TyrOH residues which could be involved: TyrOH 263, TyrOH 161 and TyrOH 319.   If residue 263 is involved then BR in the primary binding site must lie between loops 4 and 5 of the protein, whereas involvement of residue 161 would implicate loops 3 and 4 and involvement of residue 319 would implicate loops 4-6.   These interpretations are all consistent with the finding that lysine-240 is involved in the primary binding site for BR[18],[19].

As noted above photo-isomerisation of BR is the major photo-process following light absorption by BR when bound to HSA, so that the conformational change in the protein on binding to BR implied by the pulse radiolysis work may be a factor in the _in vivo_ situation.

ACKNOWLEDGEMENTS

This work was supported by grants from the Cancer Research Campaign, the Medical Research Council and the Science Research Council.   R.W.S. acknowledges an S.R.C. CASE award.

REFERENCES

1.   D.A. Lightner, T.A. Woolbridge, and A.F. McDonagh,
      "Configurational Isomerisation of Bilirubin and the
      Mechanism of Jaundice Phototherapy", Biochem. Biophys.
      Res. Commun., 86:235 (1979).
2.   D.A. Lightner, T.A. Woolbridge, and A.F. McDonagh,
      "Photobilirubin : An Early Bilirubin Photoproduct Detected
      by Absorbance Difference Spectroscopy", Proc. Natl. Acad.
      Sci. U.S.A., 76:29 (1979).
3.   A.F. McDonagh, D.A. Lightner, and T.A. Woolbridge,
      "Geometric Isomerization of Bilirubin - IX α and its Dimethyl
      Ester, J. Chem. Soc.,Chem. Commun., 110, (1979).
4.   S. Onishi, S. Itoh, N. Kawade, K. Isobe, and S. Sugiyana,
      "The Separation of Configurational Isomers of Bilirubin by
      High Pressure Liquid Chromatography and the Mechanism of
      Jaundice Phototherapy", Biochem. Biophys. Res. Commun.,
      90:890, (1979).
5.   M.S. Stoll, E.A. Zenone, D. Ostrow, and J.E. Zavembo,
      "Preparation and Properties of Bilirubin Photoisomers",
      Biochem. J., 183:139, (1979).
6.   R.W. Sloper and T.G. Truscott, "Excited States of Bilirubin",
      Photochem. Photobiol., 31:445 (1980).
7.   E.J. Land, R.W. Sloper, and T.G. Truscott, "The Radical Ions
      and Photoionization of Bile Pigments", Radiation Res., -
      in press.
8.   R.W. Sloper and T.G. Truscott, "The Quantum Yield of Bilirubin
      Photoisomerisation", Photochem. Photobiol., 35:743, (1982).
9.   A.A. Lamola, J. Flores, J. Eisinger, and F.H. Doheiden,
      "Photoisomerization of Bilirubin Bound to Human Serum
      Albumin", Ann. Meeting Am. Soc. Photobiol., 17-21 Feb.,
      Abstr. TAM D1, p.88, (1980).
10.   I.B.C. Matheson, N.U. Curry and J. Lee, "The Photochemical
      Quantum Yield for the Self-sensitized Photo-oxidation of
      Bilirubin.   Evidence for Oxygen-induced Intersystem Crossing
      at High Oxygen Concentrations", Photochem. Photobiol.,
      31:115, (1980).
11.   A.F. McDonagh, "Role of Singlet Oxygen in Bilirubin Photo-
      oxidation", Biochem. Biophys. Res. Commun., 44:1306, (1971).
12.   R. Bonnett, and J.C.M. Stewart, "Singlet Oxygen in the Photo-
      oxidation of Bilirubin in Hydroxylic Solvents", Biochem. J.,
      130:895, (1972).
13.   D.A. Lightner & A. Cu, "Wavelength Dependence of Bilirubin
      Photoreactivity", Life Sci., 20:723, (1977).
14.   W.A. Prutz, and E.J. Land, "Charge Transfer in Peptides.
      Pulse Radiolysis of One Electron Reactions in Dipeptides
      of Tryptophan and Tyrosine", Int. J. Radiat. Biol.,
      36:513, (1979).

15. W.A. Prutz, J. Butler, E.J. Land, and A.J. Swallow, "Direct Demonstration of Electron Transfer Between Tryptophan and Tyrosine in Proteins", Biochem.Biophys. Res. Commun., 96:408, (1980).

16. W.A. Prutz, E.J. Land, and R.W. Sloper, "Change Transfer in Peptides", J. Chem. Soc., Faraday 1, 77:281, (1981).

17. R.W. Sloper and E.J. Land, "Photoinitiation of One Electron Reactions in Dipeptides and Proteins Containing Tryptophan and Tyrosine", Photochem. Photobiol., 32:687, (1980).

18. C. Jacobsen, "Lysine Residue 240 of Human Serum Albumin is Involved in High Affinity Binding of Bilirubin", Biochem. J., 171:453, (1972).

19. C. Jacobsen and J. Jacobsen, "Dansylation of Human Serum Albumin in the Study of the Primary Binding Sites of Bilirubin and L-tryptophan", Biochem. J., 181:251, (1979).

IN VITRO AND IN VIVO BILIRUBIN-SENSITIZED PHOTOEFFECTS AT THE

MOLECULAR AND CELLULAR LEVELS

John D. Spikes

Department of Biology
University of Utah
Salt Lake City, Utah 84112 USA

INTRODUCTION

Phototherapy as a treatment for neonatal hyperbilirubinemia
has now been in use for approximately twenty-five years. Its
effectiveness in reducing the serum bilirubin levels in the
newborn, especially in premature infants, is well recognized.
Acute complications arising from the use of phototherapy have been
rare and none are apparently considered to be serious. Further, at
present, there does not appear to be much evidence for the development of long term complications in those individuals who have
received phototherapy.[1,2] However, it should be kept in mind that
bilirubin is a photodynamic sensitizer - a phototoxic agent -
which, although rather inefficient compared to many sensitizers,[3]
demonstrably sensitizes photodamage at the molecular and cellular
levels, both in vitro and in vivo. Thus patients should be
observed carefully during phototherapeutic treatment and should
receive only the minimum necessary light dose. In this review I
will briefly summarize a few aspects of bilirubin photochemistry
pertinent to photosensitized reactions and then examine the known
photosensitizing effects of bilirubin in biological systems.

BILIRUBIN PHOTOCHEMISTRY IN RELATION TO ITS PHOTOSENSITIZING
CAPABILITIES

The chemistry and photochemistry of bilirubin have been
extensively reviewed recently.[4-6] Bilirubin has an intense
absorption band at approximately 450 nm. On illumination at this
wavelength it goes into the lowest singlet excited state, which has
an energy of approximately 63 kcal/mole above the ground state.
Intersystem crossing from this state to the lowest lying triplet

149

state (energy = 36 kcal/mole) occurs, but with a very low
efficiency of much less than 0.1. The triplet has an absorption
maximum near 500 nm and has an unusually short lifetime for a
lowest lying triplet (9 usec, in benzene); further, the quenching
of the triplet by ground state oxygen to yield singlet oxygen is
relatively inefficient.[7,8] Bilirubin sensitizes its own photodegradation with fair efficiency in complex reactions which
apparently involve both Type II (singlet oxygen) and Type I (free
radical) pathways.[5] It is also rapidly photooxidized with typical
photodynamic sensitizers including hematoporphyrin, rose bengal,
methylene blue and flavins.[4] Self-sensitized photodegradation was
originally suggested as a major mechanistic pathway in the
decreased serum bilirubin levels observed as a result of phototherapy. It is now believed that phototherapy is mediated largely
by the conformational photoisomerization of bilirubin to more polar
isomers which are then excreted.[1,2,9] This is supported by studies
which show that the quantum yields for photoisomerization are very
much greater than those for the self-sensitized photodegradation of
bilirubin.[8,10] In summary, bilirubin is an inefficient photosensitizer because of its low yield of triplet, its poor generation
of singlet oxygen, and its continuing self-photodegradation during
illumination. Further, bilirubin quenches singlet oxygen at a rate
approaching the diffusion limit, and thus acts as a good photodynamic protective agent.[4] Even so, it can sensitize significant
photodamage to many biological systems, as described below.

BILIRUBIN-SENSITIZED PHOTOEFFECTS ON BIOMOLECULES

    As has been observed with many photodynamic sensitizers,
illuminated bilirubin forms covalent adducts with certain types of
molecules, in particular, alcohols and thiols. For example, under
anaerobic conditions, bilirubin forms photoadducts via the exo-
vinyl group with the -SH groups of N-acetylcysteine and reduced
glutathione.[11] This reaction is slow, and thus may not be
significant in vivo. As is well known, bilirubin forms 1:1 non-
covalent complexes with mammalian serum albumins by binding at a
specific high affinity site on the protein molecule. Illumination
of such a complex with bovine serum albumin (BSA) results in the
covalent binding of the bilirubin (or some bilirubin photoproduct)
to the protein; the yield of the reaction is increased under
anaerobic conditions suggesting that a free radical mechanism is
involved. Degradation studies show that the photobinding occurs at
a specific region of the molecule (the 187-397 residue segment of
the polypeptide chain), which lacks cysteine residues.[12-14]

    Illumination of the 1:1 bilirubin BSA and human serum albumin
(HSA) complexes under aerobic conditions results in the initial
destruction of approximately two histidine residues in the
molecules; there is also some tryptophan destruction, and tyrosine
is destroyed at longer illumination times. Because of the limited

radius of reaction around an illuminated photosensitizer molecule, these results suggest that the two susceptible histidine residues are located in the high affinity binding site of the albumin molecule; other lines of evidence also suggest the involvement of two histidine residues in the binding of bilirubin. Illumination of the complex causes small changes in the conformation of the albumin molecules and significantly decreases their ability to bind bilirubin.[14] Illumination of blood sera results in the oxygen-dependent inactivation of serum creatine kinase. The rate of inactivation increases progressively with increasing bilirubin levels in the sera, suggesting that the reaction is sensitized by bilirubin.[15]

Bilirubin also sensitizes the photodegradation of unsaturated phospholipids. The illumination of egg lecithin liposomes containing entrapped sodium ions and glucose-6-phosphate as markers in the presence of bilirubin results in lysis of the liposomes with the release of the entrapped markers. The reaction does not occur under anaerobic conditions, which suggests that the liposomes rupture as a result of the bilirubin-sensitized photooxidation of the unsatuated phospholipid making up the membrane. If anti-oxidants which have been shown to inhibit lipid photoperoxidation with regular photodynamic sensitizers are added, the rate of photolysis of the bilirubin loaded liposomes is markedly decreased. Bilirubin in this system is located largely in the liposomal membranes, since the bilirubin absorption peak is red shifted approximately 10 nm from that observed in an aqueous environment as would be expected when it partitions into a hydrophobic environment.[16] Membrane incorporated bilirubin is in contact with a high concentration of unsaturated lipid which might effectively compete with bilirubin for photogenerated singlet oxygen.

Bilirubin is reported to bind very strongly to DNA, apparently by intercalation between the DNA strands. Illumination of DNA under aerobic conditions in the presence of bilirubin results in characteristic patterns of nucleic acid degradation. With double stranded DNA, there is a significant change in the thermal melting profile, but no consistent change in the sedimentation pattern; the sedimentation coefficient decreases significantly after alkaline denaturation, however, indicating the production of single strand breaks in the illuminated DNA. With single stranded DNA, there is a significant increase in the sedimentation coefficient even without alkaline treatment, again indicating an extensive production of single strand breaks in the DNA as a result of the bilirubin-sensitized phototreatment. These effects on DNA are observed with a light dosage corresponding to that received by an infant during a 24 hour period of phototherapy.[17]

It is difficult to study the photochemical and photo-sensitizing properties of free bilirubin in aqueous systems at

neutrality because of its very low solubility. Thus most such
studies have been carried out in organic solvents or with the
bilirubin bound to biomolecules or incorporated into micelles or
liposomes.[18] We (J. D. Spikes, J. C. Bommer, B. F. Burnham,
unpublished results) recently initiated an examination of the
photochemical and photosensitizing properties of a highly water
soluble bilirubin derivative, bilirubin ditaurate (from Porphyrin
Products Inc., Logan, Utah). This compound has an intense
absorption peak at 451 nm as measured in pH 7.4 aqueous buffer. It
sensitizes the photooxidation of furfuryl alcohol in aqueous media
with quantum yields in the range of 0.0005 as measured by oxygen
uptake; under the same conditions, its self-sensitized photooxidation cannot be detected. This yield is roughly two orders of
magnitude lower than those found for hematoporphyrin, methylene
blue and rose bengal in the same system. Methylene blue sensitizes
the photooxidation of bilirubin ditaurate with a quantum yield of
approximately 0.003. We have covalently coupled bilirubin to 2-5
micron diameter polyacrylamide beads. This material remains in
suspension fairly well and sensitizes the photooxidation of
furfuryl alcohol under the same conditions as above with a quantum
yield of 0.0004. In organic solvents, bilirubin quenches singlet
oxygen with efficiencies approaching the diffusion controlled
limit, and thus is a protective agent against photodynamic
reactions.[1,4] We find that bilirubin ditaurate is an unusually
efficient protective agent against the methylene blue-sensitized
phootooxidation of furfuryl alcohol and the susceptible amino
acids; for example, at 33 uM it decreases the quantum yield of the
methylene blue-sensitized photooxidation of furfuryl alcohol by
50%.

BILIRUBIN-SENSITIZIED PHOTOEFFECTS ON CELLS AND SUBCELLULAR
STRUCTURES

     Almost all of the work published in this area has been carried
out with human erythrocytes. In 1908, Hausmann[19] found that rabbit
red blood cells undergo hemolysis on illumination in diluted rabbit
or cow bile. He then tested the known pigments in bile for photosensitizing activity; one sample of bilirubin available to him
sensitized photohemolysis, while biliverdin did not. Saeki, in a
series of papers, showed that the illumination of erythrocytes from
humans and a number of other mammals, as well as from the chicken,
in the presence of bilirubin results in hemolysis.[20] Somewhat
later, studies showed that the bilirubin-sensitized photohemolysis
of red blood cells from the normal human adult is preceded by an
efflux of potassium ions from the cells and a decrease in the
membrane ATPase activities; oxygen is necessary for the
reaction.[21] Red blood cells from full term infants illuminated in
the presence of added bilirubin show a significant decrease in
their content of reduced glutathione; potassium ion leakage and
hemolysis also occurs.[22] The aerobic exposure of fetal

erythrocytes to blue light in the presence of bilirubin results in a significant decrease in the affinity of the cells for oxygen; the change is not observed using erythrocytes from adult or hemolysates of fetal red blood cells. It apparently results from photosensitized damage to the erythrocyte membrane. In all studies of this type with added bilirubin, it should be recalled that this compound can act as a surfactant and, at high concentrations, produces hemolysis in the dark. The aerobic illumination of erythrocytes from newborn infants results in significant decreases in the ethanolamine and lecithin content of the cells and a significant increase in lysolecithin; it was not clearly established in these studies that bilirubin is the photosensitizer involved.[24]

The illumination of isolated red blood cell membranes ("ghosts") in the presence of bilirubin under aerobic conditions results in the free radical peroxidation of unsaturated membrane lipids, as detected by the appearance of malonaldehyde. The addition of antioxidants such as butylated hydroxytoluene or diphenyl-p-phenylenediamine inhibits bilirubin-sensitized lipid photoperoxidation in membranes. Illumination of bilirubin-treated ghosts also results in the covalent crosslinking of several different kinds of membrane polypeptides, in particular the spectrin subunits, as has been observed with other kinds of photodynamic sensitizers. The crosslinking reaction does not involve protein sulfhydryl groups, and is not inhibited by the antioxidants mentioned above. This suggests that bilirubin-sensitized lipid peroxidation and protein crosslinking occur by different mechanisms. D_2O enhances the crosslinking reaction while azide inhibits it, indicating the possible involvement of a singlet oxygen rather than a free radical process.[25,26]

As mentioned above, ATPases in red bood cells are inactivated by photodynamic treatment with bilirubin. More recent studies show that several kinds of enzymes are inactivated when bilirubin loaded red blood cell ghosts are illuminated in the presence of air. Glyceraldehyde-3-phosphate dehydrogenase (which is apparently merely bound to the interior of the membrane) is rapidly inactivated; singlet oxygen quenchers reduce the rate significantly. The integral membrane enzymes magnesium-ATPase, sodium-potassium-ATPase and acetylcholinesterase are also photoinactivated. Sodium-potassium-ATPase inactivation might be important in the initiation of photosensitized hemolysis in intact erythrocytes, since the active pumping of ions by this enzyme normally takes care of osmotic stresses on the cell. Illumination of bilirubin loaded ghosts markedly decreases the number of sulfhydryl groups in the membranes suggesting that the photooxidation of cysteine residues might be involved in the inactivation of membrane enzymes.[27]

In studies on the molecular mechanisms involved in the bilirubin-sensitized photohemolysis of red blood cells, Girotti and Deziel have exploited the use of re-sealed human erythrocyte ghosts as model systems.[16,28,29] In these preparations, essentially only the plasma membrane of the cell remains and it retains its osmotic properties. Selected molecules with different molecular weights, charge, etc. can be entrapped within the membranes during preparation, and the kinetics of the leakage of these markers during photosensitized treatment can be examined. Thus possible experimental complications due to the presence of cytoplasmic and nuclear components can be avoided. Bilirubin has a high effinity for the red blood cell membrane; once loaded into the membrane, little is removed by even extensive washing. The absorption spectrum of bilirubin in the membrane is red shifted approximately 10 A from that observed in aqueous systems indicating that bilirubin in the membrane has partitioned into a very hydrophobic environment. Bilirubin loaded resealed ghosts lyse on illumination; the rate is decreased markedly by oxygen depletion and by the presence of azide, suggesting the possible involvement of singlet oxygen in membrane photodegradation. Entrapped sodium ions start diffusing out of the bilirubin loaded membranes almost immediately after the start of illumination, while leakage of a larger marker molecule such as glucose-6-phosphate does not begin until after a considerable delay. Antioxidants which inhibit bilirubin-sensitized lipid photoperoxidation also inhibit the release of the glucose-6-phosphate, whereas they have no effect on the efflux of sodium ion. This suggests that glucose-6-phosphate release results from the photoperoxidation of membrane lipids, while sodium ion leakage results from some kind of photodamage to membrane proteins.[28] Attempts have been made to estimate the size range of the photochemically produced lesions (holes) in the erythrocyte membrane leading to the release of glucose-6-phosphate by using solutes of known molecular radii and a density flotation centrifugation technique. The results indicate that the lesions are larger than 11 A but smaller than 42 A.[29]

Very few bilirubin-sensitized photodynamic studies have been made with cells other than erythrocytes. However the effects of bilirubin-sensitized phototreatment on the transmembrane potentials of frog crystalline lens fibers have been examined using an intra-cellular microelectrode technique. Illumination of the cells under aerobic conditions causes a significant change in the transmembrane potential in the presence of bilirubin; no such change occurs in the presence of a reducing agent (ascorbic acid).[30] A few studies have appeared on bilirubin-sensitized photoeffects on isolated cell organelles. For example, illumination under aerobic conditions of isolated subunit particles from beef heart mitochondria in the presence of bilirubin results in the crosslinking of certain proteins located in the inner mitochondrial membrane. The beta subunit of the mitochondrial ATPase is much more susceptible to

bilirubin-sensitized photodynamic modification than the alpha
subunit. Such studies may provide useful information on the
molecular organization of the very complex ATPase which occurs in
mitochondria.[31]

Illumination of isolated rat hepatic microsomes in the
presence of bilirubin and air significantly and selectively
inhibits microsomal aniline hydroxylase activity and decreases the
amount of cytochrome b5 present. The treatment has no effect on
the microsomal enzymes involved in the demethylation of ethyl
morphine or on the content of cytochrome P-450. In contrast,
protoporphyrin IX selectively photoinhibits the ethyl morphine
enzymes and has little effect on the aniline hydroxylase; photosensitization by protoporphyrin IX is effectively inhibited by
biliverdin.[32] Interestingly, in other experiments, bilirubin is
found to partially inhibit the methylene blue-sensitized photodynamic inactivation of the NADPH:cytochrome c reductase and
benzopyrene hydroxylase activities of rat liver microsomes.[33]

BILIRUBIN-SENSITIZED PHOTOEFFECTS IN VIVO

In 1913 Myer-Betz attempted to demonstrate in vivo
photosensitization by bilirubin by injecting the compound sub-
cutaneously in mice and then exposing the animals to sunlight;
however, no pathological responses resulted.[34] More recently,
because of the widespread use of phototherapy, other kinds of
studies have been undertaken to determine whether bilirubin-
sensitized photodynamic effects occur in treated infants. In model
animal experiments it has been found that the exposure of shaved
jaundiced Gunn rats to standard phototherapeutic treatment leads to
the rapid development of a mild to medium anemia associated with
reticulocytosis; hematocrits gradually return toward the normal
levels with continued illumination, although some hemolysis
persists. These effects are not observed with nonicteric Gunn
rats.[35] Other studies show that exposing jaundiced Gunn rats to 18
hours of phototherapy significantly increases the osmotic fragility
of the circulating erythrocytes; again, no effects were observed
with non-jaundiced rats.[36] In contrast to these two studies, Howe
et al.[37] did not observe any damage to the red blood cells of
jaundiced Gunn rats exposed to blue fluorescent lamps, although the
treatment did effectively lower the serum bilirubin levels.

Only a very few studies indicate that phototherapeutic light
exposure produces measureable detrimental effects on the infants
involved. As described above, illumination of the 1:1 bilirubin-
HSA complex results in covalent binding of the tetrapyrrole (or
some photoproduct) to the specific binding site on the protein.
This photoadduct is also found in the blood of full term hyperbilirubinemic infants after only 7-9 hours of phototreatment. It
disappears from the blood by 15-20 days after the end of photo-

therapy, which corresponds to the normal serum albumin turnover time. The fraction of serum albumin molecules altered in this reaction is very small.[12,13,38]

The exposure of blood from normal infants to high intensity illumination alters the integrity of the red blood cell membranes slightly, but significantly, as observed by a decrease in the reduced glutathione content of the cells, by an increased rate of potassium ion leakage and cell swelling, and by increased hemolysis; all of these kinds of changes are greater in blood from jaundiced infants. These results suggest, but do not prove, that bilirubin-sensitized changes occur in erythrocytes in vivo during phototherapy.[39] Finally, it has been reported that the exposure of infants to blue light phototherapy results in a significant and consistent decrease of the sodium-potassium-ATPase activity in the erythrocytes of jaundiced infants; no effect of light treatment on in vivo hemolysis is observed, however.[39]

CONCLUDING REMARKS

All available data indicate that bilirubin in solution is a very inefficient photodynamic sensitizer. However, the studies reviewed above demonstrate unequivocally that, in vitro, bilirubin sensitizes the photodegradation of major types of biomolecules (unsaturated lipids, proteins, nucleic acids) and also mediates the photosensitized injury and killing of cells. In all of these biological systems it appears that the photochemically effective bilirubin is tightly bound to or dissolved in the material being photodegraded rather than being free in solution. Under these conditions, where the bilirubin is so closely associated with very high concentrations of photooxidizable substrates, it is possible that the substrate can compete much more efficiently for photogenerated singlet oxygen than in homogeneous solutions. Further, such a close association may also markedly increase the probability of Type I (free radical) reactions leading to degradation of the substrate.

In spite of the demonstrated capability of bilirubin to sensitize photodamage to biomolecules and cells in vitro, there is little evidence that processes of these types result in any immediate detrimental effects on the infants receiving phototherapy. Even the production of bilirubin-serum albumin adducts in vivo on illumination does not appear to have any pathological consequences. However, although the immediate risks associated with phototherapy seem extremely low, care should always be taken to properly monitor the infants being illuminated, and the minimal light dose required to produce the desired degree of therapeutic effect should be used.

The preparation of this manuscript was supported in part by

NIH Biomedical Research Support Grant No. RR07092 and by the University of Utah Research Fund.

REFERENCES

1. A.K. Brown and A.F. McDonagh, Phototherapy for neonatal hyperbilirubinemia: Efficacy, mechanism and toxicity, Adv. Pediatr. 27:341 (1980).

2. A.N. Cohen and J.D. Ostrow, New concepts in phototherapy: Photoisomerization of bilirubin IX-alpha and potential toxic effects of light, Pediatr. 65:740 (1980).

3. J.D. Spikes, Photodynamic reactions in photomedicine, p. 113 in: "The Science of Photomedicine," J.D. Regan and J.A. Parrish, eds., Plenum publishing Corp., New York (1982).

4. A.F. McDonagh, Bile pigments: bilatrienes and 5,15: biladienes, p. 293, in: "The Porphyrins," Vol. VIA, D. Dolphin, ed., Academic Press, New York (1979).

5. D.A. Lightner, Structure, photochemistry and organic chemistry of bilirubin, p. 1, in: "Bilirubin", Vol. 1, K.P.M. Heirwegh and S.B. Brown, eds., CRC Press, Boca Raton, (1982).

6. A.E. Myshkin and V.N. Sakharov, The photochemistry of bilirubin, Russ. Chem. Rev. 51:40 (1982). Transl. from Uspekhi Khimii 51:72 (1982).

7. E.J. Land, The triplet excited state of bilirubin, Photochem. Photobiol. 24:475 (1976).

8. R.W. Sloper and T.G. Truscott, The quantum yield for bilirubin photoisomerization, Photochem. Photobiol. 35:743 (1982).

9. A.F. McDonagh, L.A. Palma and D.A. Lightner, Blue light and bilirubin excretion, Science 208:145 (1980).

10. A.A. Lamola, J. Flores and F.H. Doleiden, Quantum yield and equilibrium position of the configurational photo-isomerization of bilirubin bound to human serum albumin, Photochem. Photobiol. 35:649 (1982).

11. P. Manitto, D. Monti, and E. Garbagnati, Photochemical addition of N-acetyl-L-cysteine and glutathione to bilirubin in vitro and its relevance to phototherapy of jaundice, Farmaco Ed. Sci. 27:999 (1972).

12. G. Jori, F. Rubaltelli and E. Rossi, Photoinduced modification of human serum albumin during phototherapy of jaundiced newborns, Springer Ser. Opt. Sci. 22:145 (1980).

13. G. Jori, E. Rossi, and F. F. Rubaltelli, Phototherapy-induced covalent binding of bilirubin to serum albumin, Pediatr. Res. 14:1363 (1980).

14. F.F. Rubaltelli and G. Jori, Visible light irradiation of human and bovine serum albumin-bilirubin complex, Photochem. Photobiol. 29:991 (1979).

15. D.F. Davidson, I.R. Hainsworth, R. Rowan, G. Kousourou and M.
     Colgan, Possible effect of bilirubin concentration on the
     in-vitro lability of creatine kinase during storage, Ann.
     Clin. Biochem. 18:185 (1981).

16. M.R. Deziel and A.W. Girotti, Photodynamic action of bilirubin
     on liposomes and erythrocyte membranes, J. Biol. Chem.
     255:8192 (1980).

17. W.T. Speck and H.S. Rosenkranz, The bilirubin-induced photo-
     degradation of deoxyribonucleic acid, Pediatr. Res. 9:703
     (1975).

18. A.F. McDonagh and L.A. Palma, Mechanism of bilirubin
     photodegradation: role of singlet oxygen, p. 81 in
     "Fogarty International Proceedings No. 35", P.D. Berk and
     N.I. Berlin, eds., U.S. Gov't. Printing Office,
     Washington, D.C. (1976).

19. W. Hausmann, Ueber die sensibilisierende Wirkung tierischer
     Farbstoffe und ihre physiologische Bedeutung, Biochem. Z.
     14:275 (1908).

20. K. Saeki, Studies in the photodynamic hemolytic action of
     bilirubin. I, II, III, IV, Jap. J. Gastroenterol. 4:153,
     166, 231, 244 (1932). Chem. Abstr. 27:1018, 1041 (1933).

21. G.B. Odell, R.S. Brown, and A.E. Kopelman, The photodynamic
     action of bilirubin on erythrocytes, J. Pediatr. 81:473
     (1972).

22. M.G. Blackburn, M.M. Orzalesi, and P. Pigram, Effect of light
     and bilirubin on fetal red blood cells in vitro, Biol.
     Neonate 21:35 (1974).

23. E.M. Ostrea and G.B. Odell, Photosensitized shift in the O_2
     dissociation curve of fetal blood, Acta Paediatr. Scand.
     63:341 (1974).

24. M. Castro, S.G. Tambucci, A. Panero, O. Giardini, and M.
     Orzalesi, Studio in vitro degli effetti della luce sui
     lipidi del globula rosso, Min. Pediat. 28:391 (1976).

25. A.W. Girotti, Photodynamic action of bilirubin on human
     erythrocyte membranes. Modification of polypeptide
     constituents, Biochemistry 14:3377 (1975).

26. A.W. Girotti, Bilirubin-photosensitized cross-linking of
     polypeptides in the isolated membrane of the human
     erythrocyte, J. Biol. Chem. 253:7186 (1978).

27. A.W. Girotti, Bilirubin-sensitized photoinactivation of
     enzymes in the isolated membrane of the human erythrocyte,
     Photochem. Photobiol. 24:525 (1976).

28. M.R. Deziel and A.W. Girotti, Bilirubin-photosensitized lysis
     of resealed erythrocyte membranes, Photochem. Photobiol.
     31:593 (1980).

29. M. R. Deziel and A.W. Girotti, Lysis of research erythrocyte
     ghosts by photoactivated tetrapyrroles: Estimation of
     photolesion dimension, Int. J. Biochem. 14:263 (1982).

30. T. Taura and T. Murata, Effect of bilirubin photo-oxidation on frog crystalline lens fiber membrane, Nippon Ganka Gakkai Zasshi 83:77 (1980).

31. D.D. Hackney, Photodynamic action of bilirubin on the inner mitochondrial membrane. Implications for the organization of the mitochondrial ATPase, Biochem. Biophys. Res. Commun. 94:875 (1980).

32. M.D. Maines and A. Kappas, The degradative effects of porphyrins and heme compounds on components of the microsomal mixed function oxidase system. J. Biol. Chem. 250:2363 (1975).

33. A.D. Rahimtula, F. J. Hawco and P.J. O'Brien, The involvement of $^1O_2$ in the inactivation of mixed function oxidase and peroxidation of membrane lipids during the photosensitized oxidation of liver microsomes, Photochem. Photobiol. 28:811 (1978).

34. F. Meyer-Betz, Untersuchungen ueber die biologische (photodynamische) Wirkung des Haematoporphyrins und anderer Derivate des Blut- und Gallenfarbstoffs, Deutsch. Arch. Klin. Med. 112:476 (1913).

35. S.H. Robinson and A. Schunior, Hemolytic anemia induced by light therapy in jaundiced rats, Soc. Exptl. Biol. Med. 158:81 (1978).

36. J.O. Cukier, A.C. Maglalang, and G.B. Odell, Increased osmotic fragility of erythrocytes in chronically jaundiced rats after phototherapy, Acta Paediatr. Scand. 68:903 (1979).

37. R.B. Howe, C.R. Hadland and R.R. Engel, Effect of phototherapy on serum bilirubin levels and red blood cell survival in congenitally jaundiced Gunn rats, J. Lab. Clin. Med. 92:221 (1978).

38. F.F. Rubaltelli, G. Jori and E. Rossi, Evidence of minor damage occurring during phototherapy: Photoinduced covalent binding of bilirubin to serum albumin, p. 79, in: "Intensive Care of the Newborn," Vol. III, L. Stern, F.-H. Bent and K. Paul, eds., Waverly Press, Baltimore (1981).

39. E. John, Complications of phototherapy in hyperbilirubinemia, Aust. Paediat. J. 11:53 (1975).

PHOTOOXYGENATION PRODUCTS OF BILIRUBIN IN THE URINE OF

JAUNDICED PHOTOTHERAPY NEONATES

D.A. Lightner, W.P. Linnane III, and C.E. Ahlfors

Department of Chemistry, University of Nevada
Reno, NV 89557 and Section of Neonatology
Department of Pediatrics, School of Medicine
University of California, Davis, CA 95616

Phototherapy is widely and routinely used for treating hyperbilirubinemia (jaundice) in newborn babies. Neonates are irradiated with white or blue light to enhance the elimination of the yellow, potentially cytotoxic heme metabolite, (4Z,15Z)-bilirubin-IXα (BR).[1] Under normal metabolic conditions, BR is detoxified by conjugation in the liver and excreted in bile; however, when conjugation is impaired, BR accumulates in plasma and partitions into extravascular tissues, including the brain. It has been estimated that 2.5% of the live-born in the United States received phototherapy to remove or accelerate the excretion of BR from the body and thus reduce the risk of BR encephalopathy.[1]

The molecular mechanisms[2] of BR elimination in neo-natal phototherapy have been investigated for many years. The important photochemical event was at first thought to involve accelerated catabolism of BR to water-soluble derivatives that were excreted principally in bile and, to some extent, in urine.[3] This prompted studies of BR photodegradation (photooxygenation)[3,4] wherein singlet oxygen, viz. molecular oxygen in its first electronic excited state and known to be cytotoxic,[5] was thought to be the oxidizing species.[4] The products of in vitro photooxygenation have been well characterized,[4] but recent data indicate that BR photooxygenation may involve radical intermediates.[6] Thus, singlet oxygen may not be implicated.

161

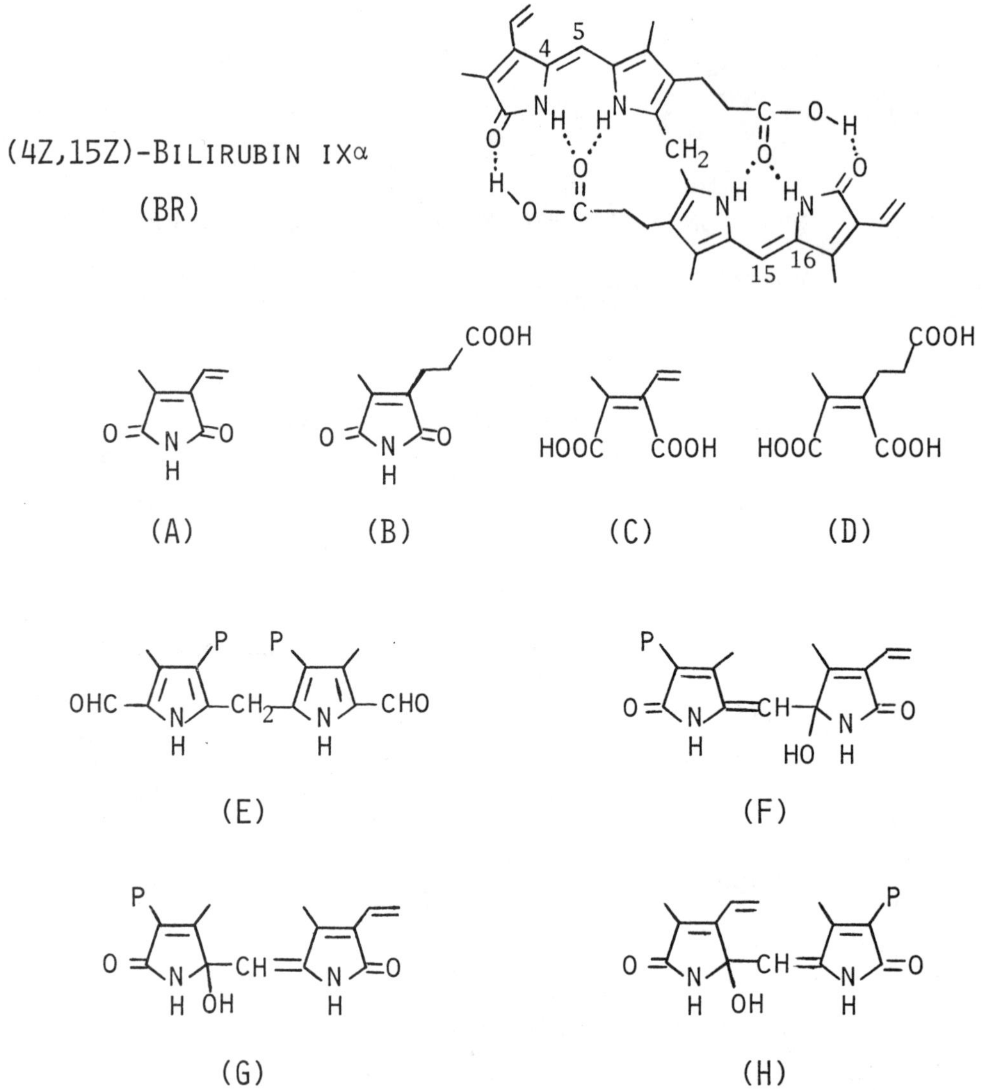

(4Z,15Z)-BILIRUBIN IXα

(BR)

Fig. 1. Structure of intramolecularly hydrogen-bonded BR and its characterized photooxygenation products (A)-(H). The latter consist of methylvinylmaleimide (A), hematinic acid imide (B), their hydrolysis products (C) and (D), respectively, a dipyrroledialdehyde (E), and the three known water-propentdyopents (F), (G) and (H). The methyl esters of (A)-(E) and the methanol-propentdyopent methyl esters of (F)-(H) were used as standards (Fig. 2) in the HPLC analyses of urine samples (Fig. 3 and Table). P = CH$_2$CH$_2$COOH

The importance of BR degradation as a molecular mechanism in neonatal phototherapy[7] began to decline with the discovery of an apparent augmented excretion of BR in the bile of Gunn rats[8] and jaundiced babies[9] undergoing light irradiation. This important discovery was also curious because BR cannot normally be excreted by the liver unless it is converted to polar conjugates, principally glucuronides.[1] To accomodate the confirmed[10,11] biliary excretion of unconjugated BR, photochemical configurational isomerization ($Z \rightleftarrows E$) at the meso carbon-carbon double bonds of (4Z,15Z)bilirubin-IXα (Fig. 1) was proposed [2,4] to give more polar and more hepatically excretable E-isomers. This hypothesis was subsequently tested[12] and confirmed in Gunn rats.[13] More recently, the structures of the E-isomers were proved,[14,15] and it has been shown that these isomers are formed in jaundiced rats exposed to blue light and in humans during phototherapy.[2,16] At present, current evidence favors the photochemical geometric configurational isomerization of BR (to E-isomers) as one of the most rapidly occurring photochemical events in phototherapy.[2]

It has remained unclear as to whether any degradation of BR occurs in vivo during phototherapy for neonatal jaundice. In early studies with Gunn rats, Ostrow[17] suggested that BR was photooxidized to smaller, more polar, water-soluble degradation products such as mono- and di-pyrroles that were easily excreted. However, there is no conclusive evidence supporting the occurrence of BR photo-oxygenation in vivo during phototherapy, and no specific photooxygenation products have been isolated and charact-erized. Callahan et al.[18] reported the presence of polar, predominantly diazo-negative BR photoproducts in bile and urine of congenitally jaundiced (Crigler-Najjar) infants undergoing phototherapy, but none of the products were identified. Ostrow[8] also reported finding BR photo-products in the bile and urine of (congenitally jaundiced) Gunn rats exposed to daylight fluorescent light. These, too, were not characterized. Significantly, however, the Gunn rat urine gave a positive pentdyopent reaction following phototherapy, suggesting the presence of di-pyrroles. Later, Onishi et al.[19] reported on unidentified BR photooxidation products in the blood, urine and stools of "bronze" babies.

Although BR photoisomerization is an important mechanism in vivo,[2] continuous irradiation is expected to lead to some photooxygenation.[20] And it seemed likely to us that photodegradation products would be excreted in

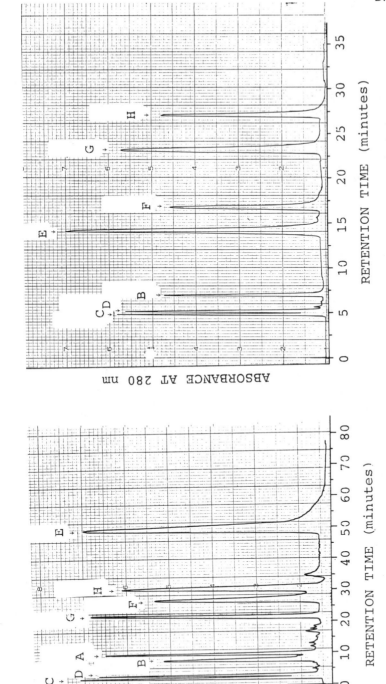

Fig. 2. HPLC (Perkin-Elmer Series 3 Analytical HPLC) scans of all reference BR photooxygenation products (see Fig. 1) using: (LEFT) A Knauer reverse phase column (25 cm x 4.6 mm i.d.) packed with 5μ ODS-C18 and an isocratic eluent of 26.9% Fisher HPLC grade acetonitrile in purified water, with a flow of 1.0 mL/min., press. 3.2 mP, and detector at 280 nm. (RIGHT) A Dupont column (25 cm x 4.6 mm i.d.) packed with Zorbax-Sil 7μ silica using an isocratic eluent of 1% acetic acid in Fisher HPLC grade chloroform, with flow 1.0 mL/min., press. 4–5.6 mP and detector at 280 nm. Methylvinylmaleimide (A) failed to appear on the silica column owing to its decomposition in the acidic solvent used as eluent.

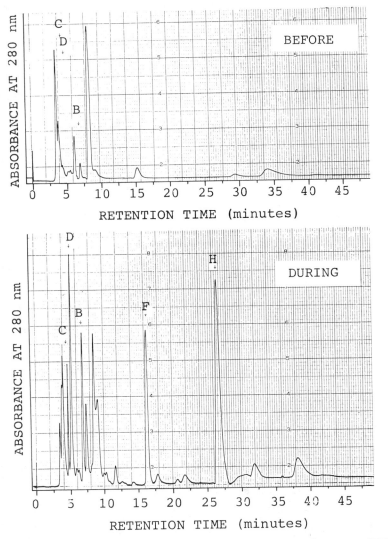

Fig. 3. HPLC (silica column) scans of urinary products. (TOP) Sample
         was taken 4 hrs after birth and before the onset of photo-
         therapy. There are essentially no BR photooxygenation pro-
         ducts detected in this voiding. (BOTTOM) Sample taken after
         4 hrs into an 8 hr phototherapy session. The intense unknown
         peak at 8.25 min. serves as an internal reference by which
         one can gauge the dramatic increase in BR photoproducts
         during phototherapy. Arrows indicate the expected positions
         of the various standards, (A)-(H). HPLC analysis of a given
         sample involved dissolving one-half of the methylated urin-
         ary material (urine samples were lyophilized, and the resi-
         due was methylated in excess ethereal-methanolic diazometh-
         ane) in 2.0 mL of chloroform (for silica column) and the
         remaining half in acetonitrile (for reverse phase column).

urine.   We therefore analyzed urine samples from jaundiced babies undergoing phototherapy.   In our analyses we used newly developed, sensitive chromatographic techniques (high performance liquid chromatography, HPLC) and well-characterized chemical standards (Fig. 1).[4]   Standard (HPLC) reference profiles were obtained by injecting the reference standards into the HPLC in order to identify retention times (Fig. 2).   Samples obtained from urine were matched with the reference standards by comparison of retention times and coinjection.   The coinjection procedure served two useful purposes: (1) to establish a high degree of confidence that an "unknown" peak in the urine sample corresponds exactly with a reference standard by coinjection on both the silica column and the reverse phase column, and (2) to allow for direct calculations of the BR photooxygenation product concentrations in the urine samples by coinjection with reference standards of known concentration and volume.   Urine was collected (protected from light) from jaundiced babies undergoing phototherapy and jaundiced control babies not receiving phototherapy. The initial voiding was frozen as soon as possible and stored protected from light.   The gestational ages of the babies ranged from 26 weeks to term, and serum BR levels ranged from 5.5 to 13.4 mg/dL.

In Fig. 3 we show typical HPLC scans to analyze for the presence of BR photooxygenation products in urine. The urine sample collected prior to phototherapy showed essentially none of the standards, either on a silica column (Fig. 3, TOP) or on a reverse phase column.   Only trace amounts of the derivatized hydrolysis products of both methylvinylmaleimide (C) and hematinic acid imide (D), and hematinic acid imide (B) were detected.   However, a urine sample collected after 4 hours of phototherapy, when the serum BR was 10.3 mg/dL, clearly showed the presence of BR photooxygenation products (Fig. 3, BOTTOM). The peaks for (B), (C) and (D) are marked enhanced, and new strong peaks appear for two propentdyopents (F) and (H).   Similar results for other jaundiced babies with hyperbilirubinemia and undergoing phototherapy are pre-sented in the Table along with control jaundiced babies with unconjugated hyperbilirubinemia and not receiving phototherapy.

We believe that our studies provide the first clear, qualitative analytical proof that BR photooxygenation products [(B), (C), (D), (F) and (H), Fig. 1] appear in urine during phototherapy of human neonates with unconju-gated hyperbilirubinemia.   These substances either do not

TABLE 1. Bilirubin photooxygenation products (see Fig. 1) found in the urine of jaundiced neonates undergoing phototherapy and jaundiced control neonates not undergoing phototherapy, and analyzed (HPLC) as their methylated derivatives. The HPLC identification was made using two different columns, silica and reverse phase ODS-C18, and the concentrations were determined by measuring HPLC peak areas and comparing them with the peak areas from sample + standard coinjections. *Means not detected. Also not detected in any of the analyses were (A), (E) and (G).

CONCENTRATIONS OF PHOTOPRODUCTS, mg/dL

Infant	(B) Silica ODS-C18	(B) Aver.	(C) Silica ODS-C18	(C) Aver.	(D) Silica ODS-C18	(D) Aver.	(F) Silica ODS-C18	(F) Aver.	(H) Silica ODS-C18	(H) Aver.	Average Conc.
No Phototherapy											
1	0.011 / 0.015	0.013	0.045 / 0.031	0.035	0.032 / 0.017	0.025	*		*		0.073
2	0.041 / 0.021	0.031	0.014 / 0.056	0.035	0.056 / 0.073	0.065	*		*		0.131
Phototherapy											
3	0.126 / 0.074	0.100	0.108 / 0.097	0.102	0.084 / 0.073	0.078	0.026 / 0.038	0.032	0.016 / 0.001	0.009	0.321
4	0.020 / 0.214	0.117	0.021 / 0.022	0.022	0.013 / 0.148	0.082	0.021 / 0.056	0.039	0.103 / 0.040	0.072	0.332
5	0.164 / 0.178	0.167	0.038 / 0.042	0.040	0.022 / 0.038	0.030	0.064 / 0.068	0.066	0.006 / 0.003	0.004	0.307

arise, or occur to a lesser extent [(B), (C), and (D)],
in jaundiced babies not undergoing phototherapy. Furthermore, except for a trace amount of (B), none of the BR
photodegradation products (Fig. 1) could be found in the
urine of a full term baby with unconjugated hyperbilirubinemia not under phototherapy. We speculate that the
origin of small quantities of (B), its hydrolysis product
(D) and the hydrolysis product (C) of (A) may arise from
BR or its metabolic precursors via enzymatic oxida-
tions.[21,22] Also, finding (C) in urine is probably
evidence for formation of its precursor methylvinylmaleimide (A) despite our failure to detect it. Methylvinylmaleimide is known to be unstable and may not survive long _in vivo_ or during the experimental processing
of the urine. The expected propentdyopent (G) and dipyrroledialdehyde (E) were not found. It is unclear
why (G) should not be found. (E) is formed in only very
small amounts during _in vitro_ BR photooxygenation,[23] and
may be formed _in vivo_ below our threshhold detection
level, if at all.

     We note, finally, that the amounts (Table) of BR
photooxygenation products excreted in urine are small,
in keeping with the distribution of excreted label
following administration of ^{14}C-BR and light irradiation[10]
and would appear to indicate that geometric configurational
isomerization and other molecular mechanisms[2] are more
important. The data confirm, nonetheless, that BR photooxygenation is a real component of phototherapy, and they
identify for the first time known BR photooxygenation
products _in vivo_.

ACKNOWLEDGEMENTS

     This work was supported by the U. S. Public Health
Service Grant HD-09026 and by the National Science
Foundation (CHE-7910133).

REFERENCES

1.   A. K. Brown and A. F. McDonagh, Phototherapy for neo-
     natal hyperbilirubinemia: Efficacy, mechanism and
     toxicity. Adv. Pediatrics 27:341 (1980).

2.   A. F. McDonagh, Molecular mechanisms of phototherapy
     of neonatal jaundice, _in_: "Proceedings of a
     Symposium on New Trends in Phototherapy", F. F.
     Rubaltelli and G. Jori, eds., Plenum Press,
     London, in press.

3. J. D. Ostrow, Photochemical and biochemical basis of the treatment of neonatal jaundice, in: "Progress in Liver Disease", vol. IV, H. Popper and D. Schaffner, eds., Grune and Stratton, New York (1972).

4. D. A. Lightner, Structure, photochemistry and organic chemistry of bilirubin, in: "Bilirubin", vol I, K. P. M. Heirwegh. and S. B. Brown, eds., CRC Press, Boca Raton, Florida (1982).

5. H. H. Wasserman and R. W. Murray, eds., "Singlet Oxygen", Academic Press, Inc., New York (1979).

6. G. L. Landen, Y-T. Park and D. A. Lightner, On the role of singlet oxygen in the self-sensitized photooxygenation of bilirubin and its pyrromethen-one models. Tetrahedron, in press.

7. A. N. Cohen and J. D. Ostrow, New concepts in photo-therapy: Photoisomerization of bilirubin IXα and potential toxic effects of light. Pediatrics 65: 740 (1980).

8. J. D. Ostrow, Photocatabolism of labelled bilirubin in the congenitally jaundiced (Gunn) rat. J. Clin. Invest. 50:707 (1971).

9. H. T. Lund and J. Jacobsen, Influence of phototherapy on the biliary bilirubin excretion pattern in new-born infants with hyperbilirubinemia. J. Pediatr. 85:262 (1974).

10. A. F. McDonagh, Photochemistry and photometabolism of bilirubin IXα, in: "Bilirubin Metabolism in the Newborn (II)", D. Bergsma and S. H. Blondheim, eds., Excerpta Medica, Amsterdam (1976).

11. J. D. Ostrow, C. S. Berry, R. G. Knodell and J. E. Zarembo, Effect of phototherapy on bilirubin excretion in man and in the rat, in: "Bilirubin Metabolism in the Newborn (II)", D. Bergsma and S. H. Blondheim, eds., Excerpta Medica, Amsterdam (1976).

12. A. F. McDonagh, L. A. Palma and D. A. Lightner, Blue light and bilirubin excretion. Science 208:145 (1980).

13. A. F. McDonagh and L. A. Palma, Hepatic excretion
     of circulating bilirubin photoproducts in the
     Gunn rat. J. Clin. Invest. 66:1181 (1980).

14. A. F. McDonagh, L. A. Palma, F. R. Trull and D. A.
     Lightner, Phototherapy for neonatal jaundice.
     Configurational isomers of bilirubin. J. Am.
     Chem. Soc. 104:6865 (1982).

15. H. Falk, N. Muller, M. Ratzenhofer and K. Winsauer,
     The structure of "photobilirubin". Monatsh. Chem.
     113:1421 (1982).

16. A. F. McDonagh, L. A. Palma and D. A. Lightner,
     Phototherapy for neonatal jaundice. Stereospecific
     and regioselective photoisomerization of bilirubin
     bound to human serum albumin and NMR characteriza-
     tion of intramolecularly cyclized photoproducts.
     J. Am. Chem. Soc. 104:6867 (1982).

17. J. D. Ostrow, Photo-oxidative derivatives of [^{14}C]
     bilirubin and their excretion by the Gunn rat,
     in: "Bilirubin Metabolism", I. A. D. Bouchier
     and B. Billings, eds., Blackwell Scientific,
     Oxford (1967).

18. E. W. Callahan, Jr., M. M. Thaler, M. Karon, K. Bauer,
     and R. Schmid, Phototherapy of severe unconjugated
     hyperbilirubinemia: formation and removal of
     labeled bilirubin derivatives. Pediatrics 46:
     841 (1970).

19. S. Onishi, M. Fujikawa, Y. Ogawa and J. Ogawa, Photo-
     degradation products of bilirubin studied by high
     pressure liquid chromatography, nuclear magnetic
     resonance and mass spectrometry, in: "Bilirubin
     Metabolism in the Newborn (II)", D. Bergsma and
     S. H. Blondheim eds., Excerpta Medica, Amsterdam
     (1976).

20. A. F. McDonagh, D. A. Lightner and T. A. Wooldridge,
     Geometric isomerization of bilirubin-IXα and its
     dimethyl ester. J. Chem. Soc. Chem. Commun. 110
     (1979).

21. R. Schmid and L. Hammaker, Metabolism and disposition
     of C^{14}-bilirubin in congenital nonhemolytic
     jaundice. J. Clin. Invest. 42:2720 (1963).

22.   R. Schmid and A. F. McDonagh, Hyperbilirubinemia,
      in: "The Metabolic Basis of Inherited Diseases",
      J. B. Stanbury, J. B. Wyngaarden and D. S.
      Frederickson, eds., McGraw-Hill, New York (1978).

23.   R. Bonnett and J. C. M. Stewart, Photooxidation of
      bilirubin in hydroxylic solvents. J. Chem. Soc.
      Perkin Trans. I 224 (1975).

MOLECULAR MECHANISMS OF PHOTOTHERAPY OF NEONATAL JAUNDICE

Antony F. McDonagh

The Liver Center and Department of Medicine
University of California, HSW 1120
San Francisco, CA 94143

INTRODUCTION

The success of phototherapy depends on photochemical transformations of bilirubin within light-exposed tissues. These reactions alter the structure of bilirubin in such a way that the intact molecule or fragments of it can be excreted via the kidney or liver without having to undergo further metabolic modification. So far three photochemical reactions of bilirubin have been shown to occur in vivo, and it is likely that these three together account for most of the effect of light on bilirubin metabolism in jaundiced newborns. The three reactions are photooxidation, configurational isomerization, and structural isomerization. In this presentation I shall discuss briefly some of our evidence for the occurrence of these reactions in vivo and speculate on their relative contributions to the net effect of phototherapy. Since the interpretation of the in vivo studies is very much dependent on knowledge gleaned from in vitro photochemical studies, I shall begin with a discussion of the latter.

PHOTOCHEMICAL STUDIES

Photooxidation

It is well known that solutions of bilirubin in equilibrium with air undergo irreversible bleaching when exposed to light.[1] This is due to photooxidation of the pigment to monocyclic imides and to bicyclic compunds of the propentdyopent type. The latter are generally isolated as adducts with water or methanol. Other products are also formed during photooxidation, but to a much lesser degree.

Recently Lightner et al.[2] have developed sensitive comple-
mentary high performance liquid chromatography (hplc) methods for
the identification and analysis of bilirubin photooxidation products.

Early studies indicated that bilirubin photooxidation is a
self-sensitized reaction involving singlet oxygen. Later work has
implicated radical intermediates and, presently, it is unclear to
what extent singlet oxygen is involved in the reaction, if at all.
Relative to configurational isomerization (see below) bilirubin
photooxidation is a slow reaction except in the presence of added
photosensitizers or high oxygen concentrations.[3]

Photoisomerization

1. _Configurational photoisomerization._ Bilirubin has the
4Z,15Z configuration.[4] When exposed to light in solution in the
vicinity of its main absorption band bilirubin undergoes very rapid
configurational isomerization to a mixture of the corresponding
4Z,15E, 4E,15Z and 4E,15E isomers (Fig. 1).[5,6] Since the reactions
are reversible and since the isomers have overlapping spectra a
photodynamic equilibrium is soon established when dilute solutions
are irradiated with polychromatic light in a closed system. All
four isomers can be separated by hplc and it has been possible, by
means of nuclear magnetic resonance (nmr) studies, to distinguish
which of the two E,Z isomers is the 4Z,15E and which is the 4E,15Z.[5]
The composition of the mixture at photoequilibrium depends on the
solvent and wavelength output of the light source,[5,7] but in
general for non-aqueous protein-free solutions:

$$[4Z,15Z-BR] \gg [4Z,15E-BR] \simeq 2x \ [4E,15Z-BR] \ggg [4E,15E-BR]$$

(For example, for photolysis in $CHCl_3/Et_3N$, 1:1, with Special Blue
light the composition at photoequilibrium is < 1% 4E,15E-BR,
$\simeq$ 8% 4E,15Z-BR, $\simeq$ 20% 4Z,15E-BR and $\simeq$ 72% 4Z,15Z-BR).

Similar photoisomerization occurs with bilirubin dimethyl ester
and with the symmetrical IIIα and XIIIα isomers of bilirubin.[3,5]
In an elegant series of studies Lugtenburg, de Groot and coworkers, using proton and ^{13}C nmr, have demonstrated identical
photochemical transformations for several synthetic model compounds
of bilirubin.[8,9] Clearly, configurational Z → E photoisomerization
is a general reaction of "rubins" and molecules containing the
dipyrromethenone chromophore.

Surprisingly, perhaps, configurational isomerization of bilirubin occurs readily even when the pigment is associated with serum
albumin.[10,11] However, protein binding does have a pronounced
effect on the stereochemistry of the reaction. For 1:1 bilirubin/
protein complexes the composition of the isomer mixture at photoequilibrium obtained using a given light source depends very much

on the identity of the protein.[10] Irradiation of the bilirubin
bound to rat serum albumin at pH 7.4 with Special Blue light gives
at photoequilibrium ≃ 3% 4E,15Z-BR, 8% 4Z,15E-BR and 89% 4Z,15Z-BR.
Under the same conditions bilirubin bound to human serum albumin
gives ≃ 31% 4Z,15E-BR and 69% 4Z,15Z-BR. Therefore, Z → E isomerization of bilirubin on human serum albumin is highly regiospecific
for the 4Z,15E isomer, which is not the case for bilirubin bound to
rat, guinea pig, horse or bovine serum albumin.[10]

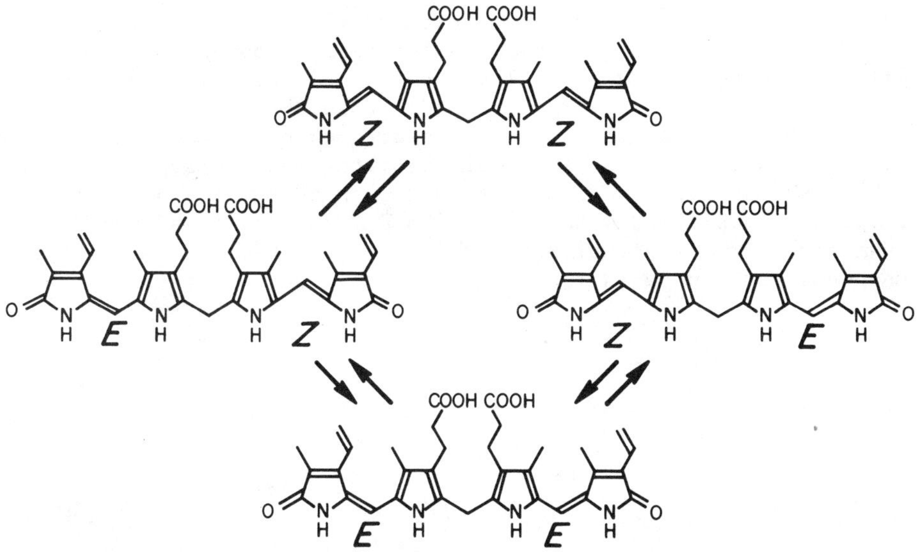

Fig. 1. Configurational isomerization of bilirubin

Isomers of bilirubin containing E double bonds revert rapidly
to the Z,Z, isomer in bile and other protic media, particularly in
the presence of acids. In 1% NH4OH/MeOH they are stable for hours
at room temperature and for days at 4°C, provided that the solutions
are kept in the dark under argon. E-Isomers bound to serum albumin
revert to the Z,Z-isomer only very slowly at room temperature and
are indefinitely stable at ≤ 4°C. Solutions containing purified
E,Z isomers of bilirubin are, however, exquisitely sensitive to
(blue) light and should be manipulated in the dark or under a red
safelight.

   Curiously, we have been able to detect only trace amounts of
configurational isomers during photolysis of bilirubin in protein-
free buffer (pH 8.5), perhaps because of rapid thermal reversion.
Under these conditions photolysis leads to marked constitutional
isomerization to bilirubins IIIα and XIIIα.

   2. Structural photoisomerization. Configurational isomerization of bilirubin is invariably accompanied by a slower reaction
which appears to involve intramolecular cyclization of the endo
vinyl group at C-3 (Fig. 2).[10,12] This reaction only becomes
clearly manifest when solutions of bilirubin are irradiated for
several times longer than is necessary to approach photoequilibration of the configurational isomers. Bilirubin XIIIα, which
has two endo vinyl groups, undergoes a similar reaction; bilirubin
IIIα and mesobilirubin IXα, which lack endovinyl groups, do not.[10]
We call the product of the cyclization reaction Z-lumirubin.[11]
Z-Lumirubin is probably the same as the main component of Photobilirubin II, described by Stoll et al.,[12,13] and "Unknown Pigment"
of Onishi et al.[14] Z-Lumirubin contains two chiral centers (at C-2
and C-7), and is presumably a mixture of four diastereoisomers (R,S,
S,R, S,S, and R,R). On thin-layer chromatography it separates into
two components with identical absorption spectra which have proton
nmr spectra consistent with the assigned structure[11] and which are
presumably pairs of enantiomers (R,S/S,R and S,S/R,R). These two
components undergo rapid equilibration and interconversion in base

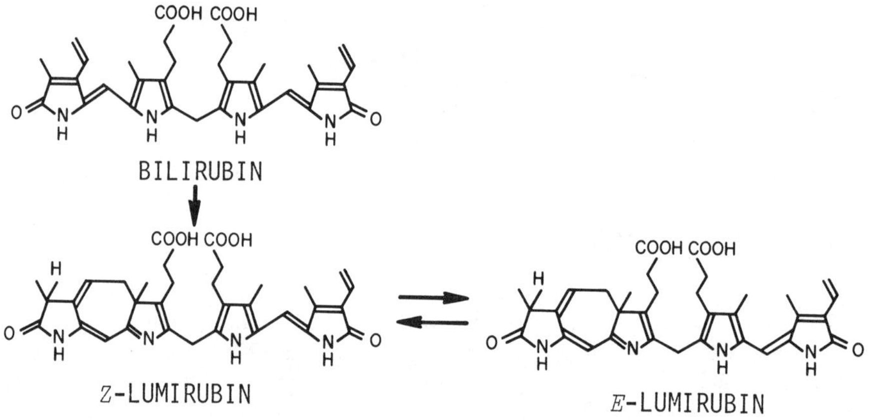

Fig. 2.   Structural photoisomerization of bilirubin. (The product
          is an equimolar mixture of epimers, Z-lumirubin and Z-iso-
          lumirubin, that differ only in configuration at C-2.
          Photolysis of each of these leads to a mixture of Z and
          E forms.[10])

due to the presence of a labile proton at C-2 which facilitates
inversion of configuration at that center.

Formation of Z-lumirubin from bilirubin is not prevented by
albumin binding. Indeed the cyclization reaction occurs more rapidly
for bilirubin bound to serum albumin than it does for bilirubin in
organic solvents such as chloroform, methanolic ammonia or dimethyl
sulphoxide. At present it is uncertain whether Z-lumirubin is
formed from bilirubin in a concerted one-photon process (4Z,15Z-BR
→ Z-Lumi) or in a sequential two-photon process with 4E,15Z-bili-
rubin as intermediate (4Z,15Z-BR → 4E,15Z-BR → Z-Lumi). However,
as noted earlier, photolysis of bilirubin on human serum albumin
(pH 7.4) results in rapid formation of the 4Z,15E configurational
isomer. This isomer cannot be a direct precursor for Z-lumirubin.
Nevertheless, on continued irradiation there is gradual formation
of Z-lumirubin and E-lumirubin without the appearance of detectable
amounts of 4E,15Z-bilirubin. Furthermore, lumirubin formation is
not markedly enhanced in systems where the configurational isomerization leads to both of the 4E,15Z and 4Z,15E bilirubin isomers.
These observations indicate that a direct one-photon mechanism may
be predominantly responsible for Z-lumirubin formation. Stoll et
al.[12] argued that the presence of an E-configuration double bond
within the seven-membered ring of Photobilirubin II provided the
first structural evidence for configurational isomerization of
bilirubin.[12] However, the possibility that a concerted one-photon
cyclization mechanism might be involved dilutes the strength of
that argument.

On exposure to blue light, purified Z-lumirubin is converted
rapidly to a photoequilibrium mixture of Z and E isomers.[10]
Continued prolonged photolysis of this mixture, or irradiation of
Z-lumirubin with very intense light, leads to slow formation of
configurational isomers of bilirubin and overall destruction of
pigment. Unlike the E,Z isomers of bilirubin, Z-lumirubin does
not undergo rapid stoichiometric photoreversion to Z,Z-bilirubin.
This observation is inconsistent with what has been reported
previously for Photobilirubin II.[13]

Brief anaerobic photolysis of bilirubin in protein-free aqueous
buffer (pH 8.5) or prolonged photolysis in a variety of other media
leads to a different type of structural or constitutional isomerization, namely disproportionation to bilirubin IIIα and bilirubin
XIIIα.[15] Aggregation (dimerization) of bilirubin probably facilitates this reaction in water. Onishi et al.[16] postulated that a
similar photochemical reaction occurs in vivo during phototherapy
and, using hplc, were able to detect bilirubins IIIα and XIIIα in
the serum of infants undergoing treatment,[14,16] In our studies we
have been unable to detect these isomers in serum from infants or
Gunn rats undergoing phototherapy. The reason for the discrepancy
is not clear.

PHOTOBIOLOGICAL STUDIES

The in vitro studies suggest that both reversible and irreversible reactions could occur during phototherapy. In vivo the initial rate for each reaction will depend on the quantum yield for the reaction and on the photon flux (light intensity) and bilirubin concentration at the site of reaction. In addition, the biological effectiveness of each reaction will be subject to the dynamics of the living organism. In considering the mechanism of phototherapy it is important, therefore, to distinguish between the photochemical mechanism and the overall mechanism.

For an irreversible reaction the overall process can be summarized symbolically as:

$$h\upsilon + BR \xrightarrow{k_1} (Products)_{site} \xrightarrow{k_2} (Products)_{excreta}$$

$$h\upsilon + BR \underset{k_{-1}}{\overset{k_1}{\rightleftharpoons}} (Products)_{site} \overset{k_2}{\rightleftharpoons} (Products)_{excreta}$$

where k_1 represents the rate constant for the photochemical reaction and k_2 the combined transport rate constants for the removal of photoproducts from the site and excretion in bile or urine. If $k_2 \gg k_1$ photoproducts will not accumulate, and, for the reversible reaction, photoequilibration between bilirubin and photoproducts would not occur. Furthermore, if the net conversion of bilirubin to photoproducts is small relative to the pool of light-accessible bilirubin, the excretion of photoproducts from either pathway would eventually reach a photostationary level which would be dependent only on the intensity of the light. Such a situation appears to occur in the Gunn rat during phototherapy (see below). On the other hand, if $k_1 > k_2$, photoproducts would accumulate in the body during phototherapy and, for the reversible reaction, photoequilibration between photoproducts and bilirubin might occur. This situation appears to prevail to some degree in the human infant (see below).

Until recently, reliable identification and analysis of bilirubin photoproducts in human and animal studies was hampered by the unavailability of well characterized standards and the lack of suitable analytical methods. The introduction of hplc and simple methods for preparing standards have made photoproduct analysis much easier. However, due to the instability of bilirubin photoproducts, special precautions are required to avoid artifacts. For example, when analysing photoproducts in bile from bile fistula animals it is imperative to collect samples close to the liver and without exposure to light. The analyses should be carried out without delay and without extraction or chemical manipulation.

And it is important to ensure that animals do not become depleted
of bile salts due to interruption of the enterohepatic circulation.
In our experience, failure to observe precautions such as these can
lead to plausible yet quite inaccurate results.

Gunn rat

The homozygous Gunn rat has lifelong unconjugated hyperbilirubinemia and responds to phototherapy in much the same way as the
jaundiced human neonate; namely, by a decrease in the concentration
of bilirubin in the blood. As a quantitative model, the Gunn rat
has some limitations. For example, rat serum albumin has a lower
affinity for bilirubin than human serum albumin.[15] Unlike humans,
rats have no gallbladder. And in most studies, adult--as opposed
to neonatal--rats have been used. Nevertheless the Gunn rat
remains very useful as a qualitative model for investigating the
photochemical mechanism of phototherapy.

When shaved bile fistula Gunn rats are exposed to Special Blue
phototherapy lights, photoproducts begin to appear in bile within
minutes (Fig. 3).[17] The total concentration of photoproducts
increases during the first 1.5-2.0 hours and then levels off to a
constant steady-state value that is maintained for at least several
hours. Altering the intensity of the light once the steady-state
has been reached results in a shift of the steady-state concentration of photoproducts to a new value. However, for a given light
source, altering the intensity does not change the relative concentrations of the individual photoproducts in the bile.[20] Therefore
the steady-state that is reached when Gunn rats are exposed to
continuous phototherapy is probably not due to a photochemical
equilibrium, but due to a dynamic balance between formation and
clearance of photoproducts.

Hplc chromatograms of bile collected during the photostationary state show a number of peaks not present in bile collected
before exposure of the animals to light (Fig. 4).[5] Using authentic standards, we have identified all of the peaks as isomers of
bilirubin. The main products are 4Z,15E- and 4E,15Z-bilirubin, with
lesser amounts of Z-lumirubin, E-lumirubin and 4E,15E-bilirubin.
Configurational isomers comprise about 85% of the photoproducts;
structural isomers (lumirubins) about 10%. Analyses of the bile by
other methods, including radioisotope methods, supports these
results and shows that significant amounts of colorless photoproducts or materials not eluted from the hplc column are not present
in the bile. Therefore, essentially all of the photoproducts in
nascent bile are isomers of bilirubin. We have found no evidence
for significant amounts of hydroxylated photoproducts of the type
proposed by Berry et al.[18] and, on chemical grounds, consider the
mechanism proposed for their formation highly unlikely.

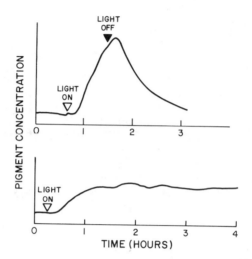

Fig. 3.   Excretion of pigment in Gunn rat bile in response to con-
          tinuous or intermittent phototherapy. Pigment concen-
          trations were measured continuously at 475 nm by
          absorption photometry.[17] The ordinates in each graph,
          which are in arbitrary linear absorbance units, are not
          drawn on the same scale.

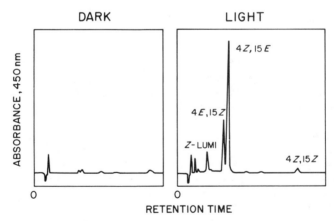

Fig. 4.   Hplc of Gunn rat bile collected before and during photo-
          therapy. Solvent system 0.1 M di-n-dodecylamine acetate
          in methanol; detector 450 nm; reverse-phase column.[10]

Hplc analysis of serum during the photostationary state revealed only traces of photoisomers. However, when the bile duct was ligated to prevent their efflux, isomers (4Z,15E; 4E,15Z; and Z-lumirubin) became readily detectable in the circulation as previously observed by other methods.[19] Therefore, transport and excretion of the photoisomers in the adult Gunn rat is very efficient, suggesting that $k_2 > k_1$, where k_2 and k_1 are as defined earlier. Interestingly, the relative concentrations of photoisomers in bile (but not the total concentration) were fairly constant from rat to rat using the same light source. This suggests that the composition of photoproducts excreted by the rat depends solely on the quantum yields of the different contributing reactions, as expected for a system in which $k_2 > k_1$.

Presumably, some photooxidation accompanies photoisomerization of bilirubin during phototherapy. Because of their low molecular weight and polar character, photooxidation products would be expected to be excreted mainly in urine. Assuming that the contribution of this pathway is small, we conclude that about 85% of the lowering of serum bilirubin levels in the bile-fistula Gunn rat during exposure to Special Blue lights is due to formation and excretion of configurational isomers of bilirubin, and about 10% to formation and excretion of lumirubins.[20] These figures may not, however, accurately represent the contribution of the two reaction pathways in the intact rat for the following reason. Configurational isomers containing Z double bonds revert spontaneously in bile to the parent Z,Z, isomer. In the intact animal a portion of this, and possibly a portion of the photoisomers themselves, may undergo enterohepatic recycling as do bile salts. Therefore, the net contribution of the two pathways, and in particular the configurational isomer pathway, to the overall effect of phototherapy may be lower in the intact animal than in the bile fistula model.

Human

Presently, the complete mechanism of phototherapy in humans is not understood. However there is now firm evidence that all three photochemical reactions discussed above (configurational isomerization, structural isomerization, and photooxidation) do occur in the jaundiced neonate undergoing phototherapy. Broadly speaking, the mechanism in humans seems to be comparable to that in the Gunn rat, but with some important differences. In humans phototherapy leads to a marked accumulation of photoproducts in the circulation (Fig. 5).[14,20] The main photoproduct that accumulates is 4Z,15E-bilirubin[10] and this is accompanied by variable, though generally relatively small, amounts of Z-lumirubin.[20] Some 4Z,15E-bilirubin may even be detectable in the serum of jaundiced patients not undergoing phototherapy, presumably because of exposure to ambient light.

The proportion of 4Z,15E-bilirubin in the blood of infants undergoing phototherapy may reach about 15-20% of the total bilirubin
present. Since this isomer is the product of a photoreversible
reaction there is probably an upper limit to the proportion that
can coexist with 4Z,15Z-bilirubin in the circulation.

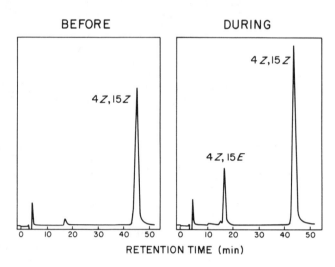

Fig. 5. Hplc of serum from an infant with neonatal jaundice before
         and after 16h of phototherapy. For conditions see Fig. 4.

It is noteworthy that very little of the 4E,15Z isomer of
bilirubin is detectable in human serum during phototherapy. This
would suggest that the 4E,15Z isomer is either excreted much more
rapidly than its twin 4Z,15E isomer or that it is hardly formed at
all. In the Gunn rat the 4E,15Z isomer is indeed excreted in bile
faster than the 4Z,15E isomer.[20] However, as already mentioned,
photoisomerization of bilirubin on human serum albumin in vitro is
highly regioselective for formation of the 4Z,15E isomer, the
isomer that accumulates in human plasma during phototherapy.
Therefore it is not certain whether the predominance of one photoisomer in the circulation in humans reflects stereospecific transport and excretion or regioselective photochemistry. Overall, our
present data favor the latter.

Although the concentration of Z-lumirubin in serum during
phototherapy is generally low, this isomer is clearly detectable in
duodenal bile.[14,20] In contrast, 4Z,15E-bilirubin (or 4E,15Z-
bilirubin) has not yet been specifically identified in human bile.
Whether this is due to impaired secretion of this isomer or to its
rapid reversion to 4Z,15E-bilirubin in bile is not yet clear.
However, it is clear that both structural and configurational isomerization of bilirubin do occur in infants during phototherapy and

that there are differences in the rates of clearance of these isomers from the circulation. In addition, there appear to be marked
differences between rats and humans in the clearance rates of
bilirubin photoisomers. Such differences may largely reflect differences in the avidity of the various photoisomers for different
serum albumins and for intrahepatic binding proteins.

Strong evidence for photooxidation of bilirubin during
phototherapy has recently been obtained by Lightner et al.[2] They
examined urine from infants undergoing phototherapy by hplc and
detected several compounds that were not present before phototherapy and that gradually disappeared when phototherapy was
stopped. By reference to authentic standards, these compounds were
identified as hematinic acid imide, hematinic acid, methyl vinyl
maleic acid and isomeric propentdyopents. Since a similar suite of
compounds is formed on photooxidation of bilirubin in vitro, it is
likely that photooxidation is also responsible for their formation
in vivo.

CONCLUSIONS

Three photochemical reactions (configurational isomerization,
structural isomerization and photooxidation) occur in jaundiced
infants undergoing phototherapy. It is likely that these three
reactions, by converting bilirubin to less lipophilic and more
readily excretable products, together account for the observed
lowering of serum bilirubin concentrations during treatment. Of
the three reactions, configurational isomerization occurs the most
rapidly, but at present the relative contribution of each of the
pathways to the overall effect of phototherapy is not known. Since
the relative contributions of the pathways may be wavelength dependent and since different types of light sources are used in phototherapy there may in fact be no single unique mechanism of phototherapy. However, the currently available data indicate that
photoisomerization reactions are invariably a major contributor.

ACKNOWLEDGEMENTS

This work was supported by Grants AM-26307, AM-11275 and
AM-26743 from the National Institutes of Health. The advice and
collaboration of Dr. D.A. Lightner, Dr. J.F. Ennever and Ms. L.A.
Palma is greatly appreciated. I thank Mr. Michael Karasik for
assistance in prepartion of the manuscript.

REFERENCES

1. D.A. Lightner, Structure, photochemistry, and organic
       chemistry of bilirubin, in: "Bilirubin", K.P.M. Heirwegh
       and S.B. Brown, eds., CRC Press, Boca Raton (1982).

2. D.A. Lightner, W.P. Linnane, and C.E. Ahlfors, Bilirubin photooxidation products in the urine of phototherapy neonates, Submitted for publication.

3. A.F. McDonagh, D.A. Lightner, and T.A. Wooldridge, Geometric isomerization of bilirubin-IXα and its dimethyl ester. J. Chem. Soc. Chem. Commun. 110 (1979).

4. R. Bonnett, J.E. Davis, M.B. Hursthouse, and G.M. Sheldrick, The structure of bilirubin, Proc. Roy. Soc. Lond. B. 202: 249 (1978).

5. A.F. McDonagh, L.A. Palma, F.R. Trull, and D.A. Lightner, Phototherapy for neonatal jaundice. Configurational isomers of bilirubin, J. Am. Chem. Soc. 102: 6865 (1982).

6. H. Falk, N. Muller, M. Ratzenhofer, and K. Winsauer, The structure of "Photobilirubin", Monatsh. Chem. 113:1421 (1982).

7. J.F. Ennever, A.F. McDonagh, and W.T. Speck, Phototherapy for neonatal jaundice: Optimal wavelengths of light, J. Pediatr. In press.

8. J.A. de Groot, R. van der Steen, R. Fokkens, and J. Lugtenburg, Synthesis and photoisomerisation of 2,3,17,18,22-penta-methyl-10,23-dihydro-1,19-[21H,24H]-bilindione, an unsymmetrical bilirubin model compound, Recl. Trav. Chim. Pays-Bas 101:219 (1982).

9. J.A. de Groot, R. van der Steen, R. Fokkens, and J. Lugtenburg, Synthesis and photochemical reactivity of bilirubin model compounds, Recl. Trav. Chim. Pays-Bas 101:35 (1982).

10. A.F. McDonagh, L.A. Palma, and D.A. Lightner, Phototherapy for neonatal jaundice. Stereospecific and regioselective photoisomerization of bilirubin bound to human serum albumin and NMR characterization of intramolecularly cyclized photoproducts, J. Am. Chem. Soc. 104:6867 (1982).

11. B.I. Green, A.A. Lamola, and C.V. Shank, Picosecond primary photoprocesses of bilirubin bound to human serum albumin, Proc. Natl. Acad. Sci. USA 78:2008 (1981).

12. M.S. Stoll, N. Vicker, C.H. Gray, and R. Bonnett, Concerning the structure of photobilirubin II, Biochem. J. 201:179 (1982).

13. M.S. Stoll, E.A. Zenone, J.D. Ostrow, and J.E. Zarembo, Preparation and properties of bilirubin photoisomers, Biochem. J. 183:139 (1979).

14. S. Onishi, K. Isobe, S. Itoh, N. Kawade, and S. Sugiyama, Demonstration of a geometric isomer of bilirubin-IX in the serum of a hyperbilirubinaemic newborn infant and the mechanism of jaundice phototherapy, Biochem. J. 190:533 (1980).

15. A.F. McDonagh, Bile Pigments: Bilatrienes and 5,15-biladienes, in: "The Porphyrins", D. Dolphin, ed., Academic Press, New York (1979).

16. S. Onishi, S. Itoh, N. Kawade, K. Isobe, and S. Sugiyama,
      The separation of configurational isomers of bilirubin by
      high pressure liquid chromatography and the mechanism of
      jaundice phototherapy, Biochem. Biophys. Res. Commun.
      90:890 (1979).
17. A.F. McDonagh, and L.M. Ramonas, Jaundice phototherapy: Micro
      flow-cell photometry reveals rapid biliary response of
      Gunn rats to light, Science 201:829 (1978).
18. C.S. Berry, J.E. Zarembo, and J.D. Ostrow, Evidence for
      conversion of bilirubin to dihydroxyl derivatives in
      the Gunn rat, Biochem. Biophys. Res. Commun. 49:1366 (1972).
19. A.F. McDonagh, L.A. Palma, and D.A. Lightner, Blue light and
      bilirubin excretion, Science 208:145 (1980).
20. A.F. McDonagh, unpublished observations.

MECHANISMS OF ACTION OF PHOTOTHERAPY: NEW CONCEPTS

John F. Ennever and William T. Speck

Department of Pediatrics
Rainbow Babies and Childrens Hospital
Case Western Reserve University School of Medicine
Cleveland, Ohio 44106   USA

INTRODUCTION

Visible light phototherapy is the most common method for treating neonatal hyperbilirubinemia. It is estimated that 2% to 6% of all infants born in the United States and Britain receive phototherapy (1,2). This treatment has long been considered both safe and effective. Reported side effects of phototherapy are generally of little clinical significance and all disappear following cessation of illumination (1,3). However, recent in vitro studies showing that light of wavelengths between 350 and 450 nm is mutagenic for procaryotic and eucaryotic cells (4,5,6), and therefore potentially carcinogenic, have caused concern because all commonly-used phototherapy lamps emit radiation in this region (7).

The design of an optimal light source for phototherapy requires knowledge of the action spectrum for the therapeutic effect of visible light. Until recently, it was assumed that photodegradation of bilirubin was responsible for the decline in serum bilirubin during phototherapy. It is now apparent that several photochemical reactions of bilirubin occur in vivo (8,9,10). The fastest reaction is configurational isomerization of the native form of bilirubin, called 4Z,15Z-bilirubin, to more polar isomers (11,12); in humans the 4Z,15E configuration predominates (11,13). Other reactions also occur in vivo, the most important being structural isomerization of bilirubin to an intramolecularly cyclized product called lumirubin (14). The relative contributions of configurational and structural isomerization to the therapeutic response to phototherapy in humans are not known; however, in the Gunn rat model, the configurational isomerization reaction is quantitatively more important (13).

187

In this paper we describe in vitro studies on the wavelength dependence for the configurational isomerization (15). In addition, we will present clinical studies performed in collaboration with Drs. R.A. Polin and A.T. Costarino at Children's Hospital of Philadelphia on the relationship between the dose of light used in phototherapy and the serum concentration of configurational and structural isomers (16). Finally, we will provide data on the rate of clearance of the configurational isomer from the serum of premature infants (17). Our clinical data suggest that configurational isomerization may not be the most important photochemical reaction occurring in jaundiced infants under phototherapy.

WAVELENGTH DEPENDENCE FOR THE CONFIGURATIONAL ISOMERIZATION OF BILIRUBIN

Most of the bilirubin in jaundiced infants is present as a complex bound to albumin (18). Recent data suggest that bilirubin undergoes configurational isomerization while bound to this protein (13). Therefore, in our in vitro studies on the wavelength dependence of this reaction we used aqueous solutions of bilirubin (44 umolar) bound to human serum albumin (88 umolar) at pH 7.4. These solutions were irradiated with narrow-band light (10 nm half-bandwidth) and the isomer composition was determined by high pressure liquid chromatography on a C-18 reversed phase column as described by McDonagh et al. (11). The results shown in Fig. 1 demonstrate that irradiation of bilirubin with any light falling within the molecule's absorption band results in the rapid conversion of the native 4Z,15Z molecule to the 4Z,15E isomer.

The configurational isomerization of bilirubin is a photochemically reversible reaction (11,12). In a closed system the isomerization of native bilirubin must compete with re-isomerization:

$$\text{4Z,15Z-bilirubin} \xrightleftharpoons[h\nu]{h\nu} \text{4Z,15E-bilirubin} \qquad (1)$$

[Bilirubin bound to a molar excess of human albumin does not isomerize at the C-4 exocyclic double bond (14).] Thus, in such a system an equilibrium is eventually reached. The amount of the 4Z,15E isomer at equilibrium is highly wavelength dependent (Fig. 1). The most efficient wavelength in vitro was 390 nm which produced greater than 40% conversion of native bilirubin to the 4Z,15E isomer at equilibrium (no increase in isomer concentration was produced by further irradiation). As the wavelength was increased from 390 to 470 nm the percent 4Z,15E at equilibrium gradually decreased. Similarly, irradiation of bilirubin-albumin solutions with wavelengths of light below 390 produced less 4Z,15E isomer at equilibrium (data not shown). Light of wavelengths greater than 490 were ineffective in the configurational

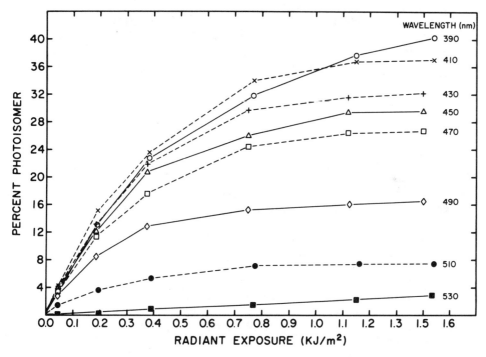

Fig. 1. Wavelength dependence for the configurational isomerization
         of bilirubin.

isomerization of bilirubin.   Not only was green (530 nm) light ineffective in the configurational isomerization of native bilirubin,
exposure of solutions containing high concentrations of the 4Z,15E
isomer (e.g., a photoequilibrium mixture generated by 450 nm light) to
green light resulted in reversion of the photoisomer back to native
bilirubin.

     These data demonstrate that the equilibrium defined by equation 1
is wavelength dependent.   In the Gunn rat the steady-state (serum)
concentration of the configurational isomers remains low (13), because
of rapid clearance of the photoproducts. Thus, in this animal model,
the influence of this wavelength dependence would not be apparent.
However, recent studies have shown that in human infants concentration
of the 4Z,15E configurational isomer in serum during phototherapy is
as high as 20% of the total bilirubin (9,10,13).   If the configurational isomerization reaction is therapeutically important in humans,
the wavelength dependence for this reaction may affect the efficacy of
phototherapy. In vivo the effectiveness of certain wavelengths may be
attenuated by light scattering or absorption by other chromophores
(19).   Despite these limitations, certain conclusions about phototherapy can be made based upon our in vitro data.   Non-geonotoxic

wavelengths of light (greater than 450 nm) are effective in the configurational isomerization of bilirubin. Furthermore, our data suggest that if configurational isomerization is a clinically important
photochemical raction, then presence of green light in the broad-
spectrum (white) phototherapy units may be counterproductive. Thus, a
phototherapy unit with spectral output limited to 460 to 480 nm, which
would be devoid of in vitro DNA-modifying activity (4,5,6), may prove
clinically effective.

CONFIGURATIONAL AND STRUCTURAL ISOMERIZATION OF BILIRUBIN: DOSE-RESPONSE RELATIONSHIP

Several investigators have demonstrated a relationship between
the "dose" of phototherapy (usually measured at 450 nm) and the therapeutic response, i.e., the rate of decline in serum bilirubin
(20,21,22). A limitation in these studies is that the decrease in
serum bilirubin represents a secondary response to light therapy.
More specific, the primary effect of light is isomerization of bilirubin to more polar configurational and structural isomers (11,12,14).
The decrease in serum bilirubin requires transport of these photoproducts from their site of formation to the liver where they are
excreted into the bile (13). The purpose of this study was to determine the effect of light dose on the production of configurational and
structural isomers of bilirubin.

The study population consisted of 20 premature infants with
physiological jaundice admitted to the Infant Intensive Care Unit of
The Children's Hospital of Philadelphia. The patients were prospectively randomized into two groups: One group received 6 uwatt/cm2-nm,
the other, 12 uwatt/cm2-nm, delivered by Cavitron model PT1400 phototherapy unit with a 250 watt tungsten halogen lamp (General Electric
type ENH). Irradiance was measured with a clinical, fixed band-width
radiometer (Air Shields PR-III). Blood samples were obtained prior to
the initiation of phototherapy, and after two hours, four hours and
eight hours of continuous treatment. During sample collection from
indwelling arterial catheters, phototherapy was briefly interrupted
and the lights in the nursery dimmed. The serum was separated by
centrifugation and stored frozen until analyzed for bilirubin and
bilirubin photoproducts by high pressure liquid chromatography (11).

The effect of light dose and treatment time on the concentration
of configurational isomers is shown Table I. Prior to the initiation
of phototherapy, a significant percent of the total bilirubin in both
groups of infants was present as configurational isomers. The percent
of these isomers increased over the first four hours of phototherapy.
No statistically significant difference was found between the two
groups in the percent of the total bilirubin converted to configurational isomers.

TABLE I. EFFECT OF LIGHT DOSE ON SERUM LEVEL OF CONFIGURATIONAL
                         ISOMER

Dose of Light (uwatt/cm2-nm)	Percent of Total Bilirubin Present As Configurational Isomers			
	hours of phototherapy			
	0	2	4	8
6	6.5 (0.8)*	9.5 (0.8)	10.8 (0.9)	11.6 (0.8)
12	6.3 (1.0)	10.5 (0.9)	12.1 (0.7)	12.5 (0.7)

* standard error of the mean.

Table II contains the data on lumirubin concentration in the serum of infants treated with high and low dose phototherapy for eight hours. Lumirubin was either absent or present in small amounts prior to the initiation of phototherapy. In both groups the lumirubin concentration increased with exposure to phototherapy, reaching maximal levels in approximately two hours in the group receiving low dose phototherapy and four hours in the high dose group. The difference between the two groups in the percent of the total bilirubin present as lumirubin was significant at both four hours ($p < .05$) and eight hours ($p < .01$).

TABLE II. EFFECT OF LIGHT DOSE ON SERUM LEVEL OF LUMIRUBIN

Dose of Light (uwatt/cm2-nm)	Percent of Total Bilirubin Present as Lumirubin			
	hours of phototherapy			
	0	2	4	8
6	0.2 (0.1)*	0.6 (0.1)	0.7 (0.1)	0.7 (0.1)
12	0.2 (0.1)	0.8 (0.1)	1.3 (0.3)	1.5 (0.4)

* standard error of the mean

These data confirm previous reports that the major bilirubin photoproducts in vivo are configurational isomers (9,10), principally the 4Z,15E isomer (13). The steady-state level of these isomers was 12%, which is comparable to the in vitro photoequilibrium of 14.5% produced by the tungsten-halogen lamp used in this study (7). Thus, the concentration of configurational isomers in the serum of premature infants receiving phototherapy approaches that found when bilirubin solutions are irradiated in a closed system (see below). Although we did not compare the clinical efficacy (i.e., rate of decline in serum bilirubin) of low vs. high dose phototherapy in this study, other investigators have demonstrated increased bilirubin elimination with higher dose phototherapy (20,21). These data indicate that this improved clinical efficacy cannot be attributed to higher production of configurational isomers.

Structural isomerization of bilirubin to lumirubin also occurs in infants exposed to phototherapy (9,13). As expected on the basis of quantum yields (12), serum levels of this isomer are less than those of the configurational isomers. We found significantly higher levels of lumirubin in the serum of patients exposed to the higher intensity phototherapy (Table II). These data suggest that the improved clinical efficacy of higher intensity phototherapy may be the result of increased production and elimination of this structural isomer of bilirubin.

IN VIVO CLEARANCE OF BILIRUBIN PHOTOPRODUCTS

Studies in a number of laboratories, including our own, have demonstrated that the principal photoproducts formed during phototherapy are configurational isomers of bilirubin (9,10,13). The therapeutic response to phototherapy (decline in serum bilirubin) requires excretion of these photoproducts. McDonagh and his co-workers have shown that the decline in serum bilirubin in the Gunn rat exposed to phototherapy is principally the result of biliary excretion of these polar isomers of bilirubin (8,13). Significant differences exist between the photochemistry of bilirubin in the Gunn rat and the human newborn infant. The most important difference is that the rate of biliary excretion of the configurational isomers in the Gunn rat is greater. In the rat, excretion is so efficient that serum levels of these photoproducts are nearly undetectable (13). As the data presented above demonstrate, in the human infant near photo-equilibrium levels of configurational isomers are found in the serum. These observations indicate that hepatic clearance of these photoisomers in the human infant is not nearly as efficient as in the Gunn rat. Moreover, the therapeutic response to phototherapy in newborn infants, in contrast to the experimental animal model, may not be as dependent on excretion of configurational isomers. The purpose of this study was to quantitate the the rate of disappearance of configurational isomers in premature infants following cessation of phototherapy.

We have studied six premature infants (mean gestational age 30 weeks) who received continuous phototherapy from a bank of eight daylight fluorescent lamps for from two to eight days. Blood samples were obtained by heel stick or venipuncture in darkened rooms and immediately placed in opaque tubes; the serum was separated by centrifugation and stored frozen until analysis. For each patient, one sample was obtained immediately following the end of phototherapy; over the next nine hours, two additional samples were drawn; and a final serum specimen was obtained twelve to twenty-four hours after phototherapy. The bilirubin isomer composition was analyzed by high pressure liquid chromatography (11). The concentration of configurational isomers in each sample was determined from the integrated area on the chromatographs. For each patient, the serum half-life of the configurational isomers was calculated from the slope of semilogarithmic plots of isomer concentration vs. time following phototherapy.

The rate of clearance for the configurational isomers from the serum was first-order over the initial eight to ten hours. Following this initial period, the concentration of the photoisomer declined more slowly. The half-life of the configurational isomers in the serum, calculated from the initial rate of disappearance, ranged from 12 to 21 hours with a mean of 15 hours. Control experiments demonstrated negligible thermal reversion of the photoisomers in buffered serum samples at 37 °C. Thus, although the disappearance of configurational isomers from the serum is slow, it most likely represents clearance rather than simple reversion of the isomers back to native bilirubin.

Our data establish that the clearance of configurational photoisomers in preterm infants is inefficient. These results contrast with that of Lamola et al. (10) who reported a serum half-life of 1.5 hours for the isomers in a three year-old girl with Crigler-Najar (I) syndrome. These disparate clearance rates may reflect differences in analytical techniques used in the two studies; alternatively, older children may excrete bilirubin configurational isomers more efficiently than premature infants. Using our clearance data, one can calculate the maximum rate of decline in serum bilirubin which can be attributed to excretion of the configurational isomers. With a total serum bilirubin concentration of 20 mg/dl, a steady-state of 20% configurational isomer and a half-life of 15 hours, the rate of bilirubin reduction would be 0.17 mg/dl/hr. This rate of decline in bilirubin is clearly an overestimate because it assumes no ongoing bilirubin production and no enterohepatic recirculation of previously excreted pigment. Since far greater therapeutic responses to phototherapy have been documented (20,22), our data indicate that alternative photochemical reactions must contribute to the clinical effectiveness of phototherapy.

Structural isomerization of bilirubin to lumirubin also occurs in infants exposed to phototherapy (see above). Although steady-state levels of lumirubin were much lower than those of the configurational isomers (0.5-2% vs. 18-20% of total bilirubin), the clearance of the structural isomer from the serum was more rapid. In all patients studied, lumirubin was detectable only in the serum samples obtained immediately following cessation of phototherapy. None was found in serum specimens obtained two to three hours after phototherapy. Thus, although lumirubin is not the principal photoisomer produced in vivo, this photoproduct may be quantitatively important in phototherapy because of its rapid excretion. Further studies are in progress to determine the contribution of lumirubin excretion to the decline in serum bilirubin concentration produced by phototherapy.

CONCLUSIONS

The principal photochemical reactions of bilirubin in vitro and in vivo are configurational and structural isomerization. In the human infant, the rate limiting step in the elimination of bilirubin is not in the formation of these polar photoproducts, but rather in their excretion. In premature infants excretion of the configurational isomers is so slow that this pathway cannot account for the therapeutic effect of phototherapy. Although quantitative data are not available, excretion of the structural isomer, lumirubin, appears to be much more rapid. Determination of the relative contributions of these two photochemical reactions to the clinically observed effect of phototherapy is needed. This information is required for the design of a more effective light source which will be devoid of DNA-modifying activity.

REFERENCES

1. A.K. Brown and A.F. McDonagh, Phototherapy for neonatal hyperbilirubinemia: Efficiency, mechanism and toxicity, Adv . Pediatr. 27:341 (1980).

2. H.M. Lewis, R.H.A. Campbell, and G. Hambleton, Use or abuse of phototherapy for physiological jaundice of newborn infants, Lancet 2:408 (1982).

3. M.J. Maisels, Neonatal jaundice, in: "Neonatology," G.B. Avery, ed., Lippincott Co., Philadelphia (1981).

4. W.T. Speck and H.S. Rosencranz, Base substitution mutations induced in Salmonella strains by visible light (450 nm), Photochem. Photobiol. 21:369 (1975).

5. R. Parshand, K.K. Sanford, G.M. Jones, and R.E. Tarone, Fluorescent light-induced chromosome damage and its prevention in mouse cells in culture, Proc. Natl. Acad. Sci. USA 75:1830 (1978).

6. E.G. Sideris, G.C. Papageorgiou, S.C. Charalampous, and E.M. Vitsa, A spectrum response study on single strand DNA breaks, sister chromatid exchanges and lethality induced by phototherapy lights, Pediatr. Res. 15:1019 (1981).

7. J.F. Ennever, M. Sobel, A.F. McDonagh, and W.T. Speck, Phototherapy for neonatal jaundice: In vitro comparison of light sources, manuscript in preparation.

8. A.F. McDonagh and L.A. Palma, Hepatic excretion of circulating bilirubin photoproducts in the Gunn rat, J. Clin. Invest. 66:1182 (1980).

9. S. Onishi, K. Isobe, S. Itoh, N. Kawade, and S. Sugiyoima, Demonstration of a geometric isomer of bilirubin IXa in the serum of a hyperbilirubinaemic newborn infant and the mechanism of jaundice phototherapy, Biochem. J. 190:533 (1980).

10. A.A. Lamola, W.E. Blumberg, R. McClead, and A. Fanaroff, Photoisomerized bilirubin in blood from infants receiving phototherapy, Proc. Natl. Acad. Sci. USA 78:1882 (1981).

11. A.F. McDonagh, L.A. Palma, F.R. Trull, and D.A. Lightner, Phototherapy for neonatal jaundice: Configurational isomers of bilirubin, J. Am. Chem. Soc. 104:6865 (1982).

12. A.A. Lamola, J.Flores, and F.H. Doleiden, Quantum yield and equilbrium position of the configurational photoisomerization of bilirubin bound to human serum albumin, Photochem. Photobiol. 35:649 (1982).

13. A.F. McDonagh, J.F. Ennever, and L.A. Palma, Phototherapy for neonatal jaundice: Configurational photoisomerization of bilirubin in babies is regioselective, manuscript in preparation.

14. A.F. McDonagh, L.A. Palma, and D.A. Lightner, Phototherapy for neonatal jaundice: Stereospecific and regioselective photoisomerization of bilrubin bound to human serum albumin and NMR characterization of intramolecularly syslized photoproducts, J. Am. Chem. Soc. 104:6867 (1982).

15. J.F. Ennever, A.F. McDonagh, and W.T. Speck, Phototherapy for neonatal jaundice: Optimal wavelengths of light, J. Pediatr. in press.

16. A.T.Costarino, J.F. Ennever, S.Baumgart, M.Paul, W.T. Speck, and R.A. Polin, Bilirubin photoisomerization in premature neonates under low and high dose phototherapy, manuscript in preparation.

17. J.F. Ennever, I.Knox, S.C. Denne, and W.T. Speck, Phototherapy for neonatal jaundice: In vivo clearance of bilirubin photoproducts, submitted for publication.

18. R. Schmid and L.Hammaker, Metabolism and disposition of C14-bilirubin in congenital nonhemolytic jaundice, J. Clin. Invest. 42:1720 (1963).

19. R.R. Anderson and J.A. Parrish, The optics of human skin, J. Invest. Dermatol. 77:13 (1981).

20. K.L. Tan, The pattern of bilirubin response to phototherapy for neonatal hyperbilirubinemia, Pediatr. Res. 16:670 (1982).

21. L. Ballowitz, G.Geutler, J.Krochmann, R. Pannitschka, G. Roemer, and I. Roemer, Phototherapy in Gunn rats - a study to assess the photobiologically most effective radiant energy and dose/response relationships, Biol. Neonate 31:229 (1977).
22. J.B. Warshaw, J.Gagliardi, and A. Patel, A comparison of fluorescent and non-fluorescent light sources for phototherapy, Pediatrics 65:795 (1980).

LASER-ORIENTED SEARCH OF THE OPTIMUM LIGHT FOR PHOTOTHERAPY

G.P.Donzelli[1], M.G.Migliorini[2], R. Pratesi[4],
G. Sbrana[3], and C.Vecchi[1]

(1) Istituto di Pediatria, Università di Firenze
(2) Istituto di Chimica-Fisica, Università di Firenze
(3) Centro di Studio dei Composti Eterociclici del
     CNR, Firenze
(4) Istituto di Elettronica Quantistica del CNR,
     · Firenze

INTRODUCTION

The availability of coherent optical sources (lasers) has
permitted a rapid development of photosurgical and photocoagu-
lative techniques during the last decade[1]. Photomedicine[2] appeared another very interesting field for laser applications in view
of the potential progresses in the already existing phototherapeutical procedures, and for the importance of laser techniques in
the photobiological field[3]. The laser photochemotherapy of tumors[4] represents a noticeable example of this prevision.

Phototherapy of hyperbilirubinemia in the newborn is a widely accepted procedure to lower bilirubin concentration in plasma.
However, despite intense clinical and experimental efforts, the
clinical procedure is still largely empirical and the mechanism
responsible for the clearance of bilirubin in light-exposed babies is not yet clearly defined[5].

Visible lasers are very convenient sources of narrow-band,
intense radiation to be used for more detailed studies of bilirubin photochemistry "in vitro" and "in vivo". For instance, the
small spectral differences among the various bilirubin photoproducts can be more easily shown using nearly-spaced laser lines or
frequency tunable lasers.

197

        In 1980 an investigation was promoted by the CNR Special
Project on Laser Applications in Medicine to explore the utiliza-
tion of longer wavelength, narrow-spectral regions in the phototherapy of hyperbilirubinemia in order to reduce the potential
side-effects associated with the near ultraviolet, violet-blue
radiation emitted by fluorescent lamps used for phototherapy[6].
Preliminary observations showed that laser photolysis of bilirubin "in vitro" could be efficiently achieved also with the 514
nm green laser line[7]. Confirmation of this result with narrow-
spectrum fluorescent green lamps "in vitro" led to clinical comparison of green and white lights. A greater efficiency of green
lamps than white fluorescent lamps was reported[8]. Further research was then devoted to compare green lamps with the "special"
blue lamps, and to understand the possible mechanisms responsible
for the observed and unexpected good efficiency of green light.

        In this paper we report in a preliminary way: "in vitro"
measurements of the influence of pH on bilirubin degradation at
various wavelengths at relatively large laser irradiances; comparative results with green and special blue fluorescent lamps in
clinical therapy; the influence of skin filtering on the spectral
efficacy of light sources for phototherapy; low irradiance investigations of bilirubin photoisomerization. In the last section,
the possible future development of solid state light-emitting de-
vices (incoherent or coherent) for phototherapy is also discussed.

LASER DEGRADATION OF BILIRUBIN "IN VITRO"

        Bilirubin (BR) supplied from Sigma (USA) was used without
further purifications. BR was dissolved in anhydrous chloroform,
phosphate buffer and phosphate buffer containing 4% human serum
albumin (HSA). The concentration of these solutions was about 10
μM. Human serum of jaundiced infants was diluted with phosphate
buffer, pH 7.5, up to a bilirubin concentration of $\approx$ 21 μM. Solutions in phosphate buffer with and without HSA were examined at
three different pH values: 6.9, 7.5, and 9.0. Standard fluorescence cells (1 cm path-length) were employed to irradiate the solutions with an Argon laser (Coherent Radiation, Model 52.A). The
light absorbed by the BR solution was evaluated by measuring the
laser input and output intensities from the cell (Coherent Radiation Power Meter Mod.210). Laser irradiances were 180, 130 and 20

mW/cm^2 for the three lines at 514.5, 488.0 and 457.9 nm used in
the experiment, respectively. The decrease of absorbance at 460 nm
has been measured as a function of the photon fluence absorbed by
BR solutions.

In chloroform the results are quite different from those previously reported in Ref.7 by considering the actual energy absorbed
by the solution. In particular, the green line (514.5 nm) is largely more efficient in BR degradation than the blue (488.0 nm) and
violet (457.9 nm) lines which give curves with a similar pattern.

The observation of the curves showing BR degradation in phosphate buffer, in phosphate buffer with HSA, and in human serum substantially confirms a comparable efficiency of the three laser lines, even if in general the green line appears to be slightly less
efficient.

The photodegradation process is faster at pH 6.9; however,
the efficiency of the laser radiation seems to be independent of
the pH. As an example in Fig.1 we report three typical plots describing the pH-dependency in phosphate buffer containing BR and
HSA.

In conclusions, these results confirm previous data[7,9], which
support the large efficiency of wavelengths longer than 490 nm "in
vitro". Our experiments also show that the relative efficiency of
the three laser lines as well as the BR photodegradation rate are
practically uneffected by different pH values.

CLINICAL COMPARISON OF SPECIAL BLUE AND GREEN LAMPS

Sources with different emission spectra, such as daylight,
blue and special blue fluorescent lamps, have been used in the
clinical procedure. However, light wavelengths between 440 nm and
470 nm are still considered most effective in reducing serum BR
level, and wavelengths outside this spectral range are considered
as having no or very little effect.

The "in vitro" experiments on laser photolysis of BR[7] allo-
wed us to employ narrow-spectrum fluorescent green lamps ($\lambda_{max} \simeq$
525 nm) in the phototherapy (PT) of neonatal hyperbilirubinemia.
Many jaundiced babies have been exposed to green lamps in our neonatal intensive care unit; since June 1981 we have replaced the
daylight tubes of our PT units with fluorescent green tubes. Our
previous investigations showed the ability of green light to induce BR degradation and we recommended the use of fluorescent
lamps instead of daylight and superblue lamps in phototherapy of

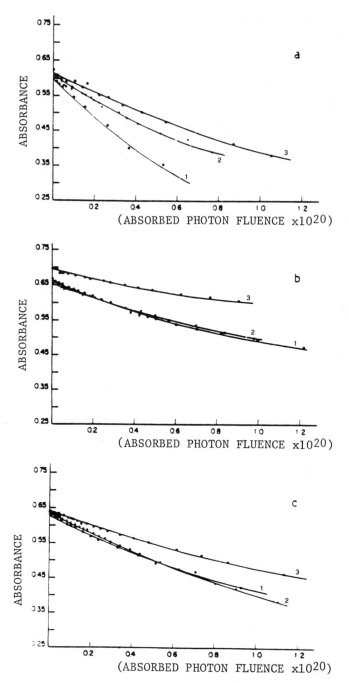

Fig. 1. Effect of different wavelength radiations on BR photodecomposition in a 4% HSA-buffer phosphate solution at
pH 6.9 (a), pH 7.5 (b) and pH 9.0 (c); λ(nm)=457.9 (1);
488.0 (2); 514.5 (3).

neonatal hyperbilirubinemia[8,10]. After the initial 24 h exposure
the mean decrement of BR was 20.3% for green lamps and 15.8% for
daylight lamps[11,12].

We report now a preliminary study comparing superblue and
green light sources. Two identical PT units, each consisting of 8
closely-spaced fluorescent lamps, have been used. Power irradiance
at the baby position was $\approx$ 3 mW/cm^2 for both PT units when equipped with Westinghouse F20T12/BB and Sylvania F20F12/G lamps (Power Meter Mod.210, Coherent Rad., USA). Twenty low-birth-weight
infants (LBWI) were randomly assigned to green lamps (10 babies)
or to superblue fluorescent lamps (10 babies). Some typical clinical features of LBWI were present in the subjects exposed to
phototherapy (hypoglicemia, hypocalcemia, etc.). No infants were
included with maternal-fetal blood group incompatibility, other
hemolytic diseases, respiratory distress and sepsis. Serum bilirubin concentration was determined by a spectrophotometric method
(Bilirubin Tester Wako) at 6,12,24 h from the beginning of PT. Birth
weight (g), gestational age (weeks), and BR concentration (mg/dl)
were 1970 (1700÷2400), 34 (31÷38) and 12.7 (11.0÷15.6), respectively for the group exposed to blue light, and 1915 (900÷2400), 35
(25÷42), 12.8 (9.6÷15.2), respectively for the group irradiated
with green light. The number of cases is too small to permit any
statistical evaluation. However, the simple comparison of the two
sets of data indicates that the evolution of BR concentration in
the two groups is similar enough. Moreover, by comparing the mean
values of BR concentration reported in Table 1 we note that blue
and green lights produce the same BR decrement after the initial
6 h irradiation, and lead to the same final values of BR concentration after 24 h exposure.

Table 1. Mean BR levels after 6,12,24 h-irradiation with
special blue and green fluorescent lamps

	Bilirubin concentration (mg/dl)							
	Special blue				Green			
T(h)	0	6	12	24	0	6	12	24
mean value	12.72	11.42	11.00	9.97	12.77	11.46	10.25	9.81

These preliminary findings, if confirmed by the complete
analysis will permit replacing white and blue lamps with green
lamps even if the latter exhibit a slightly smaller efficiency. The
possibility of using lower energy photons should be taken into account to reduce the potential side-effects of PT, including the
recently reported observations on the toxic and mutagenic effects
of 400÷450 nm light[6], and the risks of non-thermal retinal damage[13].

THE INFLUENCE OF LIGHT ABSORPTION AND SCATTERING IN SKIN ON THE
SPECTRAL EFFICIENCY OF PHOTOTHERAPY
(In collaboration with L.Ronchi, IROE-CNR, Firenze, and G.Cecchi,
  IEQ-CNR, Firenze)

The determination of the optimum peak wavelength and spectral bandwidth for phototherapy (PT) is still an open problem. Nar-
row spectrum fluorescent tubes emitting at ≈ 450 nm have been recommended for efficient PT since long time[14] on the basis of many
"in vitro" and "in vivo" action spectra of BR degradation[15]. On
the other hand, recent measurements made with monochromatic laser
light at several wavelengths in the blue-green part of the spectrum
have shown that a greater efficiency for BR degradation can be a-
chieved at wavelengths considerably longer than the peak absorption
wavelength of BR "in vitro"[7,9]. Moreover, since the relevant mechanism for BR excretion from the body is still undetermined, the spectral dependence of the various photoisomerization processes of BR
are expected to play an important role in determining the most efficient spectral region for PT[16].

The effect of the optical properties of the skin on PT efficiency has been taken into account only in a very qualitative way
due to the lack of a sufficiently accurate model of skin optics.
Recent improvements of skin optics theory[17] now make it possible
to obtain more quantitative information about the influence of
light transmission through the skin on the spectral efficiency of
PT.

In this analysis we consider the jaundiced skin as composed
of multiple layers possessing distinct optical properties. Dermal
BR is assumed to be confined within an optical thin layer underlying a 100 μm thick epidermal (ED) layer and a 200 μm thick dermal (D) layer. Values of ED and D absorption and scattering coefficients are derived from "in vitro" measurements on skin reported
in the literature[17,18]. The competing effect due to hemoglobin (HB)
absorption in the blood is taken into account by introducing a Hb-

layer of suitable thicknesses between the D-layer and BR-layer.

The rate of photon absortption, A, in the BR-layer is given by:

$$A(\nu_p) = \int T(\nu)\sigma(\nu)N(\nu,\nu_p)d\nu$$

where $T(\nu)$ denotes the transmission of the composite ED-D-HbO$_2$ layer, $\sigma(\nu)$ the absorption cross-section of BR, $N(\nu,\nu_p)$ the photon fluence rate of the light source at peak frequency ν_p in the frequency interval $\nu,\nu + d\nu$. The transmission spectra $T(\nu)$ have been computed and reported elsewhere[19].

Fig.2 shows the computed $A(\lambda_p)$ spectra of BR for a nearly

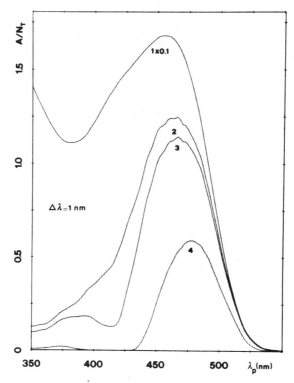

Fig.2 . $A(\lambda_p)$ spectra for nearly monochromatic light ($\Delta\lambda$=1 nm). d_{ED}= 100 µm; d_D= 200 µm; γ= 2.3(cd)$_{HbO2}$= 0,10^{-5}, 10^{-4}(curve 2,3,4 respectively) cm.M/1. The case corresponding to the "in vitro" situation is also shown for comparison (curve 1). To get absorption rates (s^{-1}) multiply A-values by 10^{-17}N$_T$ (phot./scm^2)

monochromatic ($\Delta\lambda$ = 1nm) light source as the function of the peak
wavelength λ_p between 350 nm and 600 nm for several values of the
parameter $\gamma \equiv 2.3$ (concentration x thickness) of the HbO_2-layer.
The A-value for $T(\lambda) = 1$ (which corresponds to an "in vitro" irradiation)is also shown for comparison: it simply reproduces the
absorption spectrum of BR (curve 1). The effect of the blood-free
skin layers (curve 2) is a marked reduction of the absorption rate
between 350 nm and 425 nm, and a shift $\delta\lambda$ = 12 nm of $A(\lambda_p)$ towards
longer wavelengths. This is mainly due to the strong wavelength
dependence in this region of 1) dermal scattering coefficient,
which varies[18] approximately as $\lambda^{-2.5}$; 2) epidermal absorption
coefficient which closely corresponds to the absorption spectrum
of melanin. UV-violet-blue radiation is highly absorbed and scat-
tered by the skin: therefore, the shorter wavelength part of the
absorption curve of BR is sensibly less efficient than the longer
wavelength part for BR photoisomerization. The effect of blood absorption is to further decrease A(curves 3,4) and shift the A-maxi-
mum towards longer wavelengths ($\delta\lambda \simeq 24$ nm for γ 10^{-4} cm M/1).

     Finally, Table 2 reports the A-values for several fluores-
cent lamps used in PT. A blue light-emitting diode (LED) has also
been included in view of a possible future development of LED ar-

Table 2. $A(\lambda_p)$-values for several commercial light sources and
         blood content γ. d_{ED}= 100 μm; d_D= 200 μm. To get absorp-
         tion rates (s^{-1}) multiply A-values by $10^{-19}N_T$ (phot./s.
         . cm^2)

LAMP	"IN VITRO"	$\gamma = 0$	10^{-6}	10^{-5}	10^{-4}
PHILIPS/BLU TL20WO3/T	1478.4	68.7	64.5	39.4	4.5
WESTINGHOUSE/BB F20T12/BB	1579.9	107.9	106.5	90.9	28.3
SIEMENS LED/BLU SFH 710	874.6	66.4	65.7	59.5	27.6
SYLVANIA DAYLIGHT F20F12DA	636.9	46.6	45.9	40.8	18.8
SYLVANIA GREEN F20F12G	114.2	11.0	10.9	10.4	6.2
SYLVANIA GOLD F20F12GO	16.7	1.2	1.2	1.1	0.9

rays for PT[20,21]. In the "in vitro" case (first column) the WEST/
BB ($\lambda_p \simeq 448$ nm; $\Delta\lambda \simeq 34$ nm) lamp with its peak emission matching
the absorption spectrum maximum of BR is, as expected, the most
efficient lamp to excite BR molecules. The PHIL/B ($\lambda_p \simeq 421$ nm,
$\Delta\lambda \simeq 33$ nm) lamp has the emission maximum shifted toward smaller
wavelengths, where BR absorption is lower, and results $\approx 6\%$ less
efficient than WEST/BB lamp. DAYLIGHT lamps are ≈ 2.3 times less
efficient than WEST/BB. The second column shows the effect of the
filtering action of the blood-free ED-D layers. The efficacy of
WEST/BB is reduced by a factor ≈ 15 owing to skin scattering and
absorption; the effect is more pronounced for the PHIL/B lamp, whose
efficiency is now only $\approx 63\%$ of that of WEST/BB. DAYLIGHT lamps
maintain their relative efficacy with respect to WEST/BB. When the
presence of the skin vascular system is taken into account, the
blue radiation around the Soret maximum of HbO_2 (at 418 nm) is
further attenuated. The efficiency of PHIL/B drops rapidly, while
those of SYLV/DAYL and SYLV/GR remain nearly constant and are reduced only for the highest value of $(cd)_{HbO_2}$: in this case the A-
value of the SYLV/GR lamp becomes larger than the A-value of the
PHIL/B lamp; the A-value of the SYLV/DAYL is now only $\approx 33\%$ smaller than the WEST/BB. Also the SYLV/GR has now doubled its efficacy relative to WEST/BB with respect to the case of blood-free skin.
The WEST/BB remains the most effective lamp over the entire range
examined.

It may be noted that the efficiency of the LED/BLU practically equals that of the WEST/BB lamp at a larger blood content.

In conclusion, the above results show that the upper skin
layers and hematic vascular system affect the optimum value of
the peak wavelength of the light source to be used for PT. The
balance between light losses in the skin and good light absorption
by BR molecules leads to an optimum peak wavelength for the photon
absorption rate around $\lambda \simeq 480$ nm, i.e. to a ≈ 30 nm wavelength
shift with respect to the BR absorption maximum in solution. This
result calls for clinical investigation of the comparative efficacy of new blue-green narrow-spectrum fluorescent lamps.

Finally we note that the higher efficiency of green as compared with white lamps[12], and the good efficiency of green lamp
with respect to special blue lamps reported in the preceeding section cannot be justified by this analysis: the effect of light at
still larger depths where green light becomes increasingly more
efficient than blue and white light, or a larger efficiency of the
transformation of BR and/or BR photoisomers into more easily excre-

table photoproducts at longer wavelengths could be two out of the
possible causes.

LASER INVESTIGATION OF BILIRUBIN ⇄ PHOTOBILIRUBIN CONVERSION
(In collaboration with G.Agati, F.Fusi, Istituto di Farmacologia
dell'Università, Firenze)

Any progress in the understanding of BR photochemistry may
lead to a better knowledge of the mechanisms responsible for PT
and to an improvement of phototherapeutical procedures. In this
section we report preliminary observations on the wavelength de-
pendences of photobilirubin/bilirubin (PBR/BR) photoequilibrium
(PE) and PBR → BR photoreversion.

Solutions of BR (10 μm) in HSA (115 μM phosphate-buffered
solutions at pH = 7.4) were irradiated by a continuous wave argon
laser at different wavelengths. A low-intensity white light beam
entering the BR cuvette (8 mm path length) at a right angle to the
laser beam was used to monitor the absorption spectra with a PARC
multichannel optical analyzer (OMA-2) connected to a grating poly-
chromator[22].

Wavelength Dependence of PBR Formation

Fig.3 shows the differential absorption spectra (DAS) in the
430-520 nm range taken at $1.25 \cdot 10^{15}$ phot/cm^{2}s (≈ 0.5 mW/cm^2) of
laser irradiance for three values of the laser excitation wave-
length (λ=457.9, 488.0, 501.7, 514.5 nm). An isosbestic point is
present at λ =465 nm, and the DAS maximum occurs at λ =490 nm. Similar spectral patterns have been obtained at lower and higher (15
mW/cm^2) irradiances[22]. The 457-line produces the highest value of
photoequilibrium PBR/BR mixture, while the 514-line turns out to
be quite ineffective for PBR formation. This is in agreement with
the measurements reported by Ennever[5] on isomer composition obtained by irradiating BR to PE by 10-nm-band-width light. At high irradiances PEs are reached at nearly the same corresponding values
of energy fluence; further irradiation of the solution produces a
degradation of the PBR/BR mixture, as demonstrated by the lowering
of the entire DAS.

Spectral Dependence of PBR → BR Reversion

PBRs have been observed to revert to the original BR on 510
nm irradiation[23]. We have checked PBR reversion in a greater de-

tail using different laser lines at several irradiances. Fig.(4a,
b,c/2) shows the formation of new PE values of a PBR/BR photoequilibrium mixture, obtained upon irradiation of BR at 457 nm (Fig.4a,
b,c/1) using the three lines at 488, 501 and 514 nm. It turns out
that: i) the complete reversion of PBR into BR is not achievable
with these lines; ii) the greatest reversion efficiency is associated with the 514-line, followed by the 501 and 488 lines. Interestingly the reverted DAS are now asymmetric, with the maximum
shifted towards the longer wavelength, when the 514 and 501 lines
are used. The effect is much less evident with the 488 line. This
may suggest the appearence of "additional" photoproducts, not pre-

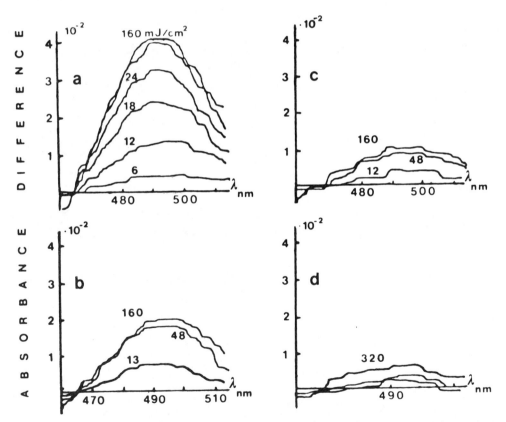

Fig.3. DAS for excitation at 457(a), 488(b), 501(c), 514(d) nm.
$P_{laser} \simeq 0.5$ mW/cm^2

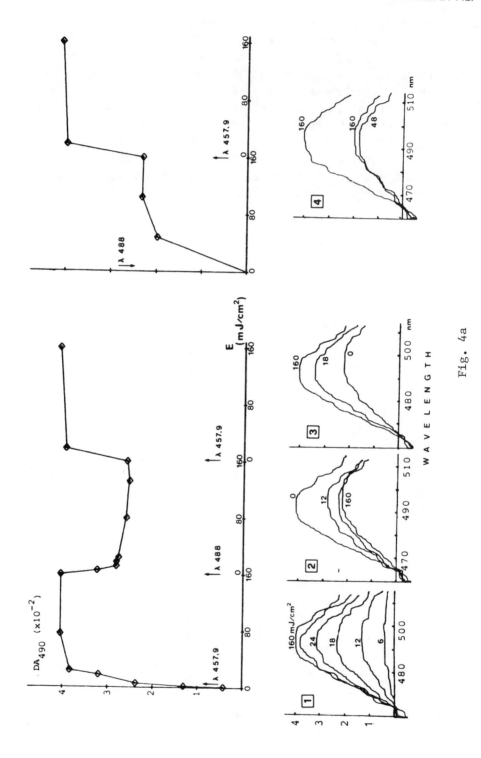

Fig. 4a

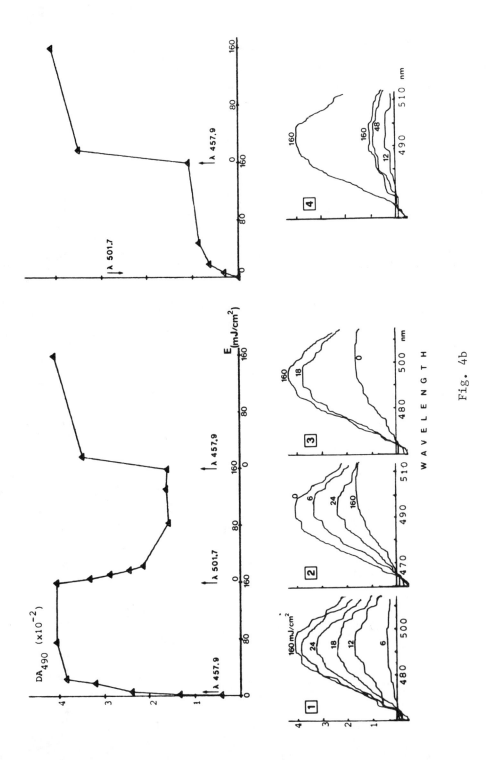

Fig. 4b

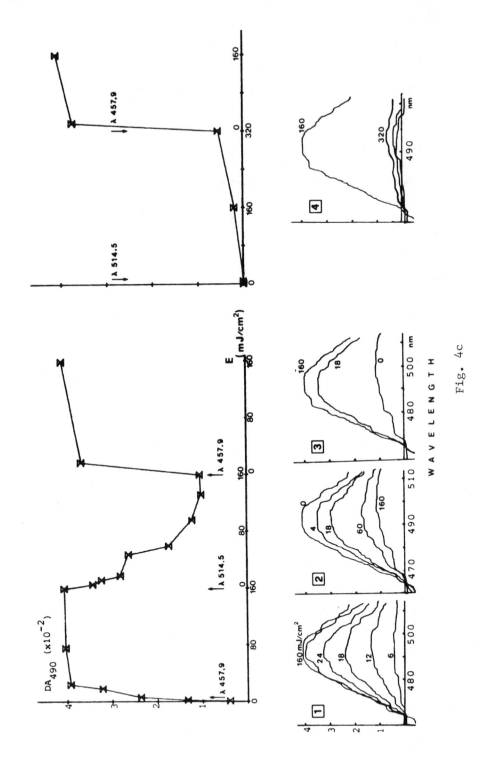

Fig. 4c

sent in the initial PBR/BR mixture.

Furthermore we checked the reversibility of the new PE mixtures to the initial PE mixture by irradiating them with the initial conversion 457-line. The same PE-values and DAS shapes have been obtained in all cases within the experimental errors. Even the "additional" products observed when irradiating with the 501 and 514 lines were reverted into the original PBR/BR mixture (Fig.4a, b,c/3).

Effect of the Irradiation Sequence

Finally we have examined the dependence of the intermediate and final PE values on the order followed in the irradiation sequence. The BR solutions have been irradiated with the 488, 501, 514 lines to give three different PE values (Fig.4a,b,c/4), and then irradiated with the 457-line up to PE (Fig.4a,b,c/4). Figs.4 a,b,c (upper part), show the value of the DAS at 490 nm as a function of the radiant exposure $E(mJ/cm^2)$ for the sequence 488/457, 501/457, 514/457 compared with the sequence 457/488/457, 457/501/ 457, 457/514/457. Clearly, the final values are equal to a good accuracy. On the contrary, the intermediate value in the case of the 457/501 sequence differs from that obtained by direct excitation at 501 nm and similarly in the case of the 514-line. Moreover, the DAS obtained with direct excitation of BR with any line are symmetric and similar in shape, while they differ from the DAS of the intermediate PE. This could suggest that the "additional" product is formed only when the PBR/BR mixture is irradiated with 501 or 514 line (the effect with the 488 line is much less evident). These preliminary results indicate the reversibility of the PBR ⇄ BR photoreaction, and the spectral dependence of the PBR/BR photoequilibrium. Possible production of BR photoproducts other than E,Z/Z,E configuration isomers (PBRs) is suggested by the observed dependence of PE values and DAS profiles on the irradiation sequence, which is not expected for the simple PBR ⇄ BR photoreaction[22].

LED-ARRAYS FOR PHOTOTHERAPY
(In collaboration with M.Scalvini, MASPEC-CNR, Parma)

The light sources currently used for PT are fluorescent lamps emitting narrow-spectrum visible radiation in the violet-blue region or broad-spectrum radiation, such as white and daylight lamps. Light power density at the body surface ranges typically from 1 to 3 mW/cm^2. These lamps are efficient and cheap; however, the high

intensity Hg lines are always present superposed on the continuous
fluorescent emission of the phosphor. The glass envelope of the
lamp cuts-off the residual UV-C and UV-B lines, while the plastic
(plexiglas-G) sheet of the illuminator or/and incubator blocks all
wavelengths below 380 nm[24]. On the other hand, the 400÷450 nm violet-blue radiation, in particular the 405 nm Hg line, has been
found to cause toxic and mutagenic effects on cultured mammalian
cells[25]. These lines cannot be easily filtered out by the available plastic materials without strongly reducing the light intensity within the useful PT spectral region. Even the recently proposed metal-vapor lamps[26] emit a large amount of power in the 400÷
430 nm range, which should be ineffective for PT according to our
computation of Section III.

Typical sources of narrow-band visible radiation are light
emitting diodes (LED), which have been available for years as in-
dicators, displays, etc. High-efficiency visible LEDs are being
increasingly developed due to requirements for a variety of optical applications. Usual peak radiation wavelengths are in the green,
yellow and red. The development of high intensity LEDs at other
wavelengths is only a technological and economical problem, and
it may be triggered by some specific application.

Blue LEDs with λ_{peak}= 480 nm and $\Delta\lambda$= 90 nm bandwidth are
already available at very low radiation power. The spectral intensity drops sharply below 440 nm and extend up to 560 nm. As shown
in Section III the phototherapeutical spectral efficiency of this
blue-LED is expected to be larger than the standard PHILIPS/BLU
fluorescent lamp and comparable to that of WESTINGHOUSE/SPECIAL
BLU lamps. As soon as the technological developments will improve
the power emission capability of this LED, a suitable shape panel
with tightly-packed arrays of LEDs could generate a sufficient
power density for PT applications, thus eliminating hazardous spectral components. Good output beam collimation can then be achieved by using the fabrication technique for the internal microlen-
sing system already available with IR-LEDs[27].

Moreover, straightforward hybrid-circuit fabrication techniques should permit the assembly of single LED chip into tightly-
packed arrays capable of producing irradiances suitable for PT, as
already proposed for photoradiation therapy of tumors[28], and recently tested using a multiple red-LED system[21]. Finally, the possible future operation of multiemitter phase-locked arrays of diode lasers in the blue-green spectral region will offer an interesting new source[23] for PT of jaundice.

REFERENCES

1. F.Hillenkamp, R.Pratesi and C.A.Sacchi, eds., "Lasers in Bio-
       logy and Medicine", Plenum Press Ltd., New York (1980).
2. J.D.Regan and J.A.Parrish, eds., "The Science of Photomedicine",
       Plenum Press Ltd., New York (1982).
3. R.Pratesi and C.A.Sacchi, eds., "Lasers in Photomedicine and
       Photobiology", Springer, Heidelberg (1980).
4. R.Cubeddu and A.Andreoni, eds., "Porphyrins in Tumor Photo-
       therapy", Plenum Press Ltd., New York in press.
5. J.F.Ennever and W.T.Speck, Mechanism of Action of Phototherapy:
       New Aspects, This volume, pp.
6. R.Parshad, R.Gantt, K.K.Sanford, G.M.Jones,and R.F. Camalier,
       Light-Induced Chromatid Damage in Human Skin Fibroblasts in
       Culture. Int.J.Cancer, 28: 335 (1982).
7. G.Sbrana, M.G.Migliorini, C.Vecchi, and G.P.Donzelli, Laser
       Photolysis of Bilirubin, Pediat.Res., 15: 1517 (1981).
8. C.Vecchi, G.P.Donzelli, M.G.Migliorini, G.Sbrana, and R.Prate-
       si, Green Light in Phototherapy of Hyperbilirubinemia, Proc.
       3rd Natl.Congr.on Quantum Electronics, Como 27-29 May 1982,
       pp.310-314 .
9. G.R.Gutcher, W.M.Yen, and G.B.Odell, The "in vitro" and "in
       vivo" Photoreactivity of Bilirubin: I. Laser-Defined Wave-
       Length Dependence, Pediat.Res, 17: 120 (1983).
10. C.Vecchi, and G.P.Donzelli, Superiority of Green Light in the
       Management of Neonatal Jaundice, 8th European Congress on
       "Perinatal Medicine", Brussels, September 7-10, 1982.
11. C.Vecchi, G.P.Donzelli, M.G.Migliorini, G.Sbrana, and R.Pratesi,
       New Light in Phototherapy, The Lancet, August 14, 390 (1982).
12. C.Vecchi, G.P.Donzelli, M.G.Migliorini and G.Sbrana, Green
       Light in Phototherapy, Pediat.Res, 17: 461 (1983).
13. W.T.Ham Jr., H.A.Mueller, and D.A.Sliney, Retinal Sensitivity
       to Damage from Short Wavelength Light, Nature, 260: 153 (1976)
14. T.R.C.Sisson, and T.P.Vogl, Phototherapy of Hyperbilirubinemia,
       in: "The Science of Photomedicine", J.D.Regan and J.A.Parrish,
       eds., Plenum Press, New York (1982).
15. D.A.Lightner, T.A.Wooldridge, S.L.Rodgers, and R.D.Norris,
       Action Spectra for Bilirubin Photodisappearence, Experientia,
       36: 380 (1980).
16. J.F.Ennever, J.F.Mc Donagh, and W.T.Speck, Phototherapy of Neo-
       natal Jaundice: Optimal Wavelengths of Light, J.Pediat, in
       press.

17. S.Wan, R.R.Anderson, and J.A.Parrish, Analytical Modeling for
    the Optical Properties of the Skin with "in vitro" and "in
    vivo" Applications, Photochem.Photobiol, 34: 493 (1981).
18. R.R.Anderson, and J.A.Parrish, The Optics of Human Skin,
    J.Invest.Dermatol, 77: 13 (1981).
19. R.Pratesi, L.Ronchi, G.Cecchi, M.G.Migliorini, G.Sbrana, G.P.
    Donzelli, and C.Vecchi, Skin Optics and Phototherapy of
    Jaundice, Submitted for publication .
20. R.Pratesi and M.Scalvini, A Solid-State Lamp (LED) Approach to
    Phototherapy, Biol.Med.Environ. 11: 467 (1983) .
21. G.Jori, R.Pratesi, and M.Scalvini, A Multi-LED Source for Pho-
    toradiation Therapy, in: "Porphyrins in Tumors Phototherapy",
    R.Cubeddu, A.Andreoni, eds., Plenum Press, in press .
22. R.Pratesi, G.Agati, F.Fusi, M.G.Migliorini, G.Sbrana, G.P.Don-
    zelli, and C.Vecchi, Laser Investigation of Bilirubin ⇄ Pho-
    tobilirubin Photoconversion, Submitted for publication.
23. D.A.Lightner, T.A.Wooldridge, and A.F.Mc Donagh, Photobilirubin:
    an Early Bilirubin Photoproduct Detected by Absorbance Diffe-
    rence Spectroscopy, Proc.Natl.Acad.Sci.(USA), 76: 29 (1979).
24. S.Yasunaga, and E.H.Kean, The effect of Plexiglas Incubators
    on Phototherapy, J.Pediat., 81: 89 (1972).
25. R.Parshad, K.K.Sanford, W.G.Taylor, R.E.Tarone, G.N.Jones, and
    A.E.Baek, Effect of the intensity and Wavelength of Fluores-
    cent Light on Chromosome Damage in Cultured Mouse Cells,
    Photochem.Photobiol., 29: 971 (1979).
26. S.Järig, D.Järig, and P.Meisel, Metal Halid Vapor Lamps in New
    Trends in Phototherapy, This volume, pp.
27. T.Ormond, Fiber-Optic Components, EDN 28: 112 (1983).
28. M.E.Mahric, M.Epstein, and R.V.Lobraico, A Proposal for Light-
    Emitting-Diode Array for Photoradiation Therapy, to be pub-
    lished.
29. D.R.Scifres, R.D.Burnham, C.Lindstrom, W.Streifer, and L.T.Paoli,
    High-Power Diode Lasers, Paper TUC5, presented at the CLEO,
    May 17-20, Baltimore, USA (1983).

This work has been supported in part by CNR Special Projects "Laser
di Potenza" and "Medicina Preventiva e Riabilitativa".

Stimulating discussions with A.A.Lamola, J.F.Ennever, A.F. Mc Donagh, T.R.C.Sisson are grateffully aknowledged.

A MATHEMATICAL DESCRIPTION OF THE PHOTOTHERAPY-EFFECT:
AN INVESTIGATION OF THE DOSE-RESPONSE RELATIONSHIP UNDER
HIGH IRRADIANCIES

G. Wiese

Children's Hospital Free University Berlin
Kaiserin Auguste Victoria Haus
Heubnerweg 6, D-1000 Berlin 19

The chief purpose of this investigation was to calculate the
dose-response relationship of phototherapy (PT) with different
effective irradiancies by using a pharmacokinetic model. The
following pharmacokinetic model for Gunn rats is used in the
calculation (clarified in figs. 1-5).

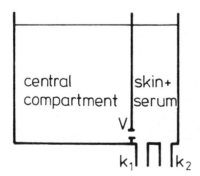

Fig. 1   Pharmacokinetic model for the mathematical description of
the PT-effect. k_1=tract for spontaneous elimination; k_2=tract
for elimination due to PT; v=intercompartmental connection.

Here the whole body is divided into two sections, a central
compartment and a skin and serum compartment. The skin/serum compartment has two bilirubin elimination tracts; one for spontaneous
elimination, k_1 and one for elimination via the photoreaction, k_2.

In the simple case k_1 is equal k_2. At first there is no connection between the two compartments (fig. 2a). After waiting a

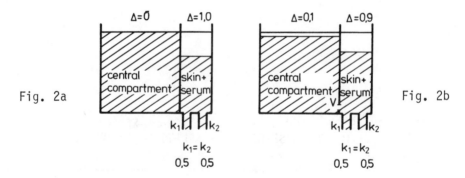

Fig. 2   Pharmacokinetic model: Dependence upon the intercompart-
           mental connection.

certain length of time, after which the content of the skin/serum
compartment has decreased arbitrarily to 1, the same amount 0.5,
must be running through both exits. In the central compartment
there is, of course, no change. However, with a connection, v
between the two compartments (fig. 2b), a transport of material
from one chamber to the other must take place, which is of course,
the natural situation. After waiting the same amount of time as in
the first example, the amount of bilirubin running through the two
openings will be the same, namely 0.5. However contrary to the
first case, the change in the levels in the skin/serum compartment
will now be significantly lower (i.e. 0.9) because bilirubin will
now flow out of the central compartment too. From this model it is
possible to deduce that:
1) The temporal change in concentration in the skin/serum compartment depends on the influx from the central compartment.

     In fig. 3a the same situation as in fig. 2a is illustrated.
In fig. 3b the exit for spontaneous elimination is reduced by half.
After waiting the same amount of time as in the first example, only
half of the previous quantity of bilirubin will run out of the

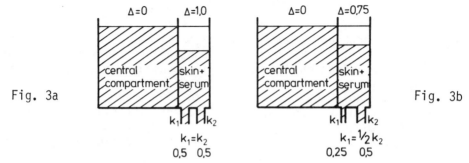

Fig. 3   Pharmacokinetic model: Dependence upon the rate of
           spontaneous elimination.

opening k_1 and therefore the total change in the skin/serum compartment will only be 0.75. From this model it can be deduced that

2) The temporal change in concentration in the skin/serum compartment depends on the rate of spontaneous elimination.

    To summarize the following result is obtained:
In order to derive the efficacy of PT one has to consider the influx v, and the spontaneous elimination k_1.

    In fig. 4a the same situation as in figs. 2a and 3a is illustrated once again. Fig. 4b demonstrates the case where there is a lower starting-amount of bilirubin. As a result of a decrease in the hydrostatic pressure, the effluent rate through both exits will also be decreased so that over the same time interval as in fig. 4a the total output will be reduced. This means:

3) The amount eliminated with time is dependant upon the starting-amount. Assuming the same efficacy of PT, higher starting-concentrations will result in larger decreases of the concentration with time. It is possible to show by calculation that a decraese in bilirubin concentration from 20 to 7 mg% requires the same PT as for a decrease from 10 to 5 mg%. Therefore, the measurement of the decrease in concentration in percent terms (as is commonly undertaken) cannot be related to the efficacy of PT.

    In addition there is a second result to be deduced from fig. 4:

4) Because the efficiency of PT is dependant upon the concentration of bilirubin in the skin and as a result of illumination the skin becomes bleached, then it follows that the efficacy will be reduced during every PT.

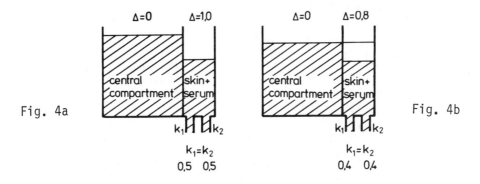

Fig. 4a   Fig. 4b

Fig. 4   Pharmacokinetic model: Dependence upon the starting concentration.

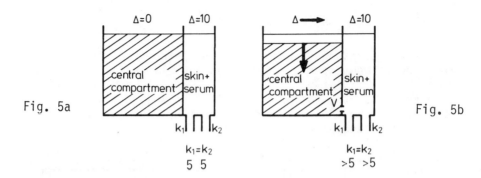

Fig. 5a

Fig. 5b

Fig. 5   Pharmacokinetic model: Situation after long-term PT.

Fig. 5 a shows the situation after a long-term PT for the case where there is no connection between the two compartments. After waiting long enough the skin/serum compartment will be emptied and k_1 and k_2 will be zero. A situation of zero flow for the opening k_2 indicates that the PT has no efficacy. However, if it is assumed that a connection between the two compartments exists (fig. 5b), then bilirubin will flow between the two and eventually a steady-state situation will envolve in the skin/serum compartment, with bilirubin being eliminated through both outflow tracts. This means that a certain efficacy of PT will remain (i.e. $k_2 > 0$). Therefore as a result mainly of PT, the amount of bilirubin in the central compartment will be reduced. This means that:

5) During long-term PT bilirubin will also be eliminated. However, once the steady-state has been reached in the skin/serum compartment, its elimination will be wholly dependant upon its rate of influx from the central compartment. This leads to the next very important conclusion. Contrary to popular belief, it follows that for every irradiance scheme during long-term PT, the rate of elimination of bilirubin will decrease. That is to say, the common postulation that a decrease in the rate of bilirubin elimination will commence above some particular irradiance level can not be upheld.
This means that during long-term, continuous PT the amount of bilirubin eliminated will fall to a level which is governed by the rate of bilirubin transfer between compartments. As a consequnce the long-term PT will appear less effective than compared to in its initial stages. Therefore, during a continuous PT treatment, it is necessary to switch to an intermittent regime once the serum bilirubin concentration has markedly decreased.

This model may be described mathematically in the following way. Bilirubin is formed by the organism according to the rate expression:

$$\frac{dc}{dt} = v \tag{1}$$

Spontaneously, (i.e. without therapy), it is eliminated with the rate:

$$\frac{dc}{dt} = -k_1 \cdot c \tag{2}$$

in which k_1 is the rate constant for spontaneous bilirubin elimination from the skin. For elimination by the photoreaction, the following expression is valid:

$$\frac{dc}{dt} = -k_2 \cdot c \tag{3}$$

in which k_2 is the rate constant for bilirubin elimination by the photoreaction. Thereby k_2 is a measure of the real PT-effect. The larger the value of k_2, the greater the amount of photobilirubin. Experiments with Gunn rats have shown the following dependence [1]:

$$k_2 = k^* \cdot c_o \cdot \frac{S}{G} \cdot E \tag{4}$$

where k^* = global photo-constant

c_o = serum bilirubin concentration prior to the PT

S = illuminated surface

G = body weight

E = effective irradiance

For the global transport equation the following is obtained:

$$\frac{dc}{dt} = v - (k_1 + k_2) \cdot c \tag{5}$$

Integration of this function gives the concentration-time equation of bilirubin in the skin during PT.

$$c = \frac{v}{k_1 + k_2} \left(1 + \frac{k_2}{k_1} \cdot e^{-(k_1+k_2) \cdot t}\right) \tag{6}$$

Fig. 6 shows the change of the bilirubin concentration in the skin for different irradiancies. The bleach-effect of PT may be observed. After a certain length of time a new steady state of bilirubin concentration in the skin is reached. This concentration

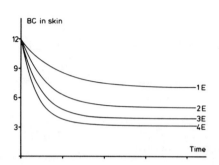

Fig. 6   Change of the bilirubin concentration (BC) in the skin
         under continuous PT (1E), doubling the energy (2E),
         threefold (3E), fourfold (4E).

is given by:

$$c_{min} = \frac{v}{k_1+k_2}$$ (7)

          and depends not only upon k_2, (i.e. the PT-regime),
but also upon the rate constant of spontaneous bilirubin elimination, k_1 and on its formation rate, v. Between these three parameters exists a complex relation. Therefore, it is impossible to
measure the efficacy of PT by the decrease of the bilirubin concentration alone.

          The derived equation, (6), describes the total change of bili-
rubin concentration in the skin, i.e. it also takes the spontaneous elimination into account. The amount a*, formed due to the
photoreaction can be calculated by:

$$\frac{da*}{dt} = k_2 \cdot V \cdot c = v*$$ (8)

where V is the distribution volume of bilirubin in the skin.
v* is the rate of eliminated bilirubin due to PT. If, at the
beginning of PT, v* is taken as 100 %, then the following equation
is obtained for the relative elimination rate, $v*_{rel}$:

$$v*_{rel} = \frac{100\ k_1}{k_1+k_2}\ (1 + \frac{k_2}{k_1} \cdot e^{-(k_1+k_2)t}$$ (9)

          Fig. 7 shows the relative elimination rate for different
irradiancies. It can be seen that the eliminated bilirubin decreases
for each irradiance. The higher the irradiance, the faster the
decrease of the relative elimination rate. In practice, this means
that the higher the irradiance, the larger the decrease in the

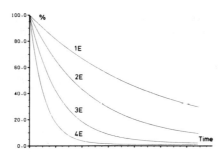

Fig. 7   Relative elimination rate under continuous PT (1E),
          doubling the energy (2E), threefold (3E), fourfold (4E).

efficacy of long-term continuous PT. However, the efficacy of the
intermittent PT is also higher, because the concentration gradient
between the skin and the central compartments increases due to the
bleach-effect.

From the derived equations the following may also be deduced.
There is no direct proportion between the effect of PT and the
decrease in bilirubin concentration over a specific time interval.
A comparison of the decrease in bilirubin concentration over a
certain time, (such as 12h or 24h), is no measure of efficacy of
the special PT-regime. Only by a quantitative examination of the
concentration-time function can reliable comparisons be made.

The model under discussion also describes the situation for
newborn babies. This can be shown from the data published by TAN 2 .
For the serum compartment, the following equation describing the
serum bilirubin concentration may be obtained:

$$c = \frac{v}{k_s+k_p} - (\frac{v}{k_s+k_p} - c_0) \cdot e^{-(k_s+k_p) \cdot t} \tag{10}$$

where k_s = rate constant for the spontaneous elimination of
            serum bilirubin

   k_p = rate constant for the elimination of serum bilirubin
          due to PT

   v = formation rate of bilirubin

   c_0 = serum bilirubin concentration prior to PT

   t = duration of illumination

For the relative change of serum bilirubin concentration the
following is obtained:

$$\Delta c_{rel} = \frac{100 \cdot (c_o - \frac{v}{k_s+k_p})}{c_o} \; (1 - e^{-(k_s+k_p) \cdot t}) \qquad (11)$$

Fig. 8 shows the relative change of the serum bilirubin concentration calculated by eq. (11) and in addition, the data published by TAN[2] (wave length range 400-480 nm). The good agreement illustrated in fig. 8 shows that the same kinetics as for Gunn rats are valid over the range of irradiances considered. The small deviations observed result from the use of a very simple model.

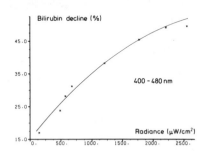

Fig. 8   Relative change of the serum bilirubin concentration calculated by eq. (11) and the data published by TAN[2] (wave length range 400-480 nm).

The decrease of the slope in this graph is the result of a change in the relation between k_1 and k_2, i.e. the relation between spontaneous elimination and the elimination due to PT. At low irradiancies, the fraction of the total eliminated bilirubin which arises spontaneously is greater than that due to the effects of PT. At higher irradiancies however these positions are reversed; that is, the relative amount of phototherapeutically eliminated bilirubin is greater. Nevertheless, a doubling of the illumination energy for example, will not result in a doubling of the total bilirubin elimination but rather, only a doubling of that fraction eliminated due to PT; the fraction spontaneously eliminates will remain constant regardless of PT scheme. Therefore, it will appear as if PT becomes less effective at higher irradiancies (fig. 8), when in fact the reverse is true.

After evaluating the concentration-time functions - by eq.10 - for maximal and moderate irradiancies as published by TAN[2], a good agreement between the calculated and the measured irradiancies was obtained, with a deviation less than 5 %!

To summarize from the quantitative consideration of this model it is possible to state the following:

CONCLUSIONS

1) A comparison of the decrease of bilirubin concentration over a defined time-period is not an adequate measure for the efficacy of a particular PT regime. Statements about the efficacy of PT can only be derived from quantitative, kinetic analyses of the concentration-time function.

2) The amount of bilirubin eliminated over a given time period will decrease during the course of a prolonged, continuous PT. For short-term PT, every irradiance will result in an adequate photoreaction, but for long-term PT however, the effects of these illuminations will be less marked.

3) As a consequence of the bleach-effect in the skin, a prolonged continuous PT will become ineffective irrespective of irradiance. Therefore, after a significant decrease in the serum bilirubin concentration, the regime has to be changed to intermittent PT.

REFERENCES

1. G. Wiese, and L. Ballowitz, Mathematical description of the temporal changes in serum bilirubin concentration during phototherapy in newborn infants, Biol. Neonate 42:222(1982).

2. K.L. Tan, The pattern of bilirubin response to phototherapy for neonatal hyperbilirubinaemia, Pediatr.Res.16:670 (1982).

THE GUNN RAT - A MODEL FOR PHOTOTHERAPY

Leonore Ballowitz, Folker Hanefeld and Günther Wiese

Children's Hospital Free University Berlin
-Kaiserin Auguste Victoria Haus-
Heubnerweg 6, D-1000 Berlin 19

For more than 15 years, neonatologists, a pediatric neurologist, illumination engineers as consultants and later on a pediatrician, formerly trained in mathematics and chemistry - are using in our hospital the Gunn rat strain as a model. Phototherapy (PT) was one of the main topics. Today, the succeeding steps of research shall be listed in short and completed by new data.*

First of all, the question of the effectiveness of PT and of possible side-effects had to be answered.

The early observation that infant rats, which were illuminated together with a lactating dam, remained smaller than littermates kept in the dark was alarming. But subsequent gavage feeding, careful observations and analyses showed that the growth retardation was mainly due to irritation of the mother rats in the unaccustomed surroundings in PT units. This provoked reduced milk production.- Retinal damage by fluorescent lights (without any changes in FiO_2) was marked and began already after a few hours of illumination in adult animals - but not so in infant rats so long as their eyelids were still closed.

---

*We have to stress that this work was continuously promoted by stimulations and fruitful discussions with many researchers from different parts of the world. We would like to express our thanks to all of them.

As for effectiveness it was not difficult to demonstrate the light induced decline of the serum bilirubin concentration (SBC). Soon it became evident that shaving or depilation of weanling and adult rats was not necessary. The fur is no essential light trap. More convincing was the proof of a protection by the lights against the detrimental effect of sulfonamides in homozygous infant Gunn rats.

Basic studies on the influence of hyperbilirubinaemia on cerebella growth, histological grading of kernicterus within the cerebellum, evaluation of neurological tests in vivo - came next - in parallel to studies on the photobiologically most effective radiant energy as well as calculations on dose/response relation-ships. It became clear that the effectiveness of PT even greatly depended on the initial SBC. With high irradiances SBC can be brought down almost to zero. The effect of different fluorescent tubes was compared. Taking the spectral energy distribution of the lamps into consideration,it was then possible to construct a special radiometer which graduates spectral energy according to its bio-logical efficiency. Digital measurements give the effective irrad-iance E_{bili} in mW/cm². The peak sensibility is set at 46o nm and half maximum sensitivities are at 435 and 488 nm. The spectral efficiency curve comes close to the bilirubin absorption curve. The Berlin radiometer differs not very much from the Olympic spectro-radiometer meanwhile developed for the control of PT.

Based on this experience we can disprove the recently pub-lished postulate of Italian investigators (4) that green light can replace fluorescent daylight lamps for PT of neonatal jaundice. Fig.1 shows the time course of SBC in a weanling Gunn rat during 48 h PT and the following rebound period. This rat was first illu-minated with blue lights (Philips BAM blue 2o W/52) E_{bili} 2.6 mW/cm², and a week later with the same blue lamps plus 4 green tubes (Osram L2oW/63). On this 2nd trial a small part of the blue tubes was screened with black tapes to compensate for blue emission which is additionally present in green fluorescent tubes (i.e. the mer-cury peak at 436 nm). E_{bili} was quite the same in both trials. Fig.2 shows the same arrangement with white fluorescent tubes in-stead of the green ones. I cannot see a different PT effect in both figures. PRATESI, one of the authors of the Italian publication, confirmed in a personal communication that the 436 and 4o5 nm peaks in the Sylvania green fluorescent lamps used by them are almost identical to those of the green Osram tubes tested by us. He is at present trying to determine the contribution of these peaks to the photoconversion of bilirubin.

On the other hand, our experiment demonstrates that the addi-tion of green does not diminish the effect of blue in the Gunn rat. ENNEVER, McDONAGH and SPECK (2), have recently shown that in vitro the bilirubin photoisomer is converted back to native bilirubin

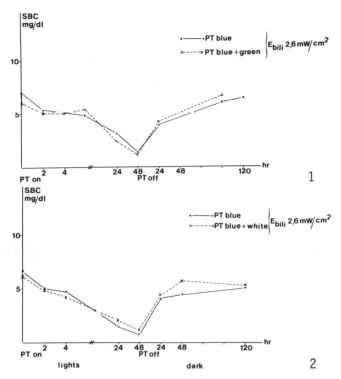

Figs. 1 and 2.   Time course of SBC in 1-mo-old homozygous Gunn rats
in 2 trials of illumination and the following rebound period.Compa-
rison of blue and blue+green PT (Fig.1) and of blue and blue+white
PT (Fig.2) in the same animal in each case.

when exposed to green (53o nm) light. In a personal communication
ENNEVER argued that our findings in Gunn rats might be due to the
extremely rapid excretion of photobilirubin in this animal. Thus,
essentially no photoisomer accumulates in the tissue, and none can
be converted to native bilirubin. This may be somewhat different in
human babies in whom under PT as much as 2o % of total bilirubin
will be present as the Z, E-isomer.

In this connection the following observation may be of interest. When hairs cliped from 1-2-mo-old jaundiced rats were illuminated for a few hours with blue lights, the reflectance of the
hairs (measured with the Minolta/Air-shield jaundice meter) distinctly changed to lower indices. After subsequent intense illumination with green fluorescent tubes from which the 436 and 4o5
mercury peaks were filtered out by corning coloured glass filters
(GG 475) the measured indices hint at a new increase - surely not
at a further decrease.

At next the enhancement of the PT effect by riboflavin has to

be mentioned. But, when high doses of riboflavin were given to the
rats as an adjunct to an intense blue PT, photodynamic reactions
with extended skin lesions appeared. Acute toxicity of riboflavin-5-
phosphate was much higher when the animals were kept under intense
PT than when they remained in the dark.

In 1979, WIESE analysed once more a good deal of our former
Gunn rat data. He was able to define with pharmaco-kinetic-methods
concentration time functions for the PT induced decrease of SBC
(and the following rebound after cessation of illumination) for any
given starting level and for any type of fluorescent tubes. The
reaction follows an e function with energy in the exponent. Equations for continuous and for intermittent PT were derived. The validity was scrutinized by a comparison of experimental data measured
by VOGL et al. (5) in Gunn rats under different PT regimens. The
conformity was striking.

A primarily not expected result was obtained when human albumin
was administered to Gunn rats under PT. The PT induced SBC decline
became distinctly enhanced. After an i.v. albumin injection about 4
times more bilirubin was eliminated under intense blue lights than
with an equally dosed PT alone.

The Gunn rat model guided the attemps of a mathematical analysis
of the PT effect in newborn humans.
This was a good deal more complicated, since in the newborn baby
we have no steady-state for SBC as we have in weanling Gunn rats.
Nevertheless, the fundamental principles revealed to be equal. An
individual prediction of SBC after a certain time of illumination
with the chosen E_{bili} (lamp) is now possible. A pertinent computer
program is available.

Knowing this, the publication of DAVIS, YEARY and LEE (1) about
"the failure of phototherapy to reduce plasma bilirubin levels in
the bile duct-ligated rat" and their statement that in bile duct-
ligated rats the renal pathway had a negligible effect was intriguing
to us - although we remembered OSTROW's data (3) on a 2-3 fold increased urine radio-activity during PT after administration of a
tracer dose of ^{14}C bilirubin to not bile duct-ligated rats. - From
the nurseries, the prompt change in colour of the urine in the beginning of PT is familiar, although the percentage of bilirubin
photoproducts excreted by this way in humans is - to my knowledge -
not yet well documented. Should here really be a profound difference in the (excretion) metabolism between Gunn rats and human
beings? We repeated the experiments of DAVIS and coworkers, with
an effective irradiance about equal to that used by the American
investigators, and in addition with an about 5-fold higher effective
irradiance. With this higher light dose a clear effect on SBC in
the bile duct-ligated group could be seen, and the excretion into
the urine (recognizable by a conspicious colour-change) increased.

We measured the colour of (single fortuitous) urine specimens in
the American Optical Bilirubinometer and came to mean values of
4,7 - 4,5 (min. 1,8 max. 8,o) during the first 24 hours of intense
PT. Corresponding values for sham operated control animals in the
dark were -o,3 up to +o,8 (readings for destill.water were set at
-o,8). (In urine specimens of human babies under PT we measured
with the AO Bilirubinometer values similar to those of sham operated rats). A mathematical analysis showed that ligation of the
bile-duct reduced elimination of bilirubin from the body during PT
by a factor 4-5. By applying a 4-5 times higher irradiance the
same effect can be seen in bile duct-ligated rats as in sham operated animals illuminated with the low (factor 1) irradiance.

Efforts to calculate the amount of enterohepatic recirculation induced some experiments in which infant rats received bilirubin by gavage feeding. A distinct rise in SBC followed. Unfortunately, the young animals did not tolerate gavage administration of bile which was collected after bile duct-canalisation from
adult heterozygous rats.

This mainly retrospective, almost historical report should be
finished with some new data on transcutaneous bilirubinometry in
Gunn rats. In 198o YAMANOUCHI and coworkers (6) described a transcutaneous bilirubinometer which allows to estimate SBC in newborn
human babies. I carried out some studies on spectral reflectance
of the skin in term and premature human babies as well as in Gunn
rats in the late sixtieth. The main idea was that the amount of
light which is not reflected by the skin should permit a calculation of the actual light dose penetrating into the skin during PT.
From these studies I knew that the reflectance differed between
homo- and heterozygous littermates. Jaundiced rats including older
animals with fur have a diminished reflectance between 43o and 5oo
nm. The differences between icteric and non-icteric rats were most
impressive in rats about 8 days of age. At this time they have
still not much fur and SBC is comparably high in the homozygous.
When the minolta apparatus became available, we supplemented these
old observations.

In Fig.3 SBC of homozygous Gunn rats and in Fig.4 TcB index
measured with the minolta apparatus are plotted against the body-
weight. Both sketches reach a peak at about 3o g i.e. at 14-16
days. Fur begins to grow at the age of 7-9 days; it becomes wooly
thick in the 3rd week and more wispy in adult rats. All Berlin Gunn
rats are albino. - Not only the light yellowish fur of the homozygous but also the white fur of the heterozygous causes a "TcB
index" by absorbing a certain amount of blue light. In Fig. 5 the
"white fur TcB values" of the heterozygous rats are plotted against
weight. It makes sense to subtract these "white fur values" from
those of the fur of homozygous animals and to plot against SBC. In
this group of animals no strict correlation was found after such a

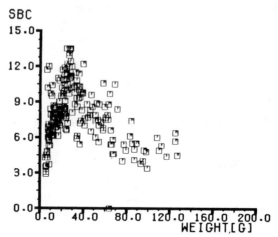

Fig.3   SBC of homozygous Gunn rats plotted against body weight.
(The correlation is somewhat better, when weight is used instead of age; 2o days ≈ 4o g)   ▥ = male   ▱ = female
rat.

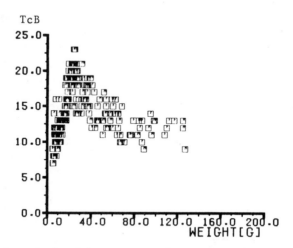

Fig.4   TcB (on fur) of homozygous Gunn rats plotted against body
weight.

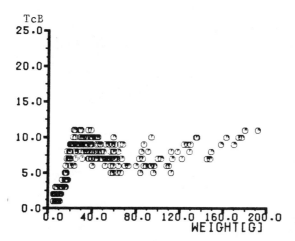

Fig.5   TcB (on fur) of heterozygous Gunn rats plotted against
         body weight   ⊙ = male   ⊙ =   female rat.

calculation. Correlation was more convincing when only littermates
were taken as a basis.

     Fig. 6 shows TcB on the fur and on a shaved area of the back
after i.v. injection of 2.5 mg bilirubin into a 1-mo-old homozygous rat (weighing 1oo g). Shortly after the injection, TcB increases distinctly in the shaved area,and it declines with declining SBC during the following days. In this age group TcB on fur is
primarily not influenced by the high artificial bilirubin load. -
It may be added that TcB on a shaved area of a weanling Gunn rat
and on the still furless skin of an infant rat showed a slight increase when the blood content of the vascular network of the skin
was reduced by bleeding the animals via carotis artery.

     Fig. 7 demonstrates SBC, fur reflectance on the back (TcB fur)
and TcB on a shaved area for a homozygous weanling rat during 48
hours illumination with blue light (E_{bili} 2,6 mW/cm²) and in the
following rebound period in the dark. The shaded broken line shows
TcB fur of a simultaneously illuminated heterozygous littermate.
Some kind of bleaching occurs in heterozygous rats under the lights,
too. The dotted line means TcB fur of the homozygous rat minus TcB
fur of the heterozygous littermate. For my opinion this sketch
demonstrates a rather good correlation between the invasive and non-
invasive measurements. Furthermore, I can see a rapid emptying of
the fur in the beginning of PT and a somewhat delayed "refilling"
in the course of the rebound period.

     New data, easily measurable and suitable for pharmaco-kinetic
studies may be the prospective result.

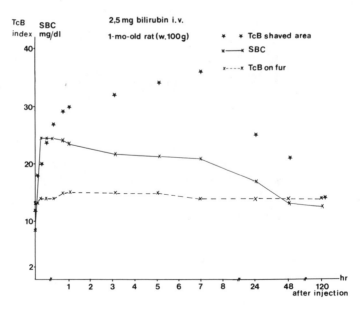

Fig.6   Time course of SBC, TcB on fur and TcB on a shaved
        area after bilirubin injection.

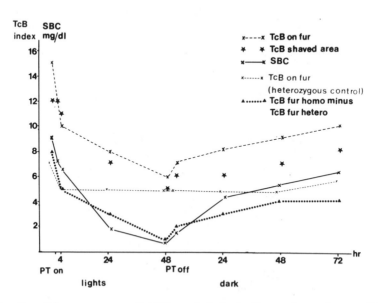

Fig.7   Time course of SBC and TcB indices in a 1-mo-old
        homozygous rat during PT and the rebound period.

REFERENCES

1. D. R. Davis, R. A. Yeary,and K. Lee, 1981, The failure of phototherapy to reduce plasma bilirubin levels in the bile duct-ligated rat, J. Pediat., 99:956.
2. J. F. Ennever, A. F. McDonagh,and W. T. Speck, Phototherapy for neonatal jaundice: Optimal wavelength of light. Submitted to J. Pediat.
3. D. Ostrow, 1969, Mechanism of phototherapy of jaundice, Soc. Pediat. Res. Atlanta City
4. C. Vecchi, G. P. Donzelli, M. G. Migliorini, G. Sbrana,and R. Pratesi, 1982, New light in phototherapy, Lancet i.i.390.
5. Th. P. Vogl, H. Cheskin, Th. A. Blumenfeld, W. T. Speck,and M. R. Koenigsberger, 1977, Effect of intermittent phototherapy on bilirubin dynamics in Gunn rats, Pediat. Res., 11:1021.
6. I. Yamanouchi, Y. Yamauchi, and I. Igarashi, 1980, Transcutaneous bilirubinometry: Preliminary studies of non-invasive transcutaneous bilirubin meter in the Okayama National Hospital, Pediatrics, 65:195

References on PT studies in Gunn rats from Kaiserin Auguste Victoria Haus - Children's Hospital Free University Berlin, can be requested from L. Ballowitz.

LIGHT DOSE-RESPONSE RELATIONSHIP IN PHOTOTHERAPY

K. L. Tan

Professor of Paediatrics, National   Univ. Singapore
Head, Neonatal Unit, Kandang Kerbau Hospital
Singapore 0821, Republic of Singapore

The Kandang Kerbau Hospital, Singapore, presently delivers about 24,000 infants per year. The proportion of infants delivered according to ethnic groups reflects the ethnic composition of the country; of the total population of 2.44 million living in an island state of 618 square kilometres, 76.6% are Chinese, 14.3% Malays, 6.1% Indians, and the rest of mixed descent or Whites.

Non-haemolytic neonatal jaundice is a common complication of newborn infants in Singapore, especially Chinese infants. This high incidence (Fig. 1) was initially ascribed to the native cultural practices especially with regard to native herbs of the different ethnic groups[1]. However, a recent survey[2] demonstrated that despite the decline of such native practices, the incidence and severity of neonatal jaundice among non-breast fed Chinese infants observed in the controlled environment of the hospital has not changed (Fig. 2). The bilirubin levels of healthy full-term infants still peak on the fourth and fifth days of life at about 10mg/dl with that of glucose-6-phosphate dehydrogenase (G6PD) deficient infants being significantly higher. Furthermore, the incidence of severe jaundice (bilirubin level $\geq$ 15mg/dl) is 9% in healthy fullterm Chinese neonates, an incidence far above those of the other ethnic groups. Obviously, the tendency to non-haemolytic jaundice in Chinese infants is an ethnic characteristic.

PHOTOTHERAPY FOR NEONATAL JAUNDICE

Phototherapy has been practised in the Kandang Kerbau Hospital for over 10 years. Its advent has virtually led to the disappearance of the need for exchange transfusions which previously had to be performed in over 300 infants yearly. Phototherapy was

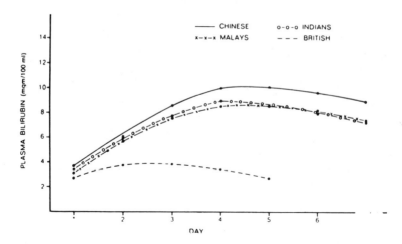

Fig. 1.   Bilirubin values in the first week of life in fullterm
           healthy neonates (1964).

initially performed with daylight lamps which still remain the
principal lamps used especially in the open ward. However,
occasional failure of phototherapy was observed especially in
haemolytic conditions. The need therefore for increased radiance
especially in the spectrum more effective for neonatal jaundice

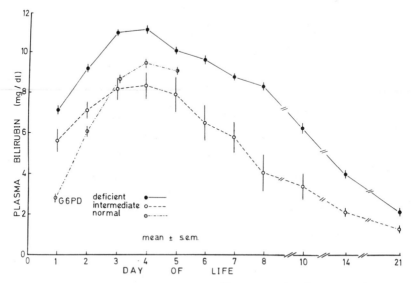

Fig. 2.   Bilirubin values in G6PD normal, intermediate and
           deficient fullterm infants (1979).

was obvious. Special blue lamps when they became available were
therefore utilised for rapidly progressive or severe jaundice.

DOSE—RESPONSE RELATIONSHIP

It was noticed previously that the effectiveness of phototherapy increased with increasing radiance[3,4]. The nature of this
dose-response relationship was later demonstrated in the neonate[5]
and the Gunn rat[6]. A later study of phototherapy for non-haemolytic
hyperbilirubinaemia[7] using a lamp with a spectral emission curve very
similar to the bilirubin absorption curve (Fig. 3) demonstrated
that although increasing radiance resulted in increasing response
(in bilirubin decline) to phototherapy, the rate of decline
progressively became less with increasing radiance (Fig. 4); a
'saturation' point was reached beyond which apparently no further
decline occurred with increase in radiance, suggesting an
asymptotic curve. At this point a decline of about 50% was observed.
There was a linear relationship between the logarithm of the dosage
and the rate of bilirubin decline (Fig. 5). By extrapolation, the
intensity for minimal effectiveness of phototherapy was about 31.85
microwatts/cm^2 (uW/cm^2) for the 440-480 nanometer (nm) range, 50.26
uW/cm^2 for the 425-475 nm range and 54.71 uW/cm^2 for the 400-480 nm
range. The results were obtained for mean bilirubin values in the
whole study exceeding 15.5mg/dl and at high radiance, 17.0mg/dl.

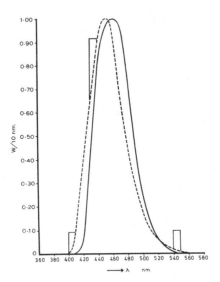

Fig. 3.   The spectral emission curve of the Philips TL20W/52 lamp
          (broken line) with the bilirubin absorption curve
          (solid line); the vertical bars are the mercury spectral
          bands. From K. L. Tan, Pediatr. Res. 16:670, 1982[7].

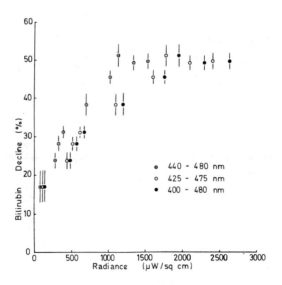

Fig. 4.   The 24-hr bilirubin decline (mean ± SE) expressed as a
           proportion of the initial bilirubin values in response
           to increasing radiance.   From K. L. Tan[7].

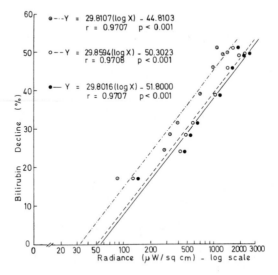

Fig. 5.   Semi-logarithmic presentation of the 24-hr decline; a
           linear relationship was observed.   From K. L. Tan[7].

When healthy fullterm infants were exposed to phototherapy at
'saturation' dose (maximal intensity phototherapy - radiance 701 uW/
cm^2 for the 440-480 nm range, 1101 uW/cm^2 for the 425-475 nm range,
and 1206 uW/cm^2 for the 400-480 nm range), a decline in bilirubin
values to about 5mg/dl occurred, after which no further decline
could be demonstrated. Comparable infants exposed to moderate
intensity phototherapy (2/3 that of maximal intensity phototherapy),
demonstrated a similar but slower decline to 5mg/dl after which no
further decline occurred. Both the responses appeared to be
exponential in nature (Fig. 6). The time required for this decline
appeared directly proportional to the logarithm of the bilirubin
value (Fig. 7). The 24-hr bilirubin decline expressed as a
proportion of the bilirubin concentration at the start of each 24-
period was proportional to the bilirubin value at the start of that
period (Fig. 8). Thus, phototherapy is more effective with high
bilirubin values, and declines in efficacy with decreasing
bilirubin values till about 5mg/dl when little further decline will
occur.

PHOTOTHERAPY IN SEVERE HAEMOLYTIC JAUNDICE

The use of phototherapy in jaundice resulting from severe
haemolytic conditions is still not clearly defined. Conflicting
views about the efficacy of phototherapy in such conditions abound.
Failure of phototherapy in severe Rhesus (Rh) haemolytic jaundice
is a common experience. However, with maximal intensity phototherapy,
such severe jaundice can also be effectively controlled as the
present data (Table) of neonates suffering from severe Rh haemolytic

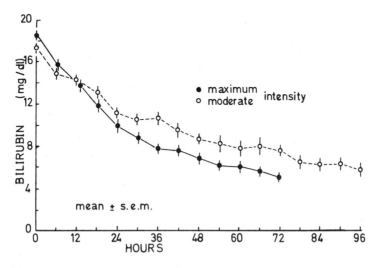

Fig. 6.   Bilirubin levels at 6-hr intervals in response to
            maximal and moderate intensity phototherapy. From K. L. Tan[7].

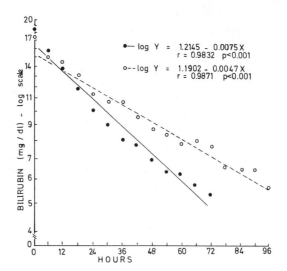

Fig. 7.   Semi-logarithmic presentation of the 6-hr decline, a
          linear relationship was observed. From K. L. Tan[7].

jaundice demonstrates. In the majority of these cases, the diagnosis
was only made after severe jaundice had occurred, the Rh status of
the mothers being not known before delivery. Maximal intensity

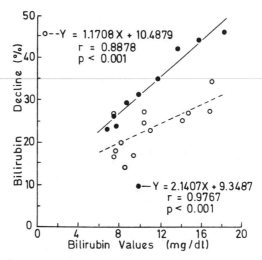

Fig. 8.   The 24-hr bilirubin decline expressed as a proportion of
          the bilirubin level at the start of the 24-hr period. A
          linear relationship was observed. From K. L. Tan[7].

Data of Infants with Rh Haemolytic Disease

Case No.	Birth wt (g)	Gest^n age (wks)	Sex	Maternal Anti-D Titre	Start of phototherapy			
					Age (hrs)	SB (mg/dl)	Hb (g/dl)	PCV (%)
1	1830	36	M	1:128 (Anti-C 1:32)	10	4.5	21.8	68
2	2400	37	F	1:256	23	10.5	17.9	55
					119	18.0	15.9	45
					252	16.5	14.1	39
3	3050	40	F	1:256	36 96-114*	18.5	17.5	50
4	2500	38	F	1:256	19	16.5	18.9	66
5	3040	39	M	1:1024	55	16.0	11.3	33
6	3450	40	F	1:512	60-70*	17.0	20.8	63
					70	20.0		
7	3000	39	F	1:512	36	17.0	23.8	75
8	2930	39	M	1:256 (Anti-C 1:6)	35	16.5	11.8	34
9	2600§	40	M	1:256	36	25.0	12.9	37
10	2260$^#$	40	F	1:512	12	17.5	10.9	35
11	2300$^#$	40	F	1:512	No phototherapy required			

*exposed to daylight lamps
#monozygous twins
§G6PD deficient

phototherapy was effective in such a situation (Fig. 9); however in one case, initial phototherapy before the diagnosis was made, with daylight lamps (radiance 140 uW/cm^2 in the 440-480 nm range, 250 uW/cm^2 in the 425-475 nm range and 295 uW/cm^2 in the 400-480 nm range) failed to control the bilirubin increase, which was later controlled when maximal intensity phototherapy was used. Associated G6PD deficiency did not affect the efficacy of phototherapy; as previously demonstrated[8], no additonal haemolysis occurred with phototherapy even when prolonged. In a pair of twins with severe Rh haemolysis, severe jaundice occurred only in one infant (Fig. 10) though rapidly progressive anaemia occurred in both; prompt response to phototherapy was observed though it had to be repeated.

Where early diagnosis was made as in three cases (Fig. 11) phototherapy was started early; it proved of minimal effectiveness at low bilirubin values. However, as the bilirubin concentration increased, the effect of phototherapy became obvious. In one case

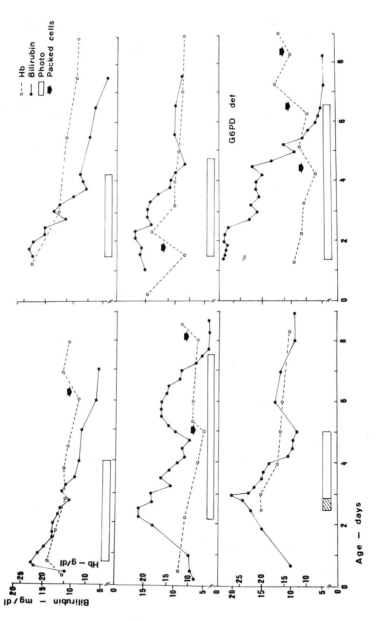

Fig. 9. Effect of phototherapy in Rh haemolytic disease. Initial use of daylight lamps in one case (hatched area) did not control the bilirubin increase.

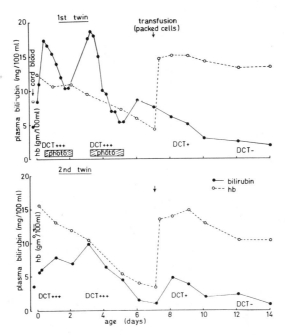

Fig. 10.   Early phototherapy in Rh haemolytic disease, in one of a
            pair of twins

temporary exposure to lower radiance from daylight lamps, after an
initial response to maximal intensity phototherapy, resulted in an
increase in bilirubin values which however again responded well to
maximal intensity phototherapy.

    With severe Rh haemolytic disease prolonged or repeated exposure
to maximal intensity phototherapy was necessary. The progressive
anaemia was easily corrected by packed cell transfusions. The
increased duration of exposure did not appear to affect the infants
adversely. Normal development was observed on followup.

    The ideal dose and duration of phototherapy has yet to be
defined. Certainly high intensity phototherapy with its greater
efficacy is indicated for severe or rapidly progressive jaundice;
even in severe haemolytic conditions it can be effective, though
prolonged or repeated exposure may be necessary. Packed cell
transfusions are necessary to correct the progressive anaemia, a
procedure far safer than repeated exchange transfusions. As the
effectiveness of phototherapy decreases with declining bilirubin
values, phototherapy is not indicated at low bilirubin
concentrations.

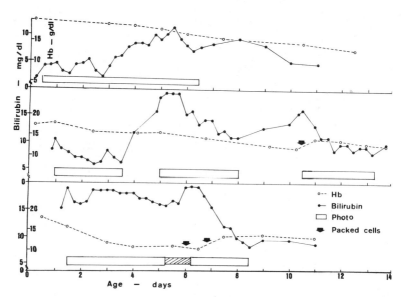

Fig. 11.   Early phototherapy in Rh haemolytic disease. Change to
           daylight lamps in one case (Hatched area) resulted in a
           rise in bilirubin concentration.

REFERENCES

1.   W. R. Brown, and H. B. Wong, Ethnic group differences in plasma
     bilirubin levels of full-term, healthy Singapore newborns,
     Pediatrics 36:745 (1965).
2.   K. L. Tan, Glucose-6-phosphate dehydrogenase status and
     neonatal jaundice, Arch. Dis. Childh. 56:874 (1981).
3.   L. C. Mims, E. Estrada, D. S. Gooden, R. R. Caldwell, and R.
     V. Kotas, Phototherapy for neonatal hyperbilirubinemia. A
     dose-response relationship, J. Pediatr. 83:658 (1973).
4.   T. C. R. Sisson, N. Kendall, A. Shaw, and L. Kechavarz-Oliai,
     Phototherapy of neonatal jaundice in the newborn: II effect
     of various light intensities, J. Pediatr. 81:35 (1972).
5.   K. L. Tan, The nature of the dose-response relationship of
     phototherapy for neonatal hyperbilirubinemia, J. Pediatr.
     90:448 (1977).
6.   L. Ballowitz, G. Geutler, J. Krachman, R. Pannitschka, G.
     Roemer, and I. Roemer, Phototherapy in Gunn rats, Biol.
     Neonate 31:229 (1977).
7.   K. L. Tan, The pattern of bilirubin response to phototherapy
     for neonatal hyperbilirubinaemia, Pediatr. Res. 16:670
     (1982).
8.   K. L. Tan, Phototherapy for neonatal jaundice in erythrocyte
     glucose-6-phosphate dehydrogenase deficient infants,
     Pediatrics 59 (suppl):1023 (1979).
Figures 3-8 are reproduced from Pediatric Research[7] with permission.

PREDICTION OF THE EFFECT OF PHOTOTHERAPY IN NEWBORNS

G.Wiese

Children's Hospital Free University Berlin
Kaiserin Auguste Victoria Haus
Heubnerweg 6, D-1ooo Berlin 19

Phototherapy (PT) is based on the interaction between light and bilirubin molecules in the skin. This photoreaction can be described by the following equation [1,2]

$$c = c_0 e^{-k\, t\,*} \qquad\qquad (1)$$

where c_0 = serum bilirubin concentration prior to PT

t^* = duration of PT

c = serum bilirubin concentration after illumination

k = photoconstant

The photoconstant can be taken as a measure of the efficacy of PT. The higher the photoconstant, the higher the efficacy. As a result of the interaction between light and bilirubin in the skin, the following dependencies of the photoconstant may be considered (fig.1).

In this diagram light is symbolizied by lines, (broken lines indicating ineffective irradiance) and bilirubin molecules by points. The following conclusions are evident [3]:

1) The change of the serum bilirubin concentration (SBC) under PT is proportional to the bilirubin concentration. A doubling of the number of bilirubin molecules results in a doubling of the number of interactions.
2) The change of the SBC under PT is proportional to the effective irradiance, E.

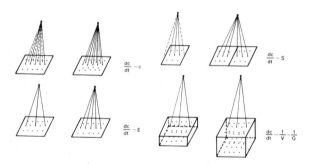

Fig.1   Representation of the dependencies of the photoconstant

3) The change of the SBC under PT is proportional to the illuminated surface area, S.
4) The change of the SBC under PT is inversely proportional to the
   volume containing the bilirubin, and therefore inversely proportional to the body weight, G.

Summarizing these statements the equation for the photoconstant is obtained :

$$k = k^* c_0 \frac{S}{G} E \qquad\qquad (2)$$

in which k^* is a general photoconstant. The so called 'photoreaction'
equation has the following form :

$$c = c_0 e^{-k^* c_0 \frac{S}{G} E t^*} \qquad\qquad (3)$$

This photoreaction equation describes the change of SBC for
Gunn rats under PT (Fig.2). The applicability of this equation for
Gunn rats is based on minor fluctuations in the SBC prior to the PT,
this means 1 month old homozygous Gunn rats are in a steady state
relative to their SBC. This is not the case for human babies (Fig.3).
Here the concentration increases during the first days of life -
phase one- and after reaching a maximum, decreases during the second
phase. When PT is begun during the first phase of normal increase,
changes in the SBC induced by the illumination may not be very impressive. In this phase it is the rate of increase in the SBC that
is diminished as a result of PT, after which the SBC will persist
for some time on a plateau, which is then followed by at first,
only a slight decrease. When PT is started during the second phase,
the normally expected decrease will be accelerated by the light.
Therefore, it is incorrect - but unfortunately common in the literature - to compare the efficacy of PT in babies with the same SBC
at the onset of therapy, but in different phases. For a mathematical

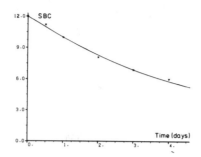

Fig.2   Comparison of the measured (*) and calculated (—) SBC in 1 month old homozygous, female Gunn rate during PT.

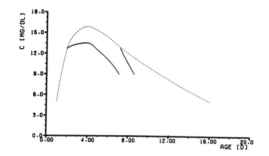

Fig.3   Calculated decline of SBC by PT in an infant in different phases with a corresponding c_i. The broken line represents SBC without PT.

analysis of PT, it proved necessary to consider the full range of observed serum bilirubin variation among infants without PT. The chief purpose of this present investigation is to express the age-dependent interactions between the influx and elimination of bili-rubin in human babies in quantitative terms. Above all I intend to clarify the diagnostic problem of when a reliable statement can be made about the postnatal course of the SBC with and without PT. Ever since the introduction of phototherapy by Cremer et al. [5], the question of efficacy with various PT regimes and other support-ive measures have been of great interest. For every investigation one needs an adequate control group. Aside from the fact that this adds a considerable amount of work to an experiment, it is diffi-cult to find access to truly comparable control groups. Therefore, a reliable prediction of the postnatal SBC would greatly reduce these requirements and make it comparable with other investigations.

Presentation of the Model and Calculations

Assuming that the bilirubin concentrations among the various compartments of the body exist in equilibrium, a change in the SBC would act as a window through which an increase or decrease in the bilirubin content of the body could be viewed. The fluctuations of the SBC lie closely connected with the maturation of the enzymes which eliminate bilirubin and with the decreasing enterohepatic circulation. Such a situation is possible to interpret pharmacokinetically. In order to do this, one combines all of the processes leading to the increase of bilirubin content under the concept of bilirubin formation; including of course, its reabsorption from the enterohepatic circulation. Likewise, one defines those processes leading to the decrease of the bilirubin content as bilirubin elimination. Then it becomes possible to describe the course of bilirubin concentration 'c' to its first approximation through the BATEMAN-function:

$$c = c_s + \frac{\hat{c}_0 \cdot k_1}{k_2 - k_1} \; (e^{-k_1 t} - e^{-k_2 t}) \tag{4}$$

in which:

c_s = the SBC (mg/dl) in the steady state (after termination of hyperbilirubinemia, i.e. $c_s \approx 1$ mg/dl)

$\hat{c}_0$ = the SBC (mg/dl) which would be formed during the period between birth and reaching the steady state, if no bilirubin were to be eliminated from the intravasal space

k_1 = the rate constant of bilirubin formation (h^{-1})

k_2 = the rate constant of bilirubin elimination (h^{-1})

t = age (h)

$\hat{c}_0$ may be calculated as follows:

$$\hat{c}_0 = \frac{100 \cdot \hat{D}}{V} \tag{5}$$

in which:

D = the amount of bilirubin (mg) formed additionally during the application of the BATEMAN function

V = the intravasal volume (ml)

If one assumes that the intravasal volume V, can be calculated with sufficient exactness by simply taking it as a proportion of the body weight, then only three parameters remain which could determine a change in the SBC: D, k_1 and k_2. Conversely the knowledge of these three parameters allows the calculation of the post-

natal SBC. In view of the fact that the change of the SBC is greatly dependent upon maturity or gestational age, it follows that
these three parameters will vary among infants and will show an
age-dependency. For the integral of function (4), i.e. the area
beneath the curve derived from the BATEMAN-function, one obtains
the following equation

$$S = c_s \cdot t_x + \frac{\hat{c}_0}{k_2} = \frac{c_s \cdot t_x \cdot k_2 + \hat{c}_0}{k_2} = \frac{100 \cdot D}{V \cdot k_2} \qquad (6)$$

in which:

t_x = period of time (h) before the steady state is reached

D = total amount of bilirubin (mg) formed during the period
between birth and reaching the steady state

Both the parameters D and k_1, are directly related by the area,
S. S is obtained by plotting SBC vs. age and then determing the area
by plane geometry. Since the course of the postnatal SBC is highly
dependent upon gestational age, the area S, must be expressed as a
function of this age. In practice one takes the birth weight, G.
Here the difficulty arises that changes in the SBC must be known
for the entire period during which the BATEMAN-function is valid.
In other words, this includes the period during which the bilirubin
concentration increases, as well as the long period afterwards
during which it decreases and finally becomes normalized. Concentrations vs. time curves of this type, i.e. for premature infants, who
often show severe and long-lasting jaundice, have been performed
all too seldomly.

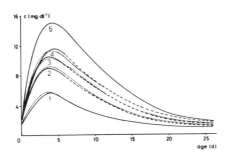

Fig.4   SBC changes with age, published by VEST [6] and WATSON [7]

1 Full-term babies [6]
2 Premature babies,birth weight 2ooo-25oo g [7]
3 Premature babies,birth weight 15oo-2ooo g [7]
4 Premature babies,birth weight 1ooo-15oo g [7]
5 Premature babies,birth weight 1ooo-15oo g [6]

In Fig.4, the SBC changes with age published by VEST [6] have been
plotted for two different weight groups (full-term and premature
babies <1500 g). These values have been measured up to the steady
state concentration of approximately 1 mg/dl. In addition, the SBC
values of other weight groups up to the sixth day have been included, obtained from WATSON et al. When these curves are extended
similary to VEST's 'complete' curves, and the area below them
determined, then it is possible to obtain the dependence between
area and birth weight G, which we had been seeking (Fig. 5).

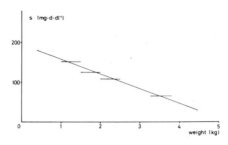

Fig.5   Area beneath the BATEMAN curve as a function of the body
         weight

By evaluating of this straight line one gets the following
equation:

$$S = 46,32 - 8,88 \text{ G} \tag{7}$$

It goes without saying that this described procedure only offers
a crude approximation of the time dependence between area and
birth weight. In the final analysis only two values are known for
the area, with two corresponding birth weights. This leaves us with
a stright line. Yet, as will be seen later, this relationship with
area shall be pragmatically sufficient for calculating the SBC.

It is assumed that 90 % of the bilirubin accounting for hyperbilirubinemia results from hemoglobin metabolism [8]. Seen over a
longer period, 0,9-1 % of postnatal extant hemoglobin is broken
down daily [6]. Accordingly, the total bilirubin D, formed during
the first three weeks after birth reaching the SBC steady state
may be calculated as follows :

$$D = 0,2 \cdot \text{Hb} \cdot 85 \cdot 35 \cdot \text{G}/100 = 5,95 \cdot \text{Hb} \cdot \text{G} \tag{8}$$

In this equation it is given that a newborn infant possesses approximately 85 ml blood per kg and that 35 mg bilirubin are formed per
1 g hemoglobin (Hb) [9].
Up to now, there are no reliable data concerning the distribution

volume V, for bilirubin in icteric newborns [1o]. In order to reach this volume, extra quantities of bilirubin would have to be injected. Therefore, it is necessary to resort to an estimation derived from experiments using Gunn rats [11]. In animals one month of age, V totals to about 27 % of the body weight. Considering that slight edema is a wide phenomenon among newborns during the first few days, V can be estimated at 1/3 of the body weight.
Solving equation (6) for k_2 with D, V, and S, we obtain for the rate constant of bilirubin elimination:

$$k_2 = \frac{5,95 \cdot 3 \cdot Hb}{S} = \frac{0,00074 \cdot Hb}{(1,93 - 0,37 \cdot G)} \qquad (9)$$

Using the time factor t_x, which varies among the different weight groups ($t_x \approx 960 - 132 \cdot G$), $\hat{c}_0$ may be calculated by combining equations (6), (7), and (9)

$$\hat{c}_0 = (S - c_s \cdot t_x) \cdot k_2 = \frac{1,78 \ (1,53 - 0,32 \cdot G) \cdot Hb}{1.93 - 0,37 \cdot G} \qquad (1o)$$

For the final calculation of the concentration vs. time function one needs the quantity k_1. This is the rate constant of bilirubin formation. With c_0 and k_2 already known, the equation for the maximal SBC can yield a conditional equation for k_1 when based upon the BATEMAN-function

$$c_{max} = c_s + \hat{c}_0 \left[\frac{k_1}{k_2} \right]^{\frac{k_2}{k_2-k_1}} \qquad (11)$$

Since this relation cannot be handled as an algebraic equation, it has more sense to determine the weight dependence of k_1 graphically for the time range under scrutiny. To this end, one establishes k_1 values for the plotted functions of concentration vs.time (Fig.4) using equation (11). These are in turn plotted against their respective birthweights (Fig.6). This function may also be described to its first approximation by taking a straight line :

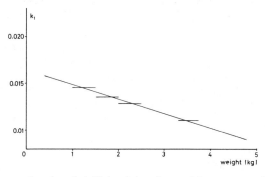

Fig.6   Rate constant of bilirubin formation as a function of the birth weight

$$k_1 = 0{,}0165 - 0{,}00162 \cdot G \tag{12}$$

When the concentration vs. time function is ascertained using equations (4), (9), (1o) and (12), there is satisfactory agreement with clinical data (Fig.4). This means that for the entire period of time under study, the deviation among all weight classes is less than 1 mg/dl. A definite disadvantage of the procedure discussed up to now, is the problem that changes of the SBC are described only as a function of the weight at birth. This implies that all newborns with the same birthweight have to show the identical changes in SBC with time. Empirically this contradicts clinical experience. A strict correlation between the SBC and body weight has not been observed in individual cases, although it has been found when different weight groups are compared. It is possible to get around this disadvantage when one dispenses with $\hat{c}_0$ (from eq. (1o)) and introduces an actual SBC c_t, at a specific point in time, t_t into the calculation. Since $\hat{c}_0$ is an expression for additionally formed bilirubin, the specific dynamics of the individual case may be taken into account - which SBC develops at which time period ? The conditional equation for SBC becomes only slightly more difficult :

One introduces the measurements c_t and t_t in equation (4), solves for $\hat{c}_0$ and introduces this once again into equation (4). The following is obtained :

$$c = c_s + \frac{c_t - c_s}{e^{-k_1 \cdot t_t} - e^{-k_2 \cdot t_t}} \left(e^{-k_1 \cdot t} - e^{-k_2 \cdot t} \right) \tag{13}$$

Using equations (9), (1o), and (13) it becomes possible to calculate changes in the SBC for every individual case. This may be seen for example, in VEST's curves (Fig.4) of premature neonates with a birthweight of less than 15oo g. If one takes $t_t = 24$ h and $c_t = 8{,}5$ mg/dl, then a good agreement is achieved (Fig.7).However, when one reduces t_t to 12 h and takes the SBC analogously at $c_t = 5{,}5$ mg/dl, then the agreement is significantly worsened (Fig.7). This arises because the accuracy of the SBC measurements is only about 1 mg/dl, so with smaller SBC's the error becomes relatively large.

This is to be expected, since the degree of agreement depends upon the exactness of the application parameters. The necessary condition for a reliable calculation of the change in bilirubin concentration is idiopathic hyperbilirubinemia. Concentration changes as a result of other illness cannot be handled by this method. In order to avoid this restriction, it is necessary to consider more measurements points, whereby the individual kinetics will be considered.

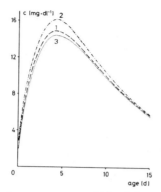

Fig.7   Comparison of the measured (1) [6] and calculated (2,3)
         SBC (G 1ooo-15oo g)
         2: t_t = 12 h, c_t = 5,5 mg/dl
         3: t_t = 24 h, c_t = 8,5 mg/dl

        The next diagram illustrates a typical example. After calcu-
lating the bilirubin concentration using only one actual experimental point it can be seen that the discrepancy between measured
and theoretical changes in concentration becomes greater with increasing age of the child. However, after considering two experimental points in the modelling the agreement is much better.
Finally, if this calculation is combined with the so-called
'photoreaction' equation (3) it is possible to reliably predict the
effects of phototherapy on newborn children. For such a prediction,
the following parameters must be known:

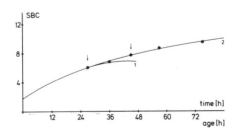

Fig.8   Comparison of the measured (*) and the predicted SBC (-)

         1 calculated with 1 experimental point
         2 calculated with 2 experimental points

Body weight - body length - hemoglobin at birth - age at the start of PT - SBC at the start of PT - effective irradiance - duration of PT.

With knowledge of these parameters, the decrease in bilirubin concentration due to the effects of PT can be accurately calculated by the following equation:

$$c = \hat{c} \cdot e^{-k_3 t^*} + \frac{(\hat{c}-c_s) \cdot k_1 \cdot e^{-k_1 \hat{t}}}{(k_3-k_1)(e^{-k_1 \hat{t}} - e^{-k_2 \hat{t}})} (e^{-k_3 t^*} - e^{-k_1 t^*})$$
$$+ \frac{(\hat{c}-c_s) \cdot k_2 \cdot e^{-k_2 \hat{t}}}{(k_2-k_3)(e^{-k_1 \hat{t}} - e^{-k_2 \hat{t}})} (e^{-k_3 t^*} - e^{-k_2 t^*}) \quad (14)$$

where

$\hat{c}$ = SBC at start of PT

$\hat{t}$ = age at the start of PT

k_3 = photoconstant (in eq. (1) $k_3 = k$)

It is possible to program this equation into a pocket calculator and thus compare the PT quantitatively as a daily clinical routine. Two predictions can be made by the use of the computer program :

1) The concentration-time function with knowledge of the called parameters. Fig.9 shows the comparison of the measured and calculated SBC.

2) The expected duration of PT to reach a certain desired limit in SBC.

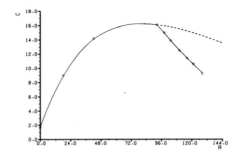

Fig.9   Comparison of the measured (o) and the predicted SBC (-) before and during PT for a newborn baby

In addition other quantities can be calculated, such as the anticipated peak either at various irradiances of PT or in the absence of illumination, or the hospital or region-specific time constant (k_1-k_3) which are probably influenced by different feeding procedures. Thus the program can aid in the selection of the optimal effective irradiance and give a rational basis for the decision - PT or exchange transfusion.

REFERENCES

1. G. Wiese,and L. Ballowitz, Phototherapy in Gunn rats, II. Further calculations on the effectivity of different irradiances (E_{bili}), Biol.Neonate 39:113 (1981).
2. G. Wiese,and L. Ballowitz, Mathematical description of the temporal changes in serum bilirubin concentration during phototherapy in newborn infants, Biol.Neonate 42:222 (1982).
3. G. Wiese,and L. Ballowitz, Vorschläge für eine rationelle Phototherapie, Pädiat.Prax.26:13 (1982).
4. G. Wiese, Phototherapy-calculations in newborns. Consequences for clinical schedules, Manuscript submitted to Stern's Intensive Care in the Newborn IV.
5. R.J. Cremer, P.W. Perryman, D.H. Richards, Influence of light on the hyperbilirubinaemia of infants, Lancet I:1o94 (1958)
6. M. Vest, Physiologie and Pathologie des Neugeborenenicterus, S. Karger, Basel-New York(1959).
7. D. Watson, T.G. Maddison, Bilirubinaemia of prematurity, Biol.Neonate 4:86 (1962).
8. J.M. London, R. West, D. Shemin, and D. Rittenberg, On the origin of bile pigment in normal man, J. biol.Chem.184:351 (1950).
9. W.B. Hawkins, and A.G. Johnson, Bile pigment and hemoglobin interrelations in anemic dogs, J.biol.Chem.126:326 (1939).
1o. D. Schmidt, E.L. Grauel, und I. Syllm-Rapoport, Bilirubin-belastung bei prämaturen Neugeborenen, Zeitschrift f. Kinderheilkunde 96:19 (1966).
11. G. Wiese, and L. Ballowitz, Mathematical analyses of the 'rebound effect' following phototherapy in hyperbili-rubinemia, Biol.Res.Pregn.1:162 (1980).

REDUCING THE DURATION OF PHOTOTHERAPY FOR NEONATAL JAUNDICE BY CHOLESTYRAMINE ADMINISTRATION

D.Nicolopoulos, E. Hadjigeorgiou,
A. Malamitsi-Puchner and N. Kalpoyannis

Neonatal Dept. of Alexandra Maternity Hospital
80 Vass. Sophias Ave., Athens 611, Greece

INTRODUCTION

In 1975 Arrowsmith et al[1] reported that, in treating a child with Crigler-Najjar syndrome, the duration of phototherapy necessary to maintain the bilirubin below certain levels was reduced by the administration of cholestyramine.

During the neonatal period, the increased production of bilirubin and the reabsorption of unconjugated bilirubin from the intestine - through its enterohepatic circulation[2] - cause loading of the hepatic cell with bilirubin. The absence of bacterial flora and the increased beta glucuronidase activity favor the intestinal absorption of bilirubin[3]. The administration of an inert absorbent with a high affinity for bilirubin (as charcoal[4], agar, polyvinylpyrrolidone[5], or cholestyramine) prevents the recirculation of bilirubin into the blood. Attempts to use agar alone[6] or as a supplement to phototherapy[7] gave no favorable results.

We tried to determine whether the combination of phototherapy and of cholestyramine administration reduced more effectively the serum bilirubin levels of jaundiced newborn infants.

MATERIAL AND METHODS

We have studied 58 fullterm and 59 premature jaundiced infants exposed to phototherapy and given 1.5

Table 1. Main data of studied newborn infants

	Phototherapy group (Control group)		Phototherapy and Cholestyramine group	
	Term infants	Premature infants	Term infants	Premature infants
Infants (n)	42	48	58	59
Ratio M:F	20/22	25/23	28/30	30/29
Gestational age (wk) (mean±SE)	39.4±0.4	33.7±0.6	38.9±0.4	33.2±0.5
Birth weight (gm) (mean±SE)	3,348±124	2.063±118	3,325±188	1,992±226
Age of beginning of treatment (hr) (mean±SE)	91.0±6.0	76.4±10	89.3±14.1	73.8±3.1
Serum bilirubin level at beginning of treatment (mg/dl) (mean±SE)	17.4±0.4	11.3±0.6	17.1±0.6	11.9±0.9
Average fluid intake (ml/kg/24hr)	120±21	117±33	125±36	119±23
Average caloric intake (Cal/kg/24hr)	82±14	79±22	85±24	81±16

Table 2. Etiology of jaundice

	Phototherapy group (control group)				Phototherapy and Cholesty-ramine group.			
	Term infants		Prematures		Term infants		Prematures	
	No	%	No	%	No	%	No	%
ABO incomp.	8	19	3	6	11	19	6	10
Rhesus "	4	10	2	4	5	8	1	2
G-6-PD def.	11	26	6	13	15	26	9	15
Varia + Unknown	19	45	37	77	27	47	43	73
Total	42	-	48	-	58	-	59	-

mg/kg/24h cholestyramine by mouth plus a 4% sodium bi-carbonate solution at a starting dose of 3 ml/kg/24 hours I.V. by continuous drip. The control group (42 full term and 48 premature jaundiced) infants were trea-ted only with phototherapy. The data on the studied new-borns are given in tables 1 and 2.

Blood pH and total CO_2 were measured daily and, using these results, the dose of sodium bicarbonate was regulated. Determination of the free fraction of indi-rect bilirubin was performed by the Sephadex method and by the more sensitive (for low densities of the free indirect bilirubin fraction) peroxidase method. Trigly-ceride and cholesterol levels were also measured, as well as Na, K and Cl.

Serum bilirubin levels for all newborns were mea-sured every 6 to 12 hours by a spectrophotometric me-thod, and phototherapy was continued until levels were lowered by at least 3 mg per deciliter from the pre-treatment levels. No infant was taken off phototherapy before treatment had been administered for at least 37 hours. The number of bowel movements and the consistency of stools were recorded.

RESULTS

Our results can be summarized as follows:

1) The duration of phototherapy required was shorter in the infants with cholestyramine. For a decrease of the bilirubin levels by 6 mg/dl in term infants of the control group 85±10 hours were needed versus 41±5 hours in the treated infants. In the premature infants for a decrease of 4 mg/dl, 74±8 hours were needed in the control group infants versus 46±6 in

Table 3. Decrease of the bilirubin levels in the jaundiced neonates.

	Phototherapy group (control group)		Phototherapy and Cholestyramine group	
	Fullterm (42)	Prematures (48)	Fullterm (58)	Prematures (59)
a) Decrease of bilirubin levels during phototherapy (mg/dl MV±SE.	6.0±0.5	4.0±0.6	6.0±0.5	4.0±0.6
b) Duration of phototherapy (hours,MV±SE)	85 ±10	74.0±8	41.0±5.0	46±6

treated ones. (Table 3).

2) There was no fall of pH in the treated infants and the Cl, Na and total CO_2 levels remained in the normal range. (Table 4). Triglyceride and cholesterol levels remained unchanged.

3) The follow-up of these infants shows that their neuromotor evolution does not differ from the evolution of the control group of infants.

DISCUSSION

The knowledge of possible complications of cholestyramine administration during childhood is still limited. Hyperchloremic acidosis, encountered in our previous study after administration of only cholestyramine, can be explained through the exchange of the Cl of cholestyramine either with glycocholic or taurocholic acid of the cholic salts in the intestine or with the bicarbonic anion of the sodium bicarbonate. From in vitro studies it is known that sodium bicarbonate is competing with bile acids for binding sites on the cholestyramine molecule[9].

Long-term administration of cholestyramine may result in steatorrhea, deficiency of fat soluble vitamins and folic acid,[10] nausea, flatulence, and constipation.[8] An other reported side effect merits a longer discussion, namely intestinal obstruction. In our study, despite a decrease of bowel movements in the cholestyramine-treated infants, we have not observed any clinical signs of partial or complete intestinal obstruction: it seems that the increase of intestinal peristalsis[11] resulting

Table 4. Electrolytes, total CO_2 and pH levels in fullterm and premature jaundiced neonates

Serum Electrolytes mEq/L		Phototherapy group (control group)		Phototherapy and cholestyramine group	
		Before phototherapy.	At end of phototherapy.	Before phototherapy.	At end of phototherapy.
Fullterms	K	5.35±0.43	5.19±0.17	5.1±0.3	5.6±0.5
	Na	140.3±1.4	138.9±0.2	137.1±0.8	136.5±1.2
	Cl	104.9±2	103.7±1.8	106±1.2	108.2±1.1
	total CO_2	24.1±0.9	23.8±0.8	22.6±1.4	20.7±1.6
	pH	7.34±0.3	7.35±0.4	7.35±0.06	7.34±0.05
Prematures	K	5.28±0.25	6.12±0.34	5.7±0.3	6.1±0.32
	Na	141.1±0.6	139.9±0.6	140.2±0.7	139.8±0.8
	Cl	110.7±1.8	106.3±2.3	109.8±1.6	107.2±2.1
	total CO_2	23.05±0.92	21.66±0.92	22.2±0.8	20.8±0.9
	pH	7.34±0.003	7.32±0.03	7.33±0.004	7.32±0.03

from phototherapy counter balances the constipating effect of cholestyramine.

Cholestyramine is a quaternary ammonium ion exchange compound with a strong affinity for bile salts.[8] The effect of cholestyramine to shorten the duration of necessary phototherapy as observed in our study, could be explained in three ways:

(1) by the formation of an inert complex of cholestyramine lipophilic unconjugated bilirubin in the intestinal lumen.

(2) by the binding of bile salts, which may participate in the reabsorption of unconjugated bilirubin.

(3) The reported[12] ineffectiveness of phototherapy in reducing plasma bilirubin concentration in the bile ductligated Gunn rat supports the recent theory of McDonagh and his coworkers[13] that during phototherapy the predominant pathway for the removal of bilirubin from the body is by biliary excretion of the water-soluble photoisomers of bilirubin. During phototherapy the stable 4Z, 15Z bilirubin IXa isomer is converted to its geometric isomers (4Z, 15E, 4E, 15Z, 4E, 15E), which are then excreted into the bile without being conjugated. Once in the bile these unstable isomers revert

back to the stable form. One could assume that cholestyramine acts by binding this stable, lipophilic isomer
and thus hinders its reabsorption from the gut.

Our experience until now is an empirical clinical
one. We have started a research project of measuring
the different compounds of cholestyramine and cholic
salts excreted in the stools of jaundiced infants subjected to phototherapy, in an attempt to explain the
pathophysiologic way by which cholestyramine acts and
reduces the duration of necessary phototherapy.

REFERENCES

1. Arrowsmith, W.A., Payne, R.B., and Littlewood, J.M.:
      Comparison of treatment for congenital nonobstruc-
      tive nonhaemolytic hypertilirubinemia, Arch Dis
      Child 50:197,(1975).
2. Poland, R.D., and Odell, G.B.:Physiologic jaundice.
      The enterohepatic circulation of bilirubin, N.
      Engl. J. Med. 284:1, (1971).
3. Brodersen, R., and Hermann L.S.:Intestinal reabsorp-
      tion of unconjugated bilirubin: A possible contri-
      buting factor in neonatal jaundice, Lancet 1:1242,
      (1963).
4. Ulstrom, R.A., and Eisenklam, E.:The enterohepatic
      shunting of bilirubin in the newborn infant. I.
      Use of oral activated charcoal to reduce normal
      serum bilirubin values, J. Pediatr. 62:27, (1964).
5. Ploussard, J.P., Foliot, A., Christoforov, B., Petite,
      J.P., Alison, F., Etienne, J.P., and Housset, E.:
      Interêt et limite de l'utilisation d'un capteur
      intestinal de la bilirubine nonconjugée (polyvi-
      nylpyrrolidone) dans l'ictère du prematuré, Arch
      Fr Pédiatr. 29:373, (1972).
6. Romagnoli, C., Polidori, M., Foschini, L., Cataldi,
      P., Turris, P. De., Tortorolo, G., and Mastrange-
      lo, R.: Agar in the management of hyperbilirubi-
      nemia in the premature baby, Arch. Dis. Child
      50:202, (1975).
7. Ebbesen, F., and Møller, J.: Agar ingestion combined
      with phototherapy in jaundiced newborn infants,
      Biol Neonate 31:7,(1977).
8. Thompson, W.G.:Cholestyramine, Can Med.Assoc.J.104:
      305,(1971).
9. Kleinman, P.K.:Cholestyramine and metabolic acidosis,
      N. Engl. J. Med. 290:861,(1974).
10. West, R.J., and Lloyd, J.K.:The effect of cholestyra-
      mine on intestinal absorption, Gut 16:93,(1975).

11. Rubaltelli, E.F., and Largajolli, G.:Effect of light
    exposure on gut transit time in jaundiced new-
    borns, <u>Acta Paediatr. Scand.</u>, 62:146, (1973).
12. Davis, D.R., Veary, R.A., and Lee, K.: The failure
    of phototherapy to reduce plasma bilirubin levels
    in the bile duct-ligated rat, <u>J. Pediatr.</u> 99:956,
    (1981).
13. Mc Donagh, A.F., Palma, L.A., and Lightner, D.A.:
    Blue light and bilirubin excretion, <u>Science</u>, 208:
    145, (1980).

BRONZE BABY SYNDROME: NEW INSIGHTS ON BILIRUBIN-PHOTOSENSITIZATION

OF COPPER-PORPHYRINS

F.F. Rubaltelli, G. Jori*, E. Rossi and G. Garbo*

Clinica Pediatrica and *Istituto Biologia Animale
Centro C.N.R. Emocianine
Università di Padova, Italy

INTRODUCTION

"Bronze" baby syndrome (**BBS**) was first described in 1972 by Kopelman et al.,[1] who observed a newborn infant with a grey-brown discoloration following phototherapy for unconjugated hyperbilirubinemia. Subsequent reports[2-6] described the clinical aspects of this syndrome while other papers attempted to clarify the biochemical mechanisms leading to the onset of BBS.[7-9] In 1982, we were able to demonstrate that a large amount of porphyrins is present in sera of BBS patients.[8] These porphyrins were identified as Cu^{2+}-uro, Cu^{2+}-copro, and Cu^{2+}-protoporphyrin.[9] In addition, large amounts of serum porphyrins and serum copper were detected in sera of adult and pediatric patients with cholestatic disorders.[10,11] On the basis of these observations and "in vitro" studies showing that, after visible light-irradiation, synthetically prepared Cu^{2+}-porphyrins added to cord blood serum exhibited spectral changes closely similar to those found upon irradiation of BBS serum, we have suggested that Cu^{2+}-porphyrins undergo photodestruction sensitized by bilirubin yielding photoproducts having generalized absorption in the near-UV and red spectral regions, hence responsible for the brown discoloration.[9]

In order to further substantiate this mechanism, we have performed a detailed study of the photosensitivity of various free base- and Cu^{2+}-porphyrins to visible light, either alone or in the presence of bilirubin. The data presented in this paper support our proposal that the simultaneous presence of copper-porphyrins, bilirubin and light is necessary for the development of BBS.

EXPERIMENTAL PROCEDURE

Materials

Bilirubin IXα was obtained from Serva in a crystal form; the sample exhibited a molar absorptivity value of 46,500 $M^{-1}cm^{-1}$ at 459 nm in good agreement with values published in the literature.[12] Human serum albumin (HSA), fraction V of Sigma, appeared to contain about 10% aggregated (essentially dimeric) material. Uroporphyrin III and coproporphyrin III were obtained from Nippon Petrochemicals (Tokyo, Japan) and were found to be homogeneous when assayed by thin layer chromatography (tlc).[13] Protoporphyrin IX and hematopor-phyrin IX, over 95% pure according to high-performance liquid chromatographic analysis, were supplied by Porphyrin Products (Logan, Utah).

Cu^{2+}, Zn^{2+} and Mg^{2+}-porphyrins were synthesized in our labora-tory by the acetate method.[14] The progress of the metalation reac-tion was followed by absorption spectroscopy in the 500-650 nm region, showing the gradual disappearance of the four-banded spec-trum typical of free base porphyrins and the appearance of the me-tallo-porphyrin two-banded (maxima at ca. 530 and 575 nm) spectrum. Quantitation of copper insertion was checked by atomic absorption spectroscopy. The following molar absorptivity values at 400 nm were estimated: Cu^{2+}-protoporphyrin IX, 107,143 ; Cu^{2+}-coproporphy-rin III, 174,074; Cu^{2+}-uroporphyrin III, 413,000 (solvent: 0.1 M phosphate buffer at pH 7.4). In all cases, porphyrin solutions were prepared by dissolving a known amount of the sample in the minimal volume of 0.1 M NaOH and then adding the desired volume of phosphate-buffered aqueous solution at pH 7.4.

Sodium azide, potassium ferricyanide and D_2O (99.9 %) were obtained from Merck.

Analytical Procedures

Tlc analyses were performed on silica gel-coated plates (ascen-ding technique); descending paper chromatography was performed using Whatman No. 1 sheets. In both cases, the binary mixture 2,6-lutidine:water (80:40, v/v) was used as the eluent; the chromato-graphic tanks were pre-saturated with the solvent mixture added with 7 M NH_4OH. The porphyrin spots were identified by illumination of the chromatograms with 254 nm- or 360 nm-light.

Absorption spectra were monitored at room temperature by means of a Perkin-Elmer mod. 576 spectrophotometer using matched quartz cuvettes of 1- cm optical path; for difference absorption spectra, double compartment cuvettes were employed. Fluorescence spectra were recorded with a Perkin-Elmer MPF 4 spectrophotofluorimeter, equipped with a red-sensitive phototube. The quartz cuvettes (1 cm

-thick) were thermostated at 20±1°C by circulating water through
the cell holder. Atomic absorption spectroscopy was performed by a
Perkin-Elmer 4000 AAS apparatus, which had been calibrated with
standard solutions of the analyzed metal ions.

Irradiation Procedures

In a typical experiment, 1.9 ml of a 33 μM porphyrin solution
in 0.1 M phosphate buffer, pH 7.4, were exposed to the light of
four 250 W tungsten lamps (Phillips) with continuous emission above
400 nm. Eventually, bilirubin and/or HSA in a 1:1 and, respectively,
2:1 molar ratio over the porphyrin were present in the irradiated
solution. In a few experiments, the irradiations were performed in
the presence of different concentrations of sodium azide or using
heavy water in the place of light water in the solvent system. The
irradiated solutions were air-equilibrated and maintained at 18±1°C.
Under our experimental conditions, the irradiance in the 400-500 nm
interval was about 1 mW/cm^2. At fixed times, suitable aliquots were
taken for spectroscopic and chromatographic analyses.

RESULTS

Irradiation of Free and HSA-Bound Porphyrins

Porphyrins having carboxyl functions in their side chains are
soluble in aqueous solutions provided they are converted to sodium
salts (see experimental). In the presence of HSA, both free base
and metallo-porphyrins yield non-covalent complexes with the protein[15] whose stoichiometry and stability depend on the porphyrin
structure and the nature of the medium. We estimated that, under
our experimental conditions, at least 60% of the porphyrin molecules
were bound with HSA.

Visible light-irradiation (15 min.) of hemato-, uro- and
copro-porphyrin, as well as their Cu^{2+}-derivatives, caused no dete=
ctable alteration of the porphyrin as judged by the invariance of
the absorption (fig. 1) and fluorescence emission spectra, as well
as by tlc and paper chromatography. The photostability of the above
mentioned porphyrins was not changed by complexation with HSA. Only
after prolonged exposure to light, we observed a slow photodegra--
dation of Cu^{2+} and free base-hematoporphyrin.

Protoporphyrin IX is intrinsically photolabile owing to a self
-sensitized photooxidative process.[16] We confirmed these observations. However, a drastic drop of the photomodification rate was noticed when the Cu^{2+} ion was coordinated with the tetrapyrrolic core.
The photosensitized reaction followed first-order kinetics (k= 0.12
s^{-1}) for short irradiation times. This phenomenon is likely to
reflect the shortening of the lifetime of porphyrin electronically
excited states caused by binding of Cu^{2+} ions [17] since the photooxi-

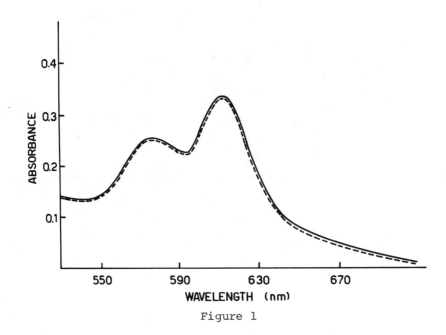

Figure 1

dation proceeds via $^1O_2$ generated from the lowest excited triplet
state of protoporphyrin.[16]

Irradiation of Free and HSA-Bound Porphyrins in the presence of Bilirubin

Hemato-, copro- and uro-porphyrin, either free or bound with
HSA, appeared to be photostable even if visible light-irradiation
was carried out in the presence of bilirubin. As known,[18] bilirubin
also binds with HSA to yield a 1:1 complex. Analogously, the addition of bilirubin had only small effects on the time-dependence of
protoporphyrin photodegradation.

On the other hand, all Cu^{2+}-porphyrins examined by us displayed
an enhanced photosensitivity when irradiated in the presence of
bilirubin. For example, the first-order rate constant for Cu^{2+}-
protoporphyrin photodegradation raised to 0.49 s^{-1} (short irradiation time). Typical patterns of spectral changes in the visible
region are shown in fig. 2: besides the decrease in the absorbance
below 450 nm, due to bilirubin photomodification, one can observe
the increased absorbance in the far-red region. Quite similar
spectral changes were shown[9] to occur upon visible light-irradiation
of sera from newborns developing BBS. The increased photolability
of Cu^{2+}-porphyrins was observed also in the presence of HSA.

Clearly, the most convenient way for following the time-depen-

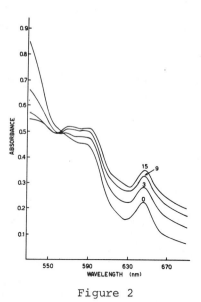

Figure 2

dence of Cu^{2+}-porphyrin photodegradation is provided by the absorbance changes above 600 nm, where bilirubin and its photoproducts
exhibit no appreciable molar absorptivity. A typical plot describing
the time-dependence of Cu^{2+}-hematoporphyrin photodegradation upon
irradiation in the presence of bilirubin is shown in fig. 3. The
plot tends to a plateau value, which suggests that stable photoproducts are formed. No significant variation of the reaction rate was
observed (fig. 3 and table 1) when the irradiation of the Cu^{2+}-hema-
toporphyrin-bilirubin system was carried out in the presence of
heither D_2O (which causes an about 14-fold increase of the lifetime
of $^1O_2$) or sodium azide concentrations as high as 0.1 M (an efficient quencher of $^1O_2$). On the other hand, addition of ferricyanide,
a known electron scavenger, induced a strong inhibition of the
photoprocess. Identical results were obtained with all other Cu^{2+}
-porphyrins.

Difference absorption studies showed no perturbation of the
visible spectrum of bilirubin upon addition of Cu^{2+}-porphyrins (and
viceversa). This observation would rule out a ground-state interaction between porphyrins and bilirubin. On the contrary, all Cu^{2+}
-porphyrins appeared to quench the fluorescence emission from
HSA-bound bilirubin. This finding might imply an interaction of Cu^{2+}
-porphyrins with the first excited singlet state of bilirubin.
However, other processes, such as electronic energy transfer and/or
inner filter, could also be responsible for the observed effect.

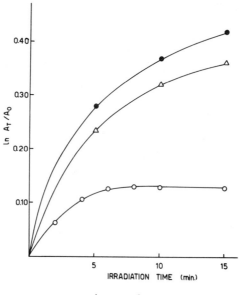

Figure 3

<u>Irradiation of Zn^{2+} and Mg^{2+}-Hematoporphyrin in the absence and in</u>
<u>the presence of Bilirubin</u>

The insertion of Mg^{2+} and, especially, Zn^{2+} into the tetrapyrrolic macrocycle usually enhances the photolability of free base
porphyrins,[16] probably as a consequence of photoinduced intramolecular electron transfer. Actually, both free and HSA-bound Zn^{2+}
-hematoporphyrin underwent readily detectable spectral changes upon
visible light irradiation (fig. 4 A); interestingly, such variations
are different from those observed in the case of Cu^{2+}-porphyrins
since there is a general decrease of the molar absorptivity throughout the visible region. In the case of Zn^{2+}-protoporphyrin, the
above described spectral changes have been ascribed to oxidative
opening of the tetrapyrrolic macrocycle.[19]

The addition of bilirubin to irradiated solutions of Zn^{2+} or
Mg^{2+}-hematoporphyrin resulted in a decreased rate of porphyrin photodegradation, the overall pattern of spectral alterations being
coincident (fig. 4 B) with that observed in the absence of bilirubin.
Hence, it is likely that bilirubin does not interfere with the photoprocesses leading to photodegradation of Zn^{2+}-porphyrins.

DISCUSSION

The lack of any detectable alteration of the spectroscopic and
chromatographic properties of uro-, copro- and hemato-porphyrin,

Table 1.   Rate constant for the bilirubin-photosensitized modifica-
           tion of 0.16 mM Cu^{2+}-protoporphyrin under different exper-
           imental conditions.

Reaction Medium	$k \cdot 10^{-4}(s^{-1})$ [a]
H_2O, pH= 7.4	9.4
" " + 10^{-4}mM N_3^-	9.1
" " + 10^{-3}mM N_3^-	9.6
" " + 10^{-2}mM N_3^-	8.7
" " + 10^{-1}mM N_3^-	7.9
D_2O, pD= 7.4	9.9
" " + HSA 0.16 mM	10.3

[a] Calculated from the initial slopes (0-5 min)

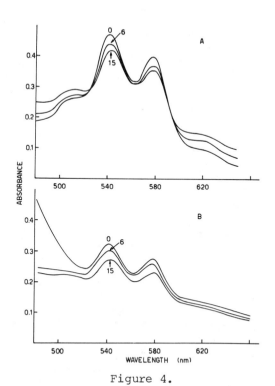

Figure 4.

both in the free base form and as copper-complexes, confirms the well-known photostability of porphyrins with aliphatic-type side chains to visible light-irradiation. Our findings indicate that the photochemical inertness of these porphyrins persists also when they are complexed with serum proteins. Analogously, the coordination of copper drastically lowers the photolability of free and HSA-bound protoporphyrin IX, almost certainly as a consequence of a shortening of the lifetime of the porphyrin excited states.[20] Therefore, although Cu^{2+}-porphyrins are present in large amounts in the sera of newborns developing BBS,[8] their direct photoinduced modification cannot be responsible for the appearence of the typical grey-brown discoloration. Further support to this conclusion is lent by the lack of photosensitivity in BBS patients, since Cu^{2+}-porphyrins are very poor photosensitizers.[17,20] Actually, the visible light-irradiation of newborn sera in the presence of various Cu^{2+}-porphyrins causes no appreciable damage of proteins,[9,10] although several amino acid residues are potentially susceptible of photosensitized degradation.[21]

On the other hand, all the Cu^{2+}-porphyrins examined in this investigation appear to be susceptible to photoinduced chemical alterations sensitized by bilirubin. We showed[9] that the presence of relatively high serum concentrations of bilirubin is necessary for the formation of bronze pigments. Once again, the spectral changes observed upon visible light-irradiation of Cu^{2+}-porphyrins and bilirubin, including the general increase of the optical density above 600 nm, are coincident with those observed upon in vitro and in vivo irradiation of sera from BBS newborns. Difference spectra indicate that the enhancement of the light-absorption properties extends to the blue and near-UV regions, although the latter process is obscured by the contemporary decrease in the absorbance of the solutions due to bilirubin photodegradation (photoisomerization and photooxidation). Such spectral changes are expected if the overall photoprocess must lead to the formation of "bronze" pigments. Therefore, we definitely propose that the photosensitizing action of bilirubin on Cu^{2+}-porphyrins represents the primary step in the onset of BBS.

Our findings allow us to gain some insights into the molecular mechanisms involved:
1) The presence of Cu^{2+} ions coordinated with the tetrapyrrolic system is required for photosensitization. This statement relies on the stability of free base uro-, copro-, and hemato-porphyrin to bilirubin-photosensitization, as well as on the drop in the photoreactivity of free base protoporphyrin when bilirubin is added to the illuminated solution (the latter phenomenon is probably a consequence of competition between the porphyrin and bilirubin for the incident light). Similarly, bilirubin protects other metalloporphyrins, such as the Zn^{2+}- and Mg^{2+}-derivatives, from photodegradation.

2) The specificity for Cu^{2+}-porphyrins of the photosensitizing action of bilirubin is possibly due to an interaction between the first excited singlet state of bilirubin it self and the ground state of Cu^{2+}-porphyrins. This interaction may involve electron transfer from or to electronically excited bilirubin, as suggested by the inhibition of the photoprocess by ferricyanide, which is an efficient electron scavenger.

3) The participation of photoexcited bilirubin in electron transfer processes has been observed by other authors.[22] In our case, the lack of reactivity of Zn^{2+} and Mg^{2+}-porphyrins could be related with their electron-acceptor or -donor properties, which are largely different from those typical of Cu^{2+}-porphyrins.[23] Photosensitization experiments involving bilirubin and metalloporphyrins with selected redox properties should clarify this point to a greater extent.

4) The redical species thus formed from Cu^{2+}-porphyrins may well initiate chain reaction causing the formation of polymeric material, in agreement with the indications of the absorption spectra of irradiated BBS sera and the stability of the bronze pigments to further visible light-irradiation. The formation of porphyrin-type polymers in BBS had been hypothesized.[23]

5) The experiments with D_2O and NaN_3 rule out any participation of $^1O_2$ in the photoprocess leading to degradation of Cu^{2+}-porphyrins. These data confirm the clinical observations indicating the absence of harmful effects due to photosensitization in BBS patients.

ACKNOWLEDGMENT

This work received financial support from Consiglio Nazionale delle Ricerche (Italy), contract No. 82.02720.04, under the Italy-USA cooperation in science.

REFERENCES

1. A. E. Kopelman, A. E. Brown, and G. B. Odell, The 'bronze' baby syndrome: A complication of phototherapy, J. Pediatr. 81: 446 (1972).

2. R. K. Sharma, G. Ente, P. J. Collip, V. T. Maddaiah, and I. Rezvani, A complication of phototherapy in the newborn: The 'bronze baby', Clin. Pediatr. 12:231 (1973).

3. C. F. Clark, S. Torii, Y. Hamamoto, and H. Kaito, The 'bronze baby' syndrome: Postmortem data, J. Pediatr. 88:461 (1976).

4. R. Weitz, Das Bronze-Baby. Eine Komplikation der Phototherapie, Padiat. Prax. 16:173 (1975).

5. E. H. Radermacher, A. Noirfalise, H. Hornchen, R. D. Maier, and K. H. Bigalke, Das Bronze-Baby Syndrom. Eine Komplikation der Phototherapie, Klin. Pädiatr. 189:1379 (1977).

6. K. L. Tan and E. Jacob, The bronze baby syndrome, Acta Paediatr. Scand. 71:409 (1982).

7. S. Onishi, S. Itoh, K. Isobe, H. Togari, H. Kitoh, and Y. Nishimurh, Mechanism of development of bronze baby syndrome in neonates treated with phototherapy, Pediatrics 69:273 (1982).

8. G. Jori, E. Reddi, and F. F. Rubaltelli, Bronze baby syndrome: Evidence for increased serum porphyrin concentration, Lancet 1:1072 (1982).

9. F. F. Rubaltelli, G. Jori, and E. Reddi, Bronze baby sindrome: A new porphyrin-related disorder, Pediatr. Res. 17:327 (1983).

10. G. Jori, E. Reddi, E. Rossi, and F. F. Rubaltelli, Porphyrin metabolism in the 'bronze' baby syndrome, in "Intensive Care in the Newborn," L. Stern, H. Bard, and B. Friis-Hansen, eds., Masson Publishing USA inc., New York (1983).

11. R. Tormo, B. Martin, B. Infante, A. Ballabriga, and C. Dominguez, Serum copper in infant cholestasis, Pediatr. Res. 15:1200 (1981).

12. R. Bonnett, J. E. Davies, M. B. Hursthouse, and G. M. Sheldrick, The structure of bilirubin, Proc. R. Chem. Soc. B. 202:249 (1978).

13. J. H. Fuhrhop and K. M. Smith, Laboratory methods, p. 757, in : "Porphyrins and Metalloporphyrins," K. M. Smith, ed., Elsevier Publishing Co., Amsterdam (1975).

14. J. W. Buchler, Static coordination chemistry of metalloporphyrins, p. 157, in: "Porphyrins and Metalloporphyrins," K. M. Smith, ed., Elsivier Publishing Co., Amsterdam (1975).

15. U. Muller-Eberhard and W. T. Morgan, Porphyrin-binding proteins in serum, Ann. N. Y. Acad. Sci. 244:624 (1975).

16. D. G. Whitten, Photochemistry of porphyrins and their metal complexes in solution and organized media, Rev. Chem. Intern. 2:107 (1978).

17. E. Reddi, E. Rossi, and G. Jori, Factors controlling the efficiency of porphyrins as photosensitizers of biological systems to damage by visible light, Med. Biol. Environ. 9:337 (1981).

18. A. K. Brown and A. F. McDonagh, Phototherapy for neonatal hyperbilirubinemia: efficacy, mechanism and toxicity, Adv. Pediatr. 27:341 (1980).

19. B. E. Horsey, F. R. Hopf, R. H. Schmehl, and D. G. Whitten, Photochemistry of free base and metalloporphyrin complexes in monolayers, p. 17, in: "Porphyrin Chemistry Advances," F. R. Longo, ed., Ann Arbor Publishers Inc., Ann Arbor (1979).

20. S. Cannistraro, A. Van de Vorst, and G. Jori, EPR studies on singlet oxygen production by porphyrins, Photochem. Photobiol. 28:257 (1978).

21. J. D. Spikes, Photodynamic reactions in photomedicine, p. 113, in: "The Science of Photomedicine," J. D. Regan and J. A. Parrish, eds., Plenum Press, New York (1982).

22. E. J. Land, R. W. Sloper and T. G. Truscott, The radical ions and photoionization of bile pigments, Radiat. Res. (1983), in the press.

23. G. B. Odell, Treatment of neonatal hyperbilirubinemia, p. 131,

in: "Neonatal Hyperbilirubinemia," G. B. Odell, ed., Grune
and Stratton, New York (1980).

EFFECT OF LIGHT AND VARIOUS CONCENTRATIONS

OF OXYGEN ON THE RETINA OF THE NEWBORN PIG

T.R.C. Sisson, S.C. and E.M. Glauser,
G. Chan and N. Romayananda
Temple University, School of Med.
Philadelphia, Pa. and
UMDNJ - Rutgers Medical School
Piscataway, N.J.

The objective of this investigation was to determine the effect of visible light, (similar to that used in phototherapy of neonatal hyperbilirubinemia) upon the retinas of newborn piglets in atmospheres of varied oxygen concentration.

Earlier studies[1] of piglet retinas exposed to standard broad-spectrum blue fluorescent light have shown profound retinal damage, with destruction of the rods and cones, inner ganglion layer, and disruption of the pigment layer. These findings have also been demonstrated by Ham, et al.[2] using a point-source laser (emitting 445 nm.) on the retinas of Rhesus monkeys and by Noell, et al., using green fluorescent light[3] in rats. This damage is not thermal, but rather photochemical.

Immature newborn infants are frequently exposed to phototherapy and to oxygen therapy at the same time, although eyes are shielded. However, the level of illumination in most intensive care nurseries is high and constant, and may be considered a significant degree of visible light irradiation. Even with eyes closed, as much as 28% of incident light will pass through the eyelid[4] or tissues even more dense and thick[5]

Materials and Methods

78 Newborn Batelle-pigs between 1850 and 2700 gms birth weight were studied between 3 and 6 days of age in groups of ten. Control animals were kept in their own cages, one in dim light another in the dark. The rest of the piglets in each group were placed in atmospheric chambers in the following schema.

	Dark		Light
	10% O_2		10% O_2
Atmospheric	21%	Atmosph.	21%
Chamber	40%	Chamber	40%
	100%		100%

Dark Cage: Room Air	Dim Light: Room Air

The study periods were for 24 hours. The spectral radiant intensity of the light source (10 fluorescent lamps F20T12/BB Westinghouse) was 34 $\mu w/cm^2/nm$ 420–475 nm., 1.4 $\mu w/cm^2$ at 445 nm. The piglets were maintained at a constant environmental temperature of 32°C. Such temperature control is known to preserve a normal body temperature in the newborn piglet.[6] Twelve animals died, two during study in 10% O_2, and ten in one group of pneumonia.

A few hours prior to study the retinas of all subjects were examined by indirect ophthalmoscopy and photographed. The piglets were returned to their cages in the animal room and after 4 weeks were re-photographed. Electroretinography was performed on 20 subjects between 4 and 5 weeks of age. At 5 weeks the animals were deeply anesthetized with Na pentothal, the eyes enucleated, and then the animals immediately sacrificed.

The eyes were placed in formalin immediately after enucleation, later bisected and photographed, then prepared for histologic sectioning and light microscopy.

Before retinal photography, the piglets' eyes were dilated with Mydriacyl 0.5% (proparacaine HCL 0.5% and phenylephrine HCL 10%). Before electroretinography, the piglets were anesthetized with intraperitoneal Na pentothal, and proparacaine 0.5% placed on each eye before application of electrodes.

Results

Indirect Ophthalmoscopy:

There was no vascular narrowing of the retinal vessels before exposures, nor was this detected in the control animals at 4 and 6 weeks of age. However, there was pallor of the fundi of those animals exposed to light, and narrowing of vascular diameters with marked constriction in the periphery, and lack of filling of some branches in those animals exposed to 21%, 40% and 100% O_2 and light, but less noticeable and uniform narrowing in those exposed to 10% O_2 and light. The eyes exposed to 10% O_2 in the dark appeared normal in comparison to the pre-exposure examination and to other post-exposure eyes.

Electroretinography:

Two control piglets, one in the dark and room air and one in dim light and room air, had normal responses to ERG before and after the study periods (Figure 1).

The two piglets exposed to light in 10% O_2 had weak responses to ERG, and the two in 10% O_2 but kept in the dark also had normal ERG patterns (Figure 2).

The other piglets exposed to light and 21, 40, and 100% O_2 had no detectable response to ERG after study. (Figures 3,4). Those in the dark in 21% and 40% O_2 had normal responses, (Fig. 5) but the two piglets in the dark but exposed to 100% O_2 had only slight ERG response.

Retinal Photography:

Ophthalmoscopic appearance of all eyes before study was considered normal, with the frequent finding of hyaloid vessels in the eyes of these neonatal pigs. It was noted that these animals, like all pigs, were afoveate, although maculae were present. Peripheral vascularization was noted similar to the development observed in the human neonate.

The retinas of two eyes of control piglets photographed immediately after enucleation showed normal number and filling of the blood vessels, and a clear pinkish transparency of the fundi overall.

The appearance of eyes just before and 4 weeks after exposure to 21% O_2 and light for 24 hours showed striking differences in the retinal vessels post-study compared with their appearance before: the calibre of the retinal vessels overlying the disks appears distinctly attenuated in the exposed eyes, and their temporal aspects show less transparency, and there are striae in the upper quadrants.

Figures 6 and 7a illustrate the appearance of a fundus in a normal eye just after enculeation. Note even calibre of vessels and full branching.

The appearance of the retina of an eye exposed to 10% O_2 in the dark for 24 hours is similar to that of a normal eye except for minimal filling of the retinal vessels, perhaps artifactual.

In contrast, the retina of an eye of one of the pigs exposed to 40% O_2 in the dark showed diffuse clouding, poor vascular filling and decreased visibility of the vessels. In many

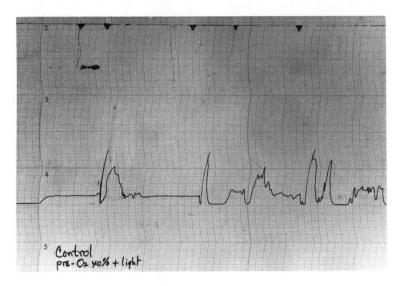

Figure 1   Electroretinogram of piglet, aged 4 days,
                  prior to exposure to 40% O_2 and phototherapy
                  light (34 μw/cm^2/nm, 420–475 nm) for 24 hrs.
                  Black triangles mark light flash.

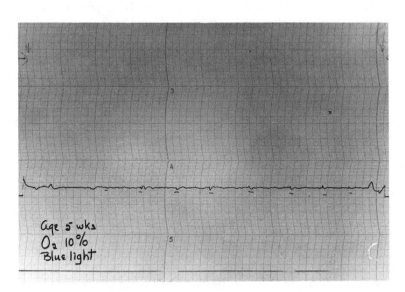

Figure 2   Electroretinogram of piglet, aged 5 weeks,
                  taken 4 weeks after 24 hr. exposure to 10%
                  oxygen and phototherapy light. (34 μw/cm^2/
                  nm, 420–475 nm).

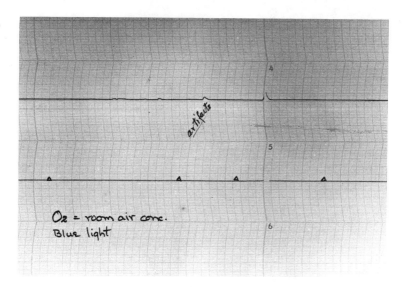

Figure 3 Electroretinogram of piglet, at 5 weeks of age, 4 weeks after 24 hr. exposure to 21% O_2 and phototherapy light (34 μw/cm^2/nm, 420-475 nm). Black triangles mark light flash.

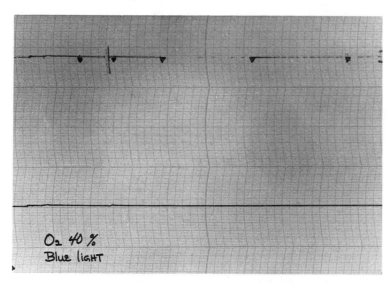

Figure 4 Electroretinogram of piglet at 5 weeks of age, 4 weeks after 24 hr. exposure to 40% O_2 and phototherapy light (34 μw/cm^2/nm, 420-475 nm). Black triangles mark light flash.

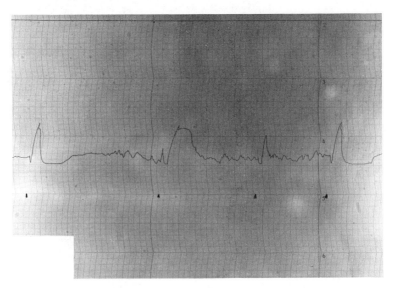

Figure 5   Electroretinogram of piglet aged 5 weeks,
                  taken 4 weeks after exposure for 24 hrs.
                  to 40% O_2 in the dark. Black triangles
                  mark light flash.

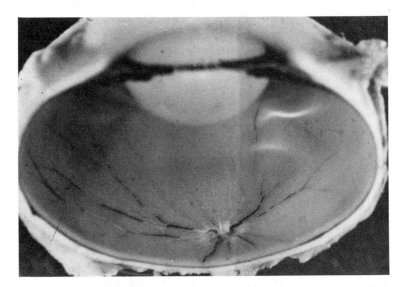

Figure 6   Fundus of a normal piglet eye at age 5 weeks.
                  There is normal calibre of all vessels, both
                  overlying the optic disk and in the peri-
                  pheral retinal structure. Branching of
                  vessels is normal.

peripheral areas, the retinal vessels were seen to have become quite attenuated and very poorly filled with blood.

The retina of an eye exposed to 10% O_2 in light for 24 hours showed vessel narrowing, relatively poor filling of the vessels and fundal edema and striation. (Figure 7b).

The retina exposed to 21% O_2 and light (Figure 7c) may be seen to demonstrate even more attenuation of the vessels, poor filling, and fundal edema.

In Figure 7d one may see the result of exposure to 40% O_2 and light. In this retina there is also obvious narrowing of the retinal vessels, loss of the clear pinkish color found in normal control fundi, and a suggestion of blurring of the disk edge.

The retina of an eye exposed to 100% O_2 in light shows even more definite vessel narrowing and changes in the appearance of the fundus due to edema. (Figure 7e)

Light Microscopy

The retinas of the control piglets were well-developed when examined at 4-5 weeks of age, with normal differentiation of the layers, regularly organized (Figure 8).

Experimentally exposed eyes demonstrated increasing damage as the oxygen concentration increased, and when this was combined with light irradiation.

In Figure 9, one may see the retina of a piglet kept in an environmental chamber, in the dark, in room air. This retina did not show vascular or other tissue damage, indicating that residence in the environmental chamber did not itself cause alteration in the structures of the retina.

Figure 10 shows the lack of significant effect on the retina by exposure to 10% O_2 in the dark.

In contrast, Figure 11 illustrates the damage occurring after exposure to 10% O_2 in the light. Here, edema may be observed with some irregularity of ganglia. The major artifactual change-separation of layers at the level of rods could not be avoided.

More obvious edema and cellular change in ganglion layers with some pykinosis may be observed in Figures 12 & 13 which is a retina exposed to room air O_2 concentration in the light.

Figure 14 illustrates the increasing damage as O_2 concentration is increased to 40% in the light.

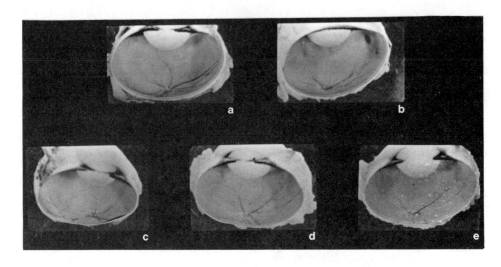

Figure 7a   Normal piglet fundus (see Figure 6)

Figure 7b   Fundus of piglet eye at 5 weeks exposed
                   for 24 hrs. to 10% O_2 and light during
                   life, 4 weeks earlier. (light exposure =
                   34 μw/cm^2/nm, 420-475 nm.)

Figure 7c   Fundus of piglet eye at 5 weeks of age,
                   exposed 4 weeks earlier for 24 hrs. to 21%
                   O_2 and light. (34 μw/cm^2/nm, 420-475 nm.)

Figure 7d   Fundus of piglet eye at 5 wks. of age,
                   exposed 4 wks. earlier for 24 hrs. to 40% O_2
                   and light (34 μw/cm^2/nm, 420-475 nm).

Figure 7e   Fundus of piglet eye at 5 wks. of age,
                   exposed 4 wks. earlier for 24 hrs. to 100%
                   O_2 and light (34 μw/cm^2/nm, 420-475 nm).

These findings are most marked in the retina pictured in Figure 15, which was exposed to 100% O_2 in the light.

Discussion

At the level of light-microscopy, the changes in retinal structures are present in increasing degree as oxygen concentrations are increased, although spectral radiant intensity of the phototherapy lights was kept constant. The changes appear to be most visible in the inner retinal layers, especially the nerve fibre and ganglion cell layers. Ganglion cells are much less compact than in the normal eye, and exhibit edema with cytoplasmic vacuolization and empty paranuclear halos.

These changes are interpreted as being due primarily to vascular phenomena, with vessel narrowing under increasing tissue O_2 tensions and from the direct effect of excess illumination on these tissues. The well-known vasoconstrictive effect on the retina of oxygen alone [shown even in the adult to cause a mean vessel diameter decrease of 11% [7]] may be exaggerated by light-induced edema of the entire retinal structure as well as a possible direct vascular effect of light.

It was clear that the piglets kept in the dark, though in low oxygen concentrations, and having histologic evidence of vascular change, could see to some degree at 4-5 weeks of age. Their acuity of vision could not be measured, however. Piglets exposed to light and in oxygen concentrations from 21% to 100% were uniformly blinded; the evidence by ERG, histologic appearance, and by simple clinical test of ability to avoid obstacles, and find food.

These studies have led us to conclude that oxygen in concentrations as low as 40% has deleterious effects upon the retinal vessels in full-term piglets in the immediate newborn period. These effects are worsened, even in room air, if there is continuous exposure to high levels of illumination, leading to blindness. The eventual recovery of such retinal damage could not be determined in this study as subjects were sacrificed at 4-5 weeks of age.

There seems to have been less damage in the combination of 10% O_2 (hypoxia) and light exposure. However, the design of this study did not permit any conclusion as to the role of initial hypoxia to later hyperoxic damage. It was apparent that the deleterious effects of light were not completely abated by low O_2 concentrations, and that some attenuation of the retinal vessels occurred also under this experimental condition.

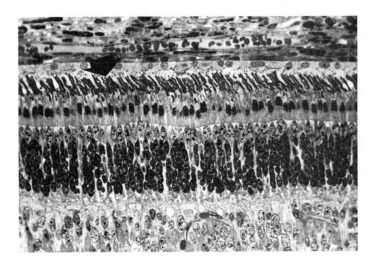

Figure 8   Retina of normal piglet eye at 5 weeks of
                        age. All layers of retina are clearly
                        formed (Mag. x400)

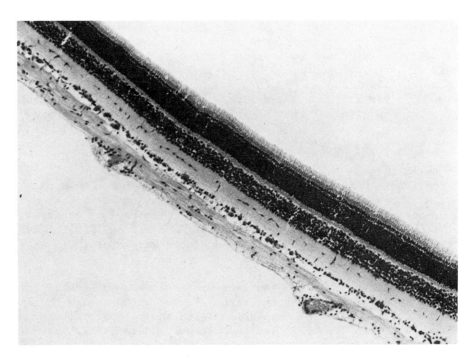

Figure 9   Retina of piglet eye at 5 weeks of age, 4 weeks
                        after exposure for 24 hrs. to room air in the
                        dark in an environmental chamber (Mag. x80)

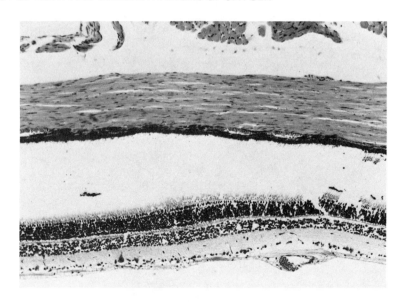

Figure 10   Retina of piglet eye 4 weeks after 24 hr.
                   exposure to 10% O_2 in dark. (Mag. 120)

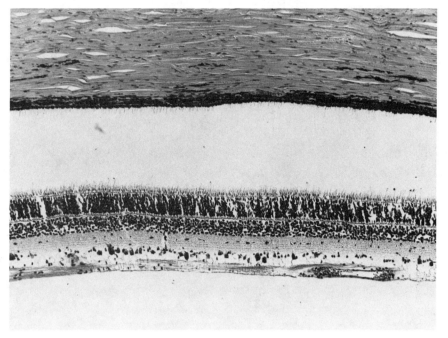

Figure 11   Retina of piglet eye 4 wks. after 24 hr.
                   exposure to room air and light (34 μw/cm^2/
                   nm, 420-475 nm.) (Mag. x80)

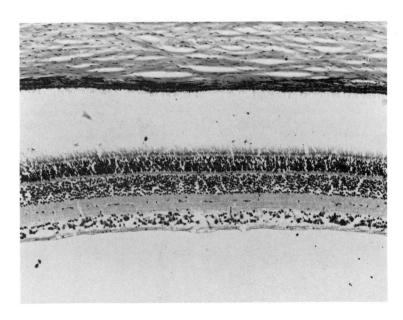

Figure 12   Retina of piglet eye 4 wks. after 24 hr.
                   exposure to room air and light (34 μw/cm^2/
                   nm, 420-475 nm.) in environmental chamber
                   (Mag. x80)

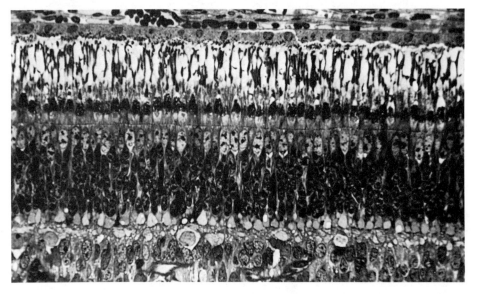

Figure 13   Retina of piglet eye 4 wks. after 24 hr.
                   exposure to room air in light (34 μw/cm^2/
                   nm, 420-475 nm.) (Mag. x400)

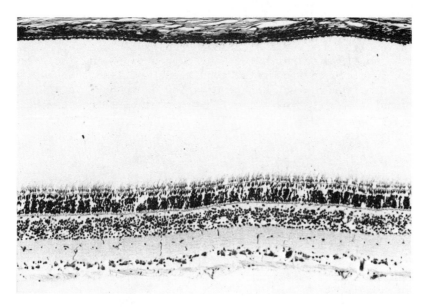

Figure 14   Retina of piglet eye 4 wks. after 24 hr. exposure to 40% O_2 in light (34 μw/cm^2/nm, 420-475 nm.)

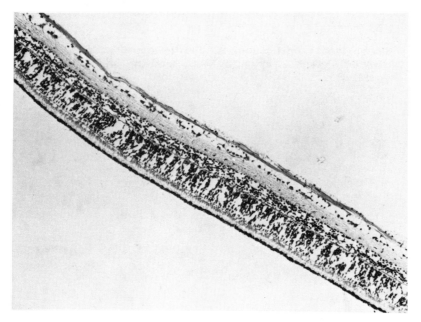

Figure 15   Retina of piglet eye 4 wks. after 24 hr. exposure to 100% O_2 in light (34 μw/cm^2/ nm, 420-475 nm.)

Our concern is that immature human neonates should be exposed to high levels of nursey illumination at a time when they are also subject to elevated levels of atmospheric oxygen concentration, and perhaps also elevated retinal tissue oxygen tensions. The effects of these combined environmental conditions, of less than physiolo= gically normal character, can be damaging as we have found in the newborn animal. It is not too difficult to accept the possibility that these same conditions may adversely affect the retinas of the more vulnerable premature human infant.

REFERENCES

1. T. R. C. Sisson, S. C. Glauser, E. M. Glauser, W. Tasman, and
       T. Kuwabara, Retinal Changes Produced by Phototherapy,
       J. Pediatr. 77:221 (1970).
2. W. T. Ham, H. A. Mueller, and A. M. Clarke, Retinal Sensitivity
       to Damage From Short Wavelength Light, in:"Sympos. on Biol.
       Effects and Meas. of Light Sources." D. G. Hazzard, ed.,
       U. S. D. H. E. W., pp. 37–45 (1976).
3. W. K. Noell, V. S. Malker, B. S. Kang, and S. Berman, Retinal
       Damage by Light in Rats, Invest. Ophthal., 5:450 (1966).
4. S. C. Glauser and T. R. C. Sisson, unpublished data.
5. T. R. C. Sisson and M. Wickler, Transmission of Light Through
       Living Tissues, Pediat. Res. 7:316 (1973).
6. L. E. Mount, Environmental Temperature Preferred by the Young
       Pig, Nature 199:1212 (1963).
7. J. E. Grunwald, S. H. Sinclair, and C. E. Reva, Effect of
       Oxygen Breathing on Retinal Flow, Ross Conference on Retino=
       pathy of Prematurity, Dec. 4–6, Washington, D. C., pp. 243–
       246 (1981).

EFFECT OF PHOTOTHERAPY ON HEPATIC MICROSOMAL DRUG

METABOLISM IN HETEROZYGOUS AND HOMOZYGOUS GUNN RATS

B. R. Sonawane*, B. Granati**, L. Chiandetti**,
F. F. Rubaltelli**, T. R. C. Sisson+, and S. J. Yaffe++
*Department of Pediatrics and Animal Biology
University of Pennsylvania, Philadelphia, Pennsylvania
U.S.A.
**Department of Pediatrics, University of Padova, Padova
Italy
+Rutgers Medical School, New Brunswick, New Jersey
U.S.A.
++Center for Research for Mothers and Children
National Institutes of Health, Bethesda, Maryland, U.S.A.

Phototherapy for the treatment and prevention of neonatal infant jaundice is widely practiced. The effectiveness of photo-therapy in reducing hyperbilirubinemia in jaundiced infants is very well established,[1,2] however, its widespread use has raised some doubts and concerns about its safety.[3] Although, the short-term effects of phototherapy for the most part are minimal[4], fluorescent light has been shown to be both toxic[5] and mutagenic[6] to mammalian cells. It has been demonstrated that visible light (450nm) is able to induce genetic changes in prokaryotic as well as eukaryotic cells[7] and that the illumination of isolated DNA in the presence of bilirubin and/or riboflavin[8-9] resulted in altera-tions in the physical and biochemical properties of this biopo-lymer. Gantt et al[10] reported that cool-white fluorescent light exposure resulted in both DNA damage and chromatid breaks in mouse cells. Futhermore, Speck and Rosenkranz[11] reported structural changes in the DNA isolated from human cells grown in culture after exposure to high intensity illumination in the absence of added photosensitizers.

An additional concern has been the lack of understanding about effects of phototherapy on a number of biochemical processes which are undergoing change in the developing newborn infant. Recently, general reviews on the subject of photoactivation of enzymes have been published[11-15] and several investigators have

291

conjugation processes. Soyka et al[22] failed to demonstrate the
effect of phototherapy on rat liver microsomal drug metabolism
while Nair et al[23] observed decreased microsomal enzyme activity
when rats were continuously illuminated. Recently, Davis et al[24]
reported that rats exposed to special blue fluorescent light had
no effect on liver microsomal cytochrome P-450 levels or mixed
function oxidase enzymes, however, a direct exposure of special
blue fluorescent light to liver microsomes caused a significant
decrease in aniline hydroxylation and p-nitroanisole-O-demethyla-
tion. In contrast, our preliminary observations suggested that
perfused livers of Gunn rats when irradiated with visible light
for one hour caused a marked increased in hepatic microsomal mono-
oxygenases and cytochrome P-450 and b_5 levels[17]. The present
report demonstrates that a direct exposure of blue light to the
isolated perfused livers or to the intact female Gunn rats increases the hepatic microsomal mixed-function oxidase enzymes.
Gunn rats, a mutant strain of Wistar rats with an inherited deficiency of bilirubin glucoronidation capability were selected as
models for the newborn infants with unconjugated hyperbilirubinemia.

MATERIAL AND METHODS

Animals

     The colony of Gunn rats used in these investigations had been
maintained at the Temple University Center for Photobiology,
Philadelphia. These Gunn rats were bred to produce homozygous (jj)
icteric (jaundiced) and heterozygous (Jj) nonicteric (non-jaundiced)
by mating homozygous males with heterozygous females Icteric rats
were identified by their yellow skins on the day of their birth
and subsequent permanent unconjugated hyperbilirubinemia which was
confirmed by measuring bilirubin concentrations in serum. The Gunn
rats were fed ad libitum with commercial pellets (obtained from
Ralston Purina Co., St. Louis, Missouri) and water. Only the
female offspring (both homozygous and heterozygous) were used in
the experimental protocol when they were 2-3 months of age.

Blue Light Exposure of Isolated Perfused Liver

     Adult female Gunn rats, icteric (jj) and nonicteric (Jj) were
used for this experiment. Both group of rats were killed by cervical dislocation, livers were removed, cannulated and perfused
with Ringer's solution. At the same time they were either exposed
to the blue light source (irradiance: 18uw/cm/nm, wavelength range
420-490nm at a distance of 24 cm) for one hour or the control livers
were only perfused but not exposed to light.

Blue Light Exposure to Intact Rats

Adult female Gunn rats, both icteric and nonicteric were shaved and deprived of food for 24 hours. Water was available ad libitum. During this period heterozygous and homozygous rats were exposed to a blue source (irradiance; 20uw/cm^2/nm, wavelength range 425–475nm at a distance of 24 cm) for 24 hours. At the end of light exposure, animals were killed by cervical dislocation and their livers were perfused in situ with ice-cold isotonic saline, removed, homogenized in 0.15M cold KCl and washed microsomal preparations were made as described below.

Preparation of Microsomes

At the end of light exposure, isolated perfused livers were flash frozen on a dry ice. While at the end of intact animal exposure to light, rats were sacrificed by cervical dislocation and their livers perfused in situ with ice-cold isotonic saline. Frozen isolated perfused as well as fresh intact animal livers were processed to prepare microsomes as described previously (25). Liver microsomal suspensions in 0.15M KCl were stored frozen at -70°C for not more than three days.

Enzyme Assays

All enzyme measurements were made on liver microsomal preparations. Enzyme measurements from at least 3 to 5 separate livers were performed in duplicate or triplicate to derive each value. Cytochrome P-450 was measured by its carbon monoxide difference spectra following reduction with dithionite, and cytochrome b5 was measured by its difference spectrum following reduction with NADH[26] with an Aminco DW-2 spectrophotometer by using the dual beam mode. p-Nitrophenol-glucuronidation was determined spectrophotometrically using 0.9mM p-nitrophenol and Triton X-100activated microsomed as described previously[27]. Benzo(a)pyrene hydroxylase activity was measured by the fluorescence method of Gielen et al[28] using authentic 3-hydroxy-benzopyrene as a reference standard with an Aminco-Bowman spectrofluorometer. Aniline hydoxylation was quantified by the method of Dixon et al[29] by monitoring the formation of p-aminophenol. Formaldehyde released by the demethylation of aminopyrine was measured by the Nash reaction as modified by Orrenius[30]. p-Nitroanisole-O-demethylase activity was measured by the method of Netter and Seidel[31]. Liver microsomal protein contents were determined by the method of Lowry et al[32] using bovine serum albumin as the standard.

Statistical analyses were done by the student's "t" test. Values were expressed as mean ± standard error and p values of <0.05 were considered significant.

RESULTS

Isolated Perfused Liver

The mean body weight (gram) of homozygous (control; 275.8 +
9.3 vs exposed; 268.4 + 13.2) and heterozygous (control; 246.5 +
18.3 vs exposed; 228.0 + 15.6) Gunn rats used in this study were
not different. Table I summarizes the data concerning the effect
of blue fluorescent light exposure to isolated perfused livers of
homozygous and heterozygous Gunn rats. The blue light exposure
for one hour during perfusion did not change the content of hepatic
microsomal protein from the non-exposed controls. However, blue
fluorescent light exposure significantly activated liver microsomal
mixed-function oxidases as well as glucuronyltrasferase activity.
Aminopyrine demethylase enzyme activity was increased by 37% in
homozygous compared to 96% in heterozygous Gunn rats by the light
exposure. Aniline hydroxlase activity increased by a factor of two
in jj and Jj Gunn rats, while glucuronyltransferase activity more
than doubled in both homozygotes and heterozygotes. The only
exception to the blue light activation of liver microsomal mixed-
function oxidases measured was benzo(a)pyrene hydroxylase in homozygous Gunn rats. Hepatic microsomal cytochrome P-450 contents
were significantly increased in homozygous (39%) as well as in
heterozygous (74%) rats. Similar light activation of cytochrome b_5
content was observed only in homozygous rats.

Intact Rats

The mean body weights (grams) of adult female Gunn rats used
in this experiment for homozygous (control; 193.8 + 14.2 vs
exposed; 182.4 + 8.8) and for heterozygous (control; 189.4 + 11.1
vs expose; 224.0 + 13.9) were not different. The effects of blue
fluorescent light exposure of intact (whole body) Gunn rats for 24
hours on their liver microsomal drug metabolizing enzymes are presented in Table II. In contrast to the light activation of liver
microsomal mixed-function oxidases in homozygous as well as heterozygous rats, significant increase in enzyme activities was observed
only in homozygous rats. Liver microsomal aminopyrene demethylase
enzyme activity was dramatically increased almost by 6 times in the
homozygous animals exposed to blue light but no significant changes
were observed in heterozygous animals. p-Nitrophenol-UDP glucuronyl transferase activity doubled in homozygous females levels
exposed to light. Cytochrome P-450 contents were also increased
by 61% in homozygous rats and 38% in heterozygotes. Cytochrome b_5
levels were not altered by light exposure to both genotypes.
Surprisingly, liver microsomal protein contents were increased by
whole body light exposure in homozygous but not in heterozygous
Gunn rats.

TABLE I

Effect of Blue Fluorescent Light Exposure of Isolated Perfused Livers of Gunn Rats on Microsomal Mixed-Function Oscication and Glucuronidation[a]

Enzyme[b]	Genotype	Control	Exposed
Aminopyrine demethylase	Homozygous (jj)	3.77 ± 0.18[c]	5.18 ± 0.24*
	Heterozygous (Jj)	2.60 ± 0.08	5.10 ± 0.16*
Benzo(a)pyrene hydroxylase	jj	0.77 ± 0.06	$.92 \pm 0.08$
	Jj	0.35 ∓ 0.09	1.20 ∓ 0.07*
Aniline hydroxylase	jj	0.15 ± 0.02	0.30 ± 0.02*
	Jj	0.19 ∓ 0.02	0.33 ∓ 0.03*
p-Nitrophenol-UDP-glucuronyltransferase	jj	6.75 ± 0.39	15.20 ± 1.05*
	Jj	10.40 ∓ 0.69	24.30 ∓ 0.04*
Cytochrome P-450	jj	$0.44 - 0.02$	0.61 ± 0.02*
	Jj	0.39 ± 0.04	0.68 ∓ 0.08*
Cytochrome b[5]	jj	0.55 ± 0.06	0.80 ± 0.04*
	Jj	0.55 ∓ 0.08	0.60 ∓ 0.21
Protein	jj	22.72 ± 2.32	19.85 ± 1.36
	Jj	18.72 ∓ 2.32	17.63 ∓ 1.58

[a]Isolated livers of adult female Gunn rats were perfused with Ringer's buffer and were also exposed to the blue light source irradiance 18um/cm^2/nm, wavelength (420-470nm) for one hour.
[b]Aminopyrine demethylase enzyme activity is expressed as nmoles HCHO formed/mg protein/10 min; benzo (a) pyrene hydroxylase activity is expressed as nmole of product formed/mg protein n/min; aniline hydroxylase activity is expressed as nmolos of p-aminophenol formed/mg protein/15 min; p-nitrophenol-UDP-glucuronyltransferase activity is expressed as nnmoles of glucuronide formed/mg protein/min. Cytochrome p-450 and cytochrome b5 content are expressed as mnmoles/mg protein and liver microsomal protein levels are expressed as mg/g liver(wet wt).
[c]All the values represent the mean $\pm$ SEM for at least 4 to 5 rats, measurements done in duplicate.
*Significantly higher from control; $P < 0.05$.

Table II

Effect of Blue Fluorescent Light Exposure of Gunn Rats on Hepatic
Microsomal Mixed-Function Oxiation and Glucuronidation[a]

Enzyme[b]	Genotype	Control	Exposed
Aminopyrine demethylase	Homozygous (jj)	6.4 ± 1.4	42.9 ± 6.9*
	Heterozygous (Jj)	10.5 ± 1.7	17.4 ± 2.6
p-Nitroanisole O-demethylase	jj	3.4 ± 0.4	8.0 ± 1.2*
	Jj	4.5 ± 1.1	6.4 ± 0.7
Aniline hydroxylase	jj	0.7 ± 0.1	2.2 ± 0.4*
	Jj	5.8 ± 1.6	9.2 ± 1.9
p-Nitrophenol-UDP-glucuronyltransferase	jj	0.6 ± 0.3	1.2 ± 0.4*
	Jj	1.7 ± 0.3	2.2 ± 0.4
Cytochrome P-450	jj	0.11 ± 0.03	0.18 ± 0.02*
	Jj	0.21 ± 0.01	0.29 ± 0.02*
Cytochrome b_5	jj	0.24 ± 0.02	0.29 ± 0.02
	Jj	0.28 ± 0.01	0.30 ± 0.01
Protein	jj	19.5 ± 0.9	24.2 ± 1.2*
	Jj	20.0 ± 0.5	19.9 ± 1.0

[a] Adult female Gunn rats were exposed to the blue light (irradiance-
$20 uw/cm^2/nm$; wavelength range-425-475nm for 24 hours).
[b] p-Nitroanisole-O-demethylase activity is expressed as nmoles of
HCHO formed/mg protein/10 min; for the expression of all other
enzyme activities, cytochromes and protein, see legend under
Table I.
[c] The values are the mean ± SEM; n=5
*Values are significantly higher than control values ($P \leq 0.05$).

DISCUSSION

The photoactivation of enzymes is an attractive concept and offers an excellent system that cannot only affect cellular metabolism but also foreign compound metabolism and disposition. Recent concern over the toxic effects of drugs in newborns, infants and children have stressed the need for better understanding of drug metabolism and action under a variety of environmental conditions. The widespread and occasionally indiscriminate use of phototherapy, an environmental agent unique to the treatment of hyperbilirubinemia in newborn infants raises some concerns about its effects on biochemical processes especially on liver endoplasmic reticular (ER) membranes.

The effects of visible light on photodecomposition of bilirubin[2, 3, 33, 34] and the consequences of whole body visible light irradiation[35] have been reported. It has been demonstrated that visible light penetrates the abdominal wall, liver and skull of adult Wistar rats as well as their newborns causing certain photochemical reactions to take place in tissues below the dermis[36]. Visible light has been shown to activate some enzyme activities in rat liver microsomes and mitochondria[17, 19]. In agreement with our previous report[17], the data presented here confirms that the direct exposure of blue light to the isolated perfused liver activates microsomal mixed-function oxidase enzymes and the activation occurs both in icteric as well as nonicteric Gunn rats. Yeary et al[16] found that rat liver microsomes when exposed to blue fluorescent light showed a significant increase in p-nitrophenol glucuronidation. However, the same authors[24] recently reported a significant decrease in aniline hydroxylase and p-nitroanisole-0-demethylase activities when liver microsomes were exposed in vitro to special blue fluorescent light. This decrease may be due to the longer time (4 hours) exposure and the use of high irradiance ($1,200 uw/cm^2$) blue fluorescent lights. It is difficult to compare their results with the data presented here since source of liver preparations as well as length and level of blue light fluorescence differs between two studies. However, Windorfer et al[37] did observe an elevation in acetylsalicylic acid esterase activity in erythrocytes of newborn rabbits and humans treated with phototherapy. When intact adult female Gunn rats (homozygous as well as heterozygous) were exposed to blue fluorescent light for 24 hours, data indicate (Table II) that liver microsomal mixed-function oxidase enzyme activities were significantly induced only in homozygous Gunn rats. The reasons for this selective genotypic induction of microsomal mono-oxygenases are unknown. The data on induction of hepatic microsomal enzymes by the blue fluorescent light exposure to whole rats presented here is in contrast to the previous reports[22-24]. The light activated induction of liver microsomal drug metabolizing enzymes in vitro and in vivo appears to be greater for some enzymes

than that produced by classical inducers such as phenobarbital.
These result suggest that visible light may act directly on liver
by activating photosensitized biomolecules such as bilirubin.
Alternatively, the site of action may be the skin in the intact
organism with circulation to the liver of a photoactivated
inducing substance.

The mechanism of photoactivation of the endoplasmic reticular
membrane enzymes remains obscure. However, it is possible to
predict that a direct response of blue light of low dosage may
excite flavins, which can interact directly with electron carriers
such as cytochromes or interact with oxygen to form oxygen radicals
or excited singlet oxygen[38]. Butler[39] has argued that specific
flavins trigger specific reactions but this model requires that
specific cytochromes be linked to a specific electron transport
system. One might also speculate that substrate activation could
well be the result of creating a redox potential or oxidized
substrates[39]. The other well documented evidence shown for green
algae[40] and euglena[41] that blue-light stimulates de novo synthesis
of enzymes, remains to be demonstrated for induction of microsomal
enzymes. Whatever the mechanism(s) involved, the data presented
here indicate that the blue fluorescent light exposure either directly to the isolated liver or to the intact animals selectively
induces hepatic microsomal drug metabolizing enzymes in the Gunn
rats, a mutant strain of Wistar rats.

The clinical significance of these findings is unknown. The
frequent usage of xenobiotics in the newborn infant, particularly
those in intensive care, warrants investigation of drug disposition in infants treated with phototherapy. It is possible that
toxicity in the neonate may result from the bioactivation of drug
molecules as a result of enhanced hepatic microsomal enzyme
activity induced via phototherapy.

REFERENCES

1. J. F. Lucey, M. Ferreiro, and J. Hewitt, Prevention of hyperbilirubinemia of prematurity by phototherapy, Pediatrics 41:
   1047-1054, 1968.
2. S. O. Porto, R. S. Pildes, and H. Goodman, Studies on the
   effect of phototherapy on neonatal hyperbilirubinemia
   among low birth weight infants, J. Pediatr. 75: 1045-1047,
   1969.
3. R. E. Behrman, A. I. Brown, M. R. Currie, J. W. Hastings,
   G. B. Odell, R. Shaffer, R. B. Setlow, T. B. Vogl,
   F. J. Wurtman, R. J. Anderson, H. J. Kostkowski, and
   A. P. Simopoulos, J. Pediatr. 84: 135, 1974.
4. J. H. Drew, K. J. Marriage, V. V. Bayle, E. Bajraszewski, and
   J. M. McNamara, Phototherapy, short- and long-term complications, Arch. Dis. Childn. 51: 454-458, 1976.

5. B. T. Noxon and R. J. Wang, Formation of photo products
    lethal for human cells in culture by daylight, fluorescent
    light and bilirubin light, Photochem. Photobiol. 26:
    589-593, 1977.
6. M. O. Bradley and N. A. Sharkey, Mutagenicity and toxicity of
    visible fluorescent light to cultured mammalian cells,
    Nature (London) 266: 724-726, 1977.
7. W. T. Speck and H. S. Rosenkranz, Base substitution mutations
    induced in Salmonella strains by visible light (450nm),
    Photochem. Photobiol. 21: 369, 1975.
8. W. T. Speck, C. C. Chen, and H. S. Rosenkranz, In vitro
    studies of the effects of light and riboflavin on DNA and
    HeLa cells, Pediat. Res. 9: 150, 1975.
9. W. T. Speck and H. S. Rosenkranz, The bilirubin induced-
    photodegradation of DNA, Pediat. Res. 9: 703, 1975.
10. R. Gantt, R. Parshad, R. A. G. Ewing, K. K. Sanford,
    G. M. Jones, R. E. Tarone, and K. W. Kohn Fluorescent
    light induced DNA Crosslinkage and chromatid breaks in
    mouse cells in culture, Proc. Natl. Acad. Sci. U.S.A. 75:
    3809-3812, 1978.
11. W. T. Speck and H. S. Rosenkranz, Intracellular
    deoxyribonucleic acid-modifying activity of phototherapy
    lights, Pediat. Res. 10: 553-555, 1976.
12. B. F. Erlanger, Photoregulation of biologically active
    macromolecules, Ann. Rev. Biochem. 45: 267-283, 1976.
13. G. Montiagnoli, Biological effects of light on proteins:
    Enzyme activity modulation, Photochem. Photobiol. 26:
    679-683, 1977.
14. D. H. Hug, The activation of enzymes with light, Photochem.
    Photobiol. Rev. 3: 1-33, 1978.
15. D. H. Hug, Photoactivation of enzymes, Photochem. Photobiol.
    Rev. 6: 87-138, 1981.
16. R. A. Yeary, K. J. Wise, and D. R. Davis, Activation of
    hepatic microsomal glucuronyltransferase from Gunn rats by
    exposure to light, Life Science 17: 1887-1890. 1976.
17. T. R. C. Sisson, B. Granati, R. Sonawane, and T. Fiorentino,
    Effect of light on enzyme activity in the perfused Gunn
    rat liver. Abstr. Am. Soc. Photobiol. 1978: 98.
18. A. W. Girotti, Bilirubin-sensitized photoinactivation of
    enzymes in the isolated membrane of the human erythrocyte.
    Photochem. Photobiol. 24: 525-532, 1976.
19. M. Orzalesi, G. Natoli, A. Panero, and M. Ciocca, Plasma
    hepatic enzyme in jaundiced newborn infants treated with
    phototherapy, Birth Defects Orig. Article Ser. 12(2):
    93-99,1976.
20. C. Dacou-Voutetakis, D. Anagnostakis, and N. Matsaniotis,
    Effect of prolonged illumination (phototherapy) on
    concentration of luteinizing hormone in human infants.
    Science 199: 1229-1231, 1978.
21. B. Lemaitre, P. L. Toubas, M. Guillot, C. Dreux, and

J. P. Relier Changes of serum gonadotropin concentrations in Premature babies submitted to phototherapy. Biol. Neonate 32: 113–118, 1977.

22. L. F. Soyka, W. G. Hunt, J. F. Lucey, Effect of phototherapy on hepatic microsomal drug metabolizing activity of rats, Ped. Res. (abstracts) 9: 287, 1975.

23. V. Nair and R. Casper, The influence of light on daily rhythm in hepatic drug metabolizing enzymes in the rat, Life Sci. 8: 1291–1298, 1969.

24. D. R. Davis, R. A. Yeary, and G. Randall, Effects of special blue fluorescent light on hepatic mixed-function oxidase activity in the rat., Pediatr. Pharmacol. 1: 313–319, 1981.

25. G. W. Lucier, O. S. McDaniel, J. R. Bend, and E. Faeder, Effects of hycanthone and two of its chlorinated analogues on hepatic microsomes, J. Pharmacol. Exp. Ther. 186: 416–424, 1973.

26. T. Omura and R. Sato, The carbon-monoxide binding pigment of liver microsomes. I. Evidence for its hemoprotein nature, J. Biol. Chem. 239: 2370–2378, 1964.

27. G. W. Lucier, B. R. Sonawane, and O. S. McDaniel, Glucuronidation and deglucuronidation reactions in hepatic and extrahepatic tissues during perinated development, Drug Metal. Dispos. 5: 279–288, 1977.

28. J. E. Gielen, F. M. Goujon, and D. W. Nebert, Genetic regulation of aryl hydrocarbon hydroxylase induction, J. Biol. Chem. 247: 1125–1137, 1972.

29. R. L. Dixon, L. G. Hart, L. A. Rogers, and J. R. Fouts, The metabolism of drugs by liver microsomes from alloxan-diabetic rats: longterm diabetes., J. Pharmac. Exp. Ther. 142: 312–319, 1963.

30. S. Orrenius, On the mechanism of drug hydroxylation in rat liver microsomes, J. Cell Biol. 26: 713–723, 1965.

31. K. J. Netter and G. Seidel, An adaptively stimulated 0-demethylating system in rat liver microsomes and its kinetic properties, J. Pharmacol. Exp. Ther. 146: 61, 1064.

32. O. H. Lowry, N. J. Rosebrough, A. L. Farr and R. J. Randall, Protein measurement with the Folin phenol reagent. J. Biol. Chem. 193: 265–275, 1951.

33. A. N. Cohn and J. D. Ostrow, New concepts in phototherapy: photoisomerization of bilirubin IX and potential toxic effects of lights, Pediatrics 65: 740–749, 1980

34. F. Rubaltelli and B. Granati, Phototherapy of neonatal hyperbilirubinemia, Med Biol. Environ. 8: 185–195, 1980.

35. T. R. C. Sisson, B. Slaven, and P. B. Hamilton, Birth Defects, Original Article Series, 6, 122, 1976.

36. T. R. C. Sisson and M. Wickler Transmission of light through living tissues (abstract) Pediat. Res. 7: 316, 1973.

37. A. Jr. Windorfer, G. Faxelius, and L. O. Boreus, Studies on

phototherapy in newborn infants. Influence on protein binding of bilirubin salicylate and on activity of acetylsalicyclate acid esterage, ACTA Pediatrica Scandinavica, 2: 293-298, 1975.

38. R. J. Strasser and W. L. Butler, Interactions of flavins with cytochrome c and oxygen in excited artificial systems, in The Blue Light Syndrome. (H. Senger, ed.), pp. 25-29, SpringerVerlag, Berlin/Heidelberg/New York, 1980

39. W. L. Butler, The mediation of redox changes by photoreceptor pigments, paper presented at the International Conference on the Effect of Blue Light in Plants and Microorganisms, Marburg, July 1979.

40. H. Senger, O. Klein, and D. Dornemann, The action of blue light on 5-aminolaevulinic acid formation, in, The Blue Light Syndrome (H. Senger, ed.), pp. 541-551, Springer-Verlag, Berlin/ Heidelberg/New York, 1980.

41. J. A. Schiff, Blue light and the photocontrol of chloroplast developement in Euglena, in, The Blue Light Syndrome (H. Senger, ed.), pp. 495-511, Springer-Verlag, Berlin/Heidelberg/New York, 1980.

LONG TERM OUTCOME OF PHOTOTHERAPY;

SELECTED ASPECTS OF THE NICHHD COOPERATIVE PHOTOTHERAPY STUDY+

Audrey K. Brown, Mae Hee Kim and Delores Bryla

Department of Pediatrics, State University of New York
Downstate Medical Center, New York

In 1974, a six-center* cooperative clinical trial of phototherapy for the treatment of neonatal hyperbilirubinemia was
initiated by the National Institute of Child Health and Human
Development (NICHHD), National Institutes of Health (NIH).
Infants were randomized into control or phototherapy groups by
a code established by the Biometry Branch of the NICHHD.
Randomization was applied to each of the birth-weight groups,
<2000 g, 2000-2499 g, and 2500 g or greater. Sex and race were also
used in cohorting for randomization. Infants entered the study
according to the following criteria:

1) All infants with birth weights <2000 g were
    entered at 24 $\pm$ 12 hours of age (922 infants).

2) Infants with birth weights 2000-2499 g were
    entered if the serum bilirubin reached 10 mg/dL
    within the first 96 hours after birth (141 infants).

+Supported in part by NICHHD Contract #N01-HD-4-2819

---

*Albert Einstein College of Medicine, Long Island Jewish Hospital,
LAC-University of Southern California Medical Center, Medical
College of Virginia, State University of New York-Downstate Medical
Center, and University of Cincinnati School of Medicine

3)   Infants with birth weights <2499 g were entered if the serum bilirubin reached 13 mg/dL in the first 96 hours after birth.   Before October 1974, the level of bilirubin for accession in this weight group was 15 mg/dL (276 infants).

When entry was completed in 1976, 672 infants**were in the phototherapy group and 667 in the control group. The phototherapy regimen stipulated that the therapy should be continuous, and the duration was set at 96 hours. A standard commercial phototherapy unit was used with a fluorescent bulb. The bulb was changed after 2000 hours of use. The study infants received standard care in the nursery. Exchange transfusion was used in both the control and phototherapy groups when the serum bilirubin exceeded the following values:

Weight(g)		1250	1250-1499	1500-1999	2000-2499	2499
Bilirubin	A	13	15	17	18	20
(Total)	B	10	13	15	17	18

Group A contained those infants who had an uncomplicated course other than hyperbilirubinemia. An infant was placed in group B when one or more of the following findings were present:

1)   Perinatal asphyxia (Apgar score less than 3 at 5 minutes).

2)   Respiratory distress (PO_2 less than 40 for more than 2 hours).

3)   Acidosis (pH 7.15 or less for more than 1 hour).

4)   Persistent hypothermia (rectal temperature at 4 cm of 35° for more than 4 hours).

5)   Low serum protein (<4 g/dL) or albumin (<2.5 g/dL), measured at least twice.

6)   Signs of clinical central nervous system deterioration.

**Protocol was breached 1 hour after entry in one infant, leaving 671 infants in the phototherapy group.

Any infant in either group could receive exchange transfusion at any time if, in the judgment of the physician, it was indicated, without regard to these criteria.

Phototherapy: Prevention and Control of Hyperbilirubinemia

Infants Weighing Less Than 2000 G

When phototherapy was instituted early, ie at 24+ 12 hours of age, in infants weighing <2000 g, hyperbilirubinemia was prevented in the majority of infants. Only 17.7% of the 462 infants treated with light had bilirubin levels >10mg/dL, compared with 62.8% of the 460 controls. Further, 24.4% of control infants in this weight group received exchange transfusions, compared with only 4.1% of infants in the phototherapy group.

Infants Weighing 2000-2499 G

In this birth-weight group, the effectiveness of phototherapy in controlling, rather than preventing, hyperbilirubinemia was tested, since the institution of phototherapy was delayed until serum bilirubin levels were 10 mg/dL. While only 18.6% of the 70 infants receiving phototherapy had serum bilirubin values >15 mg/dL, 42.3% of control infants had such levels. Fewer infants in the phototherapy group received exchange transfusions than did control infants in this weight group (4.3% v 25.4%,P=0.001).

Infants Weighing More Than 2499 G

Infants in this birth-weight group were randomized into either control or light-treated groups when the serum bilirubin reached 13 mg/dL. The mean age at entry was >60 hours in each group. Bilirubin values were moderately but significantly lower each day in the treated than in the control infants. As had been noted in the other treated infants, the major decrease in serum bilirubin occurred during the 1st day of phototherapy. A bilirubin decrement of 2.3mg/dL occurred in the phototherapy group in contrast to a decrease of only 0.47mg/dL in the first 24 hours of study in the control infants.

Phototherapy was not very effective in controlling hyperbilirubinemia secondary to hemolysis. Similar numbers of exchange transfusions were performed as in control infants. However, among infants whose jaundice was unrelated to hemolysis, phototherapy was effective in reducing the requirement for exchange.

Kernicterus in Autopsied Infants

Seventy-two (10.7%) of the 671 newborn infants who had entered
in the phototherapy group and 62 (9.3%) of the 667 infants in the
control group died during the 1st year of life. With the exception
of one infant in each group, all of the infants who died had weighed
less than 2000 g at birth. Most of the deaths in each group, ie,
67/72 in the phototherapy group and 52/62 in the control group,
occurred while the infants were still in the nursery (Table 1).
There was no significant difference in the percentage of deaths
occurring within specified time intervals, ie, 0 to 7 days, 0 to 28
days, or within the 1st year, in the phototherapy and control groups
of infants. The most frequent cause of death among newborn infants
weighing less than 2000 g was the respiratory distress syndrome
(RDS) with intracranial hemorrhage (ICH).

Four infants had evidence of kernicterus at autopsy; this
represents an incidence of 5% of the autopsied infants from the
entire group and 6% of autopsied infants who weighed less than
1500 g. All the kernicteric infants were in that weight group.
None of the phototherapy-treated infants had evidence of kernicterus (Table 2). Kernicterus (KI) was defined as grossly
visible yellow staining of specific nuclei of the brain.

Some of the characteristics of the infants with kernicterus
were as follows: Three of the four infants were males. Two infants weighed less than 1000 g at birth and expired on the 2nd
day of life. One of these very small infants was the only female
in the group; she weighed 980 g. Although female, she was deficient in glucose-6-phosphate dehydrogenase and had a sharp drop
in hemoglobin on the 2nd day of life. Her peak bilirubin was 6.5

Table 1. Total Number of Deaths in Phototherapy and Control
Infants

	Phototherapy Group	Control Group	Total
Total deaths (in nursery)	67	52	120*
Total autopsied	48 (72%)	37 (71%)	86*
Kernicterus	0	3+(8%)	4* (5%)

*There was an additional case of kernicterus in which study
protocol was breached (no phototherapy)
+P=0.079 (Fisher exact test)

Table 2. Cooperative Phototherapy Study, Kernicterus at Autopsy; Infants <1500 G.

	Phototherapy Group	Control Group	Total
Infants <1500 g	215	195	411*
Deaths in nursery (<1500 g) (<60 days)	51 (24%)	41 (21%)	93* (23%)
Autopsied (<1500 g) (<60 days)	40	29	70*
Kernicterus	0	3+ (10%)	4* (6%)

* There was an additional case of kernicterus in which study protocol was breached (no phototherapy)
+P=0.07 (Fisher exact test)

Table 3. NICHHD Cooperative Phototherapy Study: Bilirubin and Binding Studies in Infants With Kernicterus.

Case #	IQ0017	BQ0033	GN220012	BQ0044
Weight (g)	760	980	1220	1270
Exchange Transfusion	No	No	Yes (X4)	Yes (X1)
Peak bilirubin (mg/dL)	8.6	6.5	14.2	14.0
Lowest albumin(g/dL)	1.4	2.9	2.9	2.0
Lowest hydroxybenzene azobenzoic acid binding (HABA)(%)	19.6	68.4	34.8	23.8
Kernlute	Pos	Neg	Neg	Neg
Salicylate index	5.2	3.0	8.1	7.0

mg/dL on the 1st day. Her hydroxybenzene azobenzoic acid (HABA) binding was inappropriately low (68%) for that low serum bilirubin concentration. Table 3 shows the bilirubin binding studies in these infants.

There was deep yellow staining of the thalamus bilaterally as well as of the dentate nucleus, the inferior colliculus, and the periaqueductal area. In addition, there was an acute hemorrhage in the germinal matrix extending into the ventricle and to the subarachnoid space.

The other very small infant with KI weighed 760 g at birth and was the first of twins. His peak bilirubin level of 8.6 mg/dL was associated with a very low HABA binding of only 19.6%. The Sephadex test was positive for "free" bilirubin (see Table 3). He was edematous and had a serum albumin level of only 1.4 g/dL.

At autopsy there was yellow staining of the thalamus and focal staining of the 3rd cranial nucleus as well as other cranial nerve nuclei. There was hemorrhage in the left temporo-occipital area. It is of interest that his twin (who survived), who had less severe RDS with episodes of bradycardia and apnea, is now neurologically impaired and has a defect in language processing. The twin's bilirubin had peaked at 10 mg/dL but his HABA had been higher than the first twin's, at 46%.

The third infant with evidence of kernicterus (protocol breached in this child) weighed 1220 g at birth and died at 7 days of age with RDS. His peak serum bilirubin was 14.2 mg/dL at 48 hours of life. HABA binding was 34.8% and the salicylate index was high, 8.1. He had, in error, received 1 hour of phototherapy at 48 hours of life just before receiving the first of four exchange transfusions, but was not part of the phototherapy study group. In addition to gross yellow staining of the basal ganglia there was periventricular leukomalacia as well as intraventricular hemorrhage.

The fourth infant with evidence of kernicterus weighed 1270 g at birth at 33 weeks' gestation. He died at 55 days of age with evidence of severe liver failure. He had had perinatal asphyxia, had developed RDS, and had an ICH. There had been a sudden rise in the serum bilirubin on the 4th day of life. The serum bilirubin peaked at 14 mg/dL on the 5th day of life, at which time an exchange transfusion was performed. Some bilirubinemia persisted throughout his course. At autopsy, the brain showed focal yellow discoloration of the right thalamus and focal and severe loss of neurons with astrocytosis of the right thalamus, base of pons, and inferior olivary nuclei.

The neuropathologist[+] has carefully reviewed these findings and has no question that they represent kernicterus, chronic phase.

There was in addition extremely severe hypoxic encephalopathy with characteristic perinatal telencephalic leukoencephalopathy, acute and chronic, with leukomalacia. There was also hemorrhage, subacute, in the right lateral ventricle and evidence of an old subependymal germinal matrix hemorrhage.

Table 4. Clinical Characteristics of Infants With Kernicterus.

Sex	3 male, 1 female
Spontaneous vaginal delivery	4/4
Apgar $\leq$5	4/4
Weight <1500 g	4/4
Respiratory distress syndrome	4/4
Sepsis or infection	0/4

Table 5. Laboratory Findings: Comparison of Laboratory Findings in Infants in the Control Group Who Died With (KI) and Without (Non-KI) Kernicterus.

		KI	Non-KI
Bilirubin	<10 mg/dL	2/4	37/43
	>15 mg/dL	0/4	2/43
HABA*	<37%	3/4	5/43+
Hematocrit	<40%	4/4	37/43
Acidosis	pH<7.15	4/4	37/43
Hypoxia	PaO_2 <40	4/4	33/43

*hydroxybenzene azobenzoic acid
+P=0.01 (Fisher exact test)

+We wish to thank Dr. Joanna Sher, Professor of Pathology at SUNY-Downstate Medical Center, who reviewed the brain pathology in these cases.

Table 6. Clinical and Laboratory Data in Infants With
Low HABA* With (KI) and Without (Non-KI) Kernicterus.

	Low HABA	
	KI	Non-KI
Male	3/4	3/5
Phototherapy	0/4	2/5
<1500 g	4/4	5/5
Total bilirubin <10	2/4	3/5
>15	0/4	0/5
Hematocrit <40%	4/4	5/5
Acidosis	4/4	5/5
Hypoxia	4/4	4/5
Apgar ≤5	4/4	3/5
Respiratory distress syndrome	4/4	5/5
Sepsis	0/4	4/5

*hydroxybenzene azobenzoic acid

Summary of Clinical and Laboratory Characteristics of the Infants With Kernicterus

Clinical characteristics of the infants with kernicterus are
summarized in Table 4. All weighed less than 1500 g at birth;
all had Apgar scores less than 3 at 1 minute and less than 5 at
5 minutes. All had RDS. All were products of spontaneous
vaginal deliveries. None had proven septicemia. All had poor Moro
and grasp reactions and two had poor sucking reactions as well.
Two had seizures.

The laboratory findings in infants with and without
kernicterus are summarized in Table 5. Two infants with kernicterus had serum bilirubin levels less than 10 mg/dL. None had
levels in excess of 15 mg/dL. All had laboratory confirmation
of anemia, hypoxia, and acidosis. HABA binding was low or inappropriate in all four infants with KI but in only 5/43 without
KI in whom HABA binding studies were done (P=0.001).

Comparison With Nonkernicteric Infants

Since three of the four infants had low HABA binding and all
weighed less than 1500 g, we compared the data from the KI infants
with those with no KI and these same two characteristics. The
data in Table 6 indicate that there were no significant differences.

Table 7.   Neurologic Outcome at 1 Year - Infants > 2000 g

BIRTH WT.		NORMAL	SUSPICIOUS	ABNORMAL	TOTAL
2000-2499g.	P	48	6	1	55
	C	58	0	1	59
≥2500g.	P	117	3	1	121
	C	114	3	0	117

Cooperative PhotoRx Study
1983

Table 8.   Neurologic Outcome at 1 Year - Infants ≤ 2000 g

Bilirubin mg/dl		<10			10-14.9			15-19.9			≥20			Total
		N	S	A	N	S	A	N	S	A	N	S	A	
	P	208	30	21	44	7	4	5	0	1	-	0	-	320
	C	93	14	4	115	22	10	37	8	7	1	1	1	313

		Suspicious		Abnormal	
	P	37/320	N.S.	26/320	N.S.
	C	45/313		22/313	

N = Normal

S = Suspicious

A = Abnormal

Cooperative PhotoRx Study
1983

We examined the autopsy data with regard to the incidence
of intracranial hemorrhage in all infants and found no significant
difference from the KI infants.

Thus far analysis of the autopsy data allows us to conclude
that use of phototherapy was not associated with the development
of kernicterus, whereas 10% of control infants <1500 g who were
autopsied had evidence of kernicterus. The latter infants were
managed under strict protocol for the use of exchange transfusion
to control hyperbilirubinemia. None of the infants with kernicterus had bilirubin levels >15 mg/dL.

The HABA binding was significantly lower in the group of
infants who developed kernicterus than in those who died with no
evidence of kernicterus. Of the nine who had had HABA binding
values <37%, four developed kernicterus. No other distinguishing
feature was identified.

Long Term Follow Up

I.   Neurologic outcome at one year

Preliminary analysis of the neurological outcome at one year
has been made and the relationship between this outcome and peak
serum bilirubin levels in the neonatal period in the phototherapy
(P) and control (C) groups are outlined in table 7 and table 8.

When the phototherapy and control outcomes were compared,
there was no statistically significant difference in the overall
incidence of abnormal or suspicious neurological findings at one
year. Further, preliminary analysis reveals no significant
relationship between neurological outcome at one year and peak
serum bilirubin levels in the neonatal period.

II.   Visual Functions in Children Enrolled in the
      NIH Cooperative Phototherapy Study*+
      (Preliminary Findings)

In 1982 visual functions were tested in 45 children originally enrolled in the cooperative phototherapy study at Downstate
Medical Center; 19 children from the "light" treatment group and
26 from the "control" group. The studies were performed in the

*Louise Hainline, Ph.D., Israel Abramov, Ph.D., Elizabeth Lemerise,
M.A., Joseph Turkel, Ph.D., Brooklyn College of CUNY and,
Audrey K. Brown, M.D., Downstate Medical Center of SUNY

+Supported in part by: TSC- CUNY Grant #663209 (I.A.)

Infant Study Center at Brooklyn College of CUNY*.   20 "normal"
children not enrolled in the original study were also tested; they
were full-term, healthy infants who were matched in age to the study
groups.

The following examinations were performed:

(i) spatial resolution (Snellen acuity as well as contrast
sensitivity at different spatial frequencies), (ii) receptor
functions (color screening as well as two-color increment thresholds
with stimuli chosen to isolate short-wavelength ("blue") cones,
long-wavelength ("red") cones, and rods), (iii) binocular vision
(stereoacuity), and (iv) temporal resolution (critical flicker
fusion).   Most tests were run under both photopic and scotopic
adaptation states.   To secure cooperation from the children, all
tests were disguised as "space games".

Analysis of the data is not complete but the following
preliminary statements can be made:

On all tests the phototherapy group as a whole does not
differ from the control group as a whole, and neither is different
from the normal population.   However, in the control group a significant number of children (5 out of 26) failed color vision
screening; some of these color-anomalous children failed only
monocularly.   All of the failures were of an unusual "mixed" variety, but included a clear tritanopia-like component (i.e., a
deficity in sensitivity of short wavelength cones).   Data from these
control subjects were segregated and treated separately.   The
remainder of the results shows that this sub-group differs from
the rest of the children tested on many cone functions, but not on
rod functions.

Specifically, the color-anomalous children had slightly lower
Snellen acuity; more importantly, their photopic contrast
sensitivity was 20-40% lower than normal at all spatial frequencies
(from 0.5 to 32 cycles/degree).   Consistent with the ways in which
they failed standard color screening tests, their blue cone thresholds were about 3 times higher (i.e., less sensitive) than those
of the other children and their red cone thresholds were about 2
times higher (less sensitive); rod thresholds, however, were the
same as for the other children.   Only in the color-anomalous group
did we find children with no demonstrable stereopsis (3 of 5);
the remaining 2 children had stereopsis but poor stereoacuity.
On all other tests this subgroup did not differ from the other
children.   Some of these deficits (e.g., cone increment thresholds)
are consonant with losses at the receptor level. However, such losses
cannot account for all the data; the small acuity deficit could
be due to receptor damage, but in that case, there should not be
deficits at the lower spatial frequencies.   The over-all deficits

in spatial contrast sensitivity point to neural changes at post-
receptoral levels. The stereopsis deficits indicate cortical
involvement as well.

At this stage in the analysis of the data collected from the
Downstate Medical Center study group, we do not have enough
information to answer the question of why a significant proportion
of the control subjects show damage. The following possibilities
are under consideration. Prolonged illumination, even at moderate
levels, can damage the visual system, especially short-wavelength
cones. Children in the "light" group had their eyes shielded
from phototherapy lights while they were in the hospital as infants. Control group children did not have eye shielding. Light
levels in neonatal intensive care units are quite high, and lights
are often on continuously. The color anomalous control subjects
may thus be exhibiting damage due to the phototoxic effects of
hospital illumination. Alternatively, high bilirubin levels
may directly effect the visual system, as may variations in oxygen
tension caused by respiratory problems or exchange transfusions.

In an effort to identify the factor(s) that may be responsible,
an analysis of some of the neonatal variables was made. Preliminary
assessment of the neonatal clinical characteristics of the color
anomalous patients reveals an interesting constellation of features.
5/5 were in the control (or non-phototherapy) group; 4/5 were anemic
(Hct values 30-41%). 3/5 had 1 minute Apgar scores <5; 4/5 had
serum bilirubin values >12 mg/dL (2 of these infants had serum
bilirubin values in excess of 15 for 3 days); 4/5 weighed <2000 g
at birth (three of these infants were pre-term but one infant
weighing only 1595 g was a very small for gestational age term
infant). It is of interest that this undergrown infant was the
only one who was not anemic but his poor development and relatively
high hematocrit at birth (62%) clearly suggests intra-uterine
hypoxia due to placental inadequacy for delivery of oxygen.

The only infant of birth weight greater than 2000 g suffered
from erythroblastosis fetalis with attendant marked anemia and
hyperbilirubinemia.

The clinical features in this group of patients can be
summarized as being clearly abnormal with the possible common
feature of hypoxia. In 4/5 this was evidenced by the very low Apgar
score and/or anemia and in the fifth infant by the marked failure
to grow in utero and the relative (compensatory?) polycythemia.

INDEX

315

THE LIBRARY
UNIVERSITY OF CALIFORNIA
San Francisco
(415) 476-2335

THIS BOOK IS DUE ON THE LAST DATE STAMPED BELOW

Books not returned on time are subject to fines according to the Library Lending Code. A renewal may be made on certain materials. For details consult Lending Code.